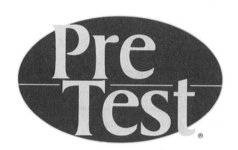

Pediatrics

PreTest® Self-Assessment and Review

Notice

Medicine is an ever-changing science. As new research and clinical experience broaden our knowledge, changes in treatment and drug therapy are required. The authors and the publisher of this work have checked with sources believed to be reliable in their efforts to provide information that is complete and generally in accord with the standards accepted at the time of publication. However, in view of the possibility of human error or changes in medical sciences, neither the authors nor the publisher nor any other party who has been involved in the preparation or publication of this work warrants that the information contained herein is in every respect accurate or complete, and they disclaim all responsibility for any errors or omissions or for the results obtained from use of the information contained in this work. Readers are encouraged to confirm the information contained herein with other sources. For example and in particular, readers are advised to check the product information sheet included in the package of each drug they plan to administer to be certain that the information contained in this work is accurate and that changes have not been made in the recommended dose or in the contraindications for administration. This recommendation is of particular importance in connection with new or infrequently used drugs.

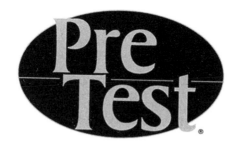

Pediatrics

PreTest® Self-Assessment and Review

Fifteenth Edition

Robert J. Yetman, MD
Professor of Pediatrics
Director, Division of Community and General Pediatrics
Assistant Chief Medical Officer, Children's Memorial Hermann Hospital
Department of Pediatrics
McGovern Medical School at The University of Texas Health Science Center at Houston
Houston, Texas

Mark D. Hormann, MD
Associate Professor of Pediatrics
Vice Chair for Education and Training
Division of Community and General Pediatrics
Department of Pediatrics
McGovern Medical School at The University of Texas Health Science Center at Houston
Houston, Texas

New York   Chicago   San Francisco   Athens   London   Madrid   Mexico City
Milan   New Delhi   Singapore   Sydney   Toronto

Pediatrics: PreTest® Self-Assessment and Review, Fifteenth Edition

PreTest® is a registered trademark of McGraw Hill.

1 2 3 4 5 6 7 8 9   LCR   24 23 22 21 20 19

ISBN 978-1-260-44033-1
MHID 1-260-44033-8

This book was set in Minion pro by Cenveo® Publisher Services.
The editors were Bob Boehringer and Christina M. Thomas.
The production supervisor was Richard Ruzycka.
Project management was provided by Megha Bhardwaj, Cenveo Publisher Services.

This book is printed on acid-free paper.

Library of Congress Cataloging-in-Publication Data

Names: Yetman, Robert, editor. | Hormann, Mark, editor.
Title: Pediatrics : PreTest self-assessment and review / [edited by] Robert
  J. Yetman, Mark D. Hormann.
Other titles: Pediatrics (Lipman)
Description: Fifteenth. | New York, New York : McGraw-Hill, 2019. |
  Includes bibliographical references and index. | Summary: "The PreTest Clinical Science
  Series prepares medical students for the USMLE Step 2 CK, which assesses students'
  medical knowledge of core clinical topics with USMLE style review questions. Useful as
  reviews for clerkship exams following core clinical rotations, each PreTest book contains
  500 questions with comprehensive, targeted answers and rationale. Discussions review
  correct and incorrect answer options to reinforce learning. The 15th edition of Pediatrics:
  PreTest simulates the USMLE Step 2 CK test-taking experience by including vignette-style
  questions and updates on the latest treatments and therapies for infants, children and
  adolescents. To ensure that questions are representative of the style and level of difficulty of
  the exam, each PreTest book is reviewed by students who either recently passed Step 2CK
  or completed their Pediatrics rotation"—Provided by publisher.
Identifiers: LCCN 2019033830 | ISBN 9781260440331 (paperback) |
  ISBN 9781260440348 (ebook)
Subjects: MESH: Pediatrics | Examination Question
Classification: LCC RJ48.2 | NLM WS 18.2 | DDC 618.9200076—dc23
LC record available at https://lccn.loc.gov/2019033830

Student Reviewer

Blake Arthurs, MD
Resident
University of Michigan Family Medicine Residency Program

Contents

Infectious Diseases and Immunology

Hematologic and Neoplastic Diseases

Endocrine, Metabolic, and Genetic Disorders

The Adolescent

Introduction

Pediatrics: PreTest® Self-Assessment and Review, Fifteenth Edition, provides comprehensive self-assessment and review within the field of pediatrics. The 455 questions in the book have been designed to be similar in format and degree of difficulty to the questions in Step 2 CK of the United States Medical Licensing Examination (USMLE). They may also be a useful study tool for Step 3 or clerkship examinations.

For multiple-choice questions, the one best response to each question should be selected. For matching sets, a group of questions will be preceded by a list of lettered options. For each question in the matching set, select one lettered option that is most closely associated with the question. Each question in this book has a corresponding answer, a reference to a text that provides background to the answer, and a short discussion of various issues raised by the question and its answer.

To simulate the time constraints imposed by the qualifying examinations for which this book is intended as a practice guide, the student or physician should allot about 1 minute for each question. After answering all questions in a chapter, as much time as necessary should be spent in reviewing the explanations for each question at the end of the chapter. Attention should be given to all explanations, even if the examinee answered the question correctly. Those seeking more information on a subject should refer to the reference materials listed in the bibliography or to other standard texts in medicine.

Bibliography

Hay WW, Levin MJ, Deterding RR, Abzug MJ, eds. *Current Diagnosis and Treatment in Pediatrics*. 24th ed. New York, NY: McGraw-Hill Education; 2018.

Kliegman RM, Stanton BF, St Geme JW, Schor NF, eds. *Nelson Textbook of Pediatrics*. 20th ed. Philadelphia, PA: Elsevier; 2016.

Rudolph CD, Rudolph AM, Lister GE, eds. *Rudolph's Pediatrics*. 22nd ed. New York, NY: McGraw-Hill Education; 2011.

General Pediatrics

Questions

1. A 9-year-old boy is seen in the pediatrician's office with a several days' history of weakness of his mouth. He reports that he had a viral upper respiratory tract infection (URI) about 2 weeks prior. He denies headache, fever, vomiting, constipation, or other weakness. He has been a healthy child without serious previous illnesses. On physical examination the vital signs are normal. The left side of his mouth droops, he is unable to completely close his left eye, and his smile is asymmetric (Photograph). The mucous membranes are pink, moist, and without lesions. Extraocular eye movement and fundoscopic examinations are normal. Gait, sensation, and deep tendon reflexes are normal. Which of the following is the most likely diagnosis?

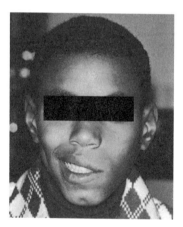

(Reproduced with permission from Knoop KJ, Stack LB, Storrow AB: Atlas of Emergency Medicine, 2nd ed. New York, NY: McGraw-Hill Education; 2002.)

a. Guillain-Barré syndrome
b. Botulism
c. Cerebral vascular accident
d. Brainstem tumor
e. Bell palsy

2. A 13-year-old boy is seen in the pediatrician's office for a 3-day history of pain in the right knee and a limp. The pain began as dull and deep in the right thigh, and over the previous 2 days he developed pain in the right knee and a limp on that side. He reports that he has been unable to participate in sports due to pain. Over-the-counter ibuprofen and acetaminophen have been minimally helpful. He has had no fever, nausea, vomiting, or trauma. He denies alcohol, drugs, or sexual activity. His past medical history is positive for mild hypertension noted on the previous year's well-child examination. On physical examination his height is 170 cm (5'7"), weight 100 kg (220 lb), and body mass index (BMI) 34.5 kg/m². The right leg shows reduced internal rotation, reduced abduction, and reduced flexion. Upon flexion of the right hip the right thigh and leg rotate externally. Which of the following is the most likely diagnosis?

a. Legg-Calvé-Perthes disease
b. Slipped capital femoral epiphysis
c. Osteomyelitis
d. Septic arthritis of the hip
e. Transient synovitis

3. A 4-year-old child is seen in the emergency department (ED) for limp. The mother reports no fever, vomiting, or change in behavior. She notes that the child had a URI about 1 week prior; the illness seemed to self-resolve. On physical examination the temperature is 37°C (98.5°F), heart rate is 99 beats per minute, respiratory rate is 21 breaths per minute, and blood pressure is 90/56 mm Hg. The mucous membranes are moist and without lesions. The chest is clear. Heart has a normal S1 and S2 without murmur. All joints have full range of motion with mild tenderness noted with manipulation of the right hip. A limp is noted with ambulation. Plain radiographs of the hips are normal. Laboratory data reveal the following:

  Hemoglobin: 14.2 g/dL
  Hematocrit: 41.5%
  White blood count (WBC): 7500/mm^3
  Segmented neutrophils: 49%
  Band forms: 0%
  Lymphocytes: 51%
  Platelet count: 138,000/mm^3
  Erythrocyte sedimentation rate (ESR): 23 mm/h
  High-sensitivity C-reactive protein: 2.5 mg/L

Which of the following is the most likely mechanism for these findings?
a. Loss of blood flow to the joint
b. Direct inoculation of the joint space with bacteria
c. Hematogenous spread of bacteria to the joint space
d. Infiltration of the joint by leukemic blasts
e. Transient inflammation of the joint space

4. A 4-year-old girl is seen by the pediatrician for a 1-month history of limp and swollen right knee. The grandmother reports that the child has had intermittent limping and a swollen right knee, but denies fever, bruising, fatigue or weight loss. She has been a healthy child without serious previous illnesses. She takes a daily multivitamin. On physical examination she has a temperature of 37°C (98.5°F), heart rate of 90 beats per minute, respiratory rate of 22 breaths per minute, and blood pressure of 100/62 mm Hg. The left knee is slightly swollen, warm, and has decreased range of motion. An ophthalmologic examination reveals findings as depicted in the photograph. Which of the following is the most likely diagnosis?

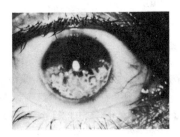

a. Juvenile idiopathic arthritis (JIA)
b. Slipped capital femoral epiphysis
c. Henoch-Schönlein purpura (HSP)
d. Legg-Calvé-Perthes disease
e. Osgood-Schlatter disease

5. A 4-year-old child is admitted to the hospital for fever and rash. The mother reports the child had been well until about 2 days prior when she developed a fever of 40°C (104°F) and a bright red rash all over her body. The mother denies medication usage, exposure to toxins, sick contacts, and travel. On physical examination she has a temperature of 38.9°C (102.1°F), a heart rate of 115 beats per minute, a respiratory rate of 22 breaths per minute, and a blood pressure of 100/60 mm Hg. The mucous membranes are moist with crusting and fissuring around the eyes, mouth, and nose. The skin is edematous and red, especially in the folds of the joints. Desquamation of skin occurs with gentle traction (Photographs). Which of the following is the most likely diagnosis?

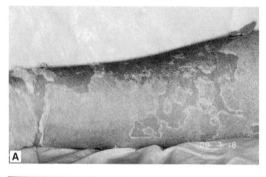

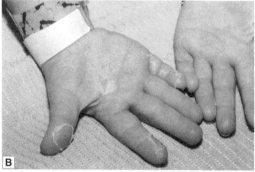

(Used with permission from Adelaide Hebert, MD.)

a. Epidermolysis bullosa
b. Staphylococcal scalded skin syndrome
c. Erythema multiforme
d. Drug eruption
e. Scarlet fever

6. A representative from an infant formula company uses the following sales aid to promote their product. From the sales aid you can conclude that which of the following statements is correct?

a. About 75% of infants fed this company's infant formula will experience no symptoms of colic.

b. The mixture of probiotics and whey protein results in an immune system equal to that of the breast-fed infant.

c. Infants with a strong family history of colic should be fed this brand of formula rather than breast milk.

d. Four published studies were utilized to draw conclusions presented in the sales presentation.

e. This brand of infant formula is proven to be gentle on an infant's stomach.

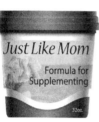

7. A 9-year-old girl is seen in the pediatrician's office in follow-up after having been admitted to the hospital for a 3-weeks' history of fever and positive blood cultures due to *Staphylococcus aureus*. The hospital evaluation ultimately demonstrated vegetations on the mitral valve. She is now in her sixth week of a planned 6-week course of intravenous antibiotics. She denies fever, vomiting, headache, or change in behavior. On physical examination she has a temperature of 37°C (98.5°F), a heart rate of 105 beats per minute, a respiratory rate of 18 breaths per minute, and a blood pressure of 95/59 mm Hg. The mucous membranes are moist and without lesions. The chest is clear. Heart has a normal S1 and S2 without murmur. The extremities are without edema or splinter hemorrhages. Future planning for this child would include which of the following?

a. Restrict the child from all strenuous activities.
b. Give the child a no-salt-added diet.
c. Provide the child with antibiotic prophylaxis for dental procedures.
d. Test all family members in the home with repeated blood cultures.
e. Avoid allowing the child to get upset or agitated.

8. A mother contacts the on-call physician line reporting that her 4-year-old son bit the hand of her 2-year-old son 2 days prior. She states that the area around the injury has become red, swollen, and tender. Over the previous 12 hours the child has developed a temperature of 39.4°C (103°F). She denies any previous serious illness or medication intake. The child is drinking well, eating less than normal, and his activity is decreased. Which of the following is the most appropriate next step in managing this child?

a. Arrange for a plastic surgery consultation at the next available appointment.
b. Refer the child to the hospital for likely surgical debridement and antibiotic treatment.
c. Prescribe penicillin over the telephone and have the mother apply warm soaks for 15 minutes four times a day.
d. Suggest purchase of bacitracin ointment to apply to the lesion three times a day.
e. Send the patient to a local urgent care center to suture the laceration.

9. A 14-year-old boy is seen in the pediatric office with a 14-day history of rash. He reports that the first lesion (Photograph A) began on his lower abdomen and then additional lesions developed a few days later on his back (Photograph B). He reports the rash is slightly pruritic but denies fever, nausea, vomiting, headache, or musculoskeletal symptoms. His past history is positive only for mild seasonal allergic rhinitis for which he occasionally takes over-the-counter antihistamines. His vaccines are current. On physical examination he has a temperature of 37°C (98.5°F), a heart rate of 92 beats per minute, a respiratory rate of 16 breaths per minute, and a blood pressure of 110/69 mm Hg. The mucous membranes are moist and without lesions. The rash on the abdomen and back are slightly raised at the edges with a somewhat scaly appearance in the center. Which of the following is the most likely diagnosis?

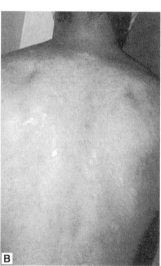
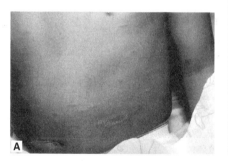

(Used with permission from Adelaide Hebert, MD.)

a. Contact dermatitis
b. Pityriasis rosea
c. Seborrheic dermatitis
d. Lichen planus
e. Psoriasis

10. A father brings his 6-month-old son into the pediatric office for a well-child visit. The father has no concerns other than thinking that the boy's penis is inadequate in length. The boy was a 4200-g product of a term pregnancy, was delivered vaginally, and was discharged at about 48 hours of life. He was exclusively breast-fed for the first 4 months of life, and now gets supplements to those feedings with infant formula and solid foods. He takes vitamin D and fluoride drops daily. On physical examination the weight is at the 95th percentile, the length at the 50th percentile, and the head circumference at the 50th percentile. He is a happy, alert infant without abnormalities on examination. The genitourinary examination is shown in the photograph. Which of the following is the most appropriate first step in management of this child?

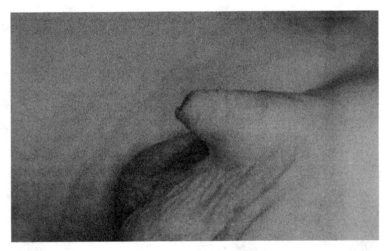

(*Used with permission from Michaelene R. Ribbeck, NP, PhD.*)

a. Surgical consultation
b. Evaluation of penile length after retracting the skin and fat lateral to the penile shaft
c. Ultrasound of the abdomen for uterus and ovaries
d. Chromosome analysis
e. Serum testosterone levels

11. A previously healthy 5-year-old boy is seen in the ED with a 1-day history of low-grade fever, colicky abdominal pain, and a rash. His mother reports no vomiting, diarrhea, sick contacts, recent illnesses or change in behavior. He has had no previous serious illnesses and takes no medications. His immunizations are current. On physical examination he has a temperature of 38°C (100.5°F), a heart rate of 101 beats per minute, a respiratory rate of 20 breaths per minute, and a blood pressure of 100/58 mm Hg. He is awake, alert, active, and in no distress. The skin has diffuse erythematous maculopapular and petechial lesions on the buttocks and lower extremities (Photograph). Laboratory data demonstrate:

CBC:
    Hemoglobin: 14 g/dL
    Hematocrit: 42%
    WBC: 8000/mm³
        Segmented neutrophils: 60%
        Band forms: 1%
        Lymphocytes: 39%
    Platelet count: 135,000/mm³
Urinalysis:
    30 red blood cells (RBCs) per high-powered field, 2+ protein
Stool:
    Occult blood positive

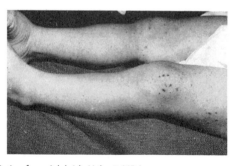

(Used with permission from Adelaide Hebert, MD.)

Which of the following is the most likely mechanism for these findings?
a. IgA-mediated vasculitis
b. Bacterial infection
c. Inflicted injury
d. Infiltrate of skin by blasts
e. Coagulation disorder

12. A 4-month-old infant is brought via ambulance to the ED intubated and with CPR in progress. Despite 30 minutes of resuscitation, the infant is pronounced dead. The parents report that he had been healthy and that they put him to bed as usual for the night at about 8 PM. He did not awaken for his normal nightly feeding. When they next saw him in the morning, he was not breathing. Physical examination in the ED shows only evidence of resuscitation including an endotracheal tube from the mouth, an intraosseous line in the left leg, and redness over the chest at the sternum where chest compressions were administered. A film of the right leg from a routine skeletal survey is shown in the photograph. Which of the following is the most likely diagnosis?

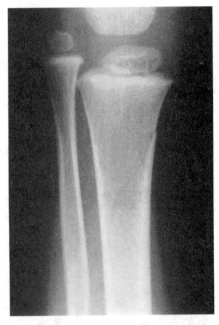

(Used with permission from Susan John, MD.)

a. Scurvy
b. Congenital syphilis
c. Sudden infant death syndrome (SIDS)
d. Osteogenesis imperfecta
e. Abuse

13. A healthy 6-year-old boy is seen in the pediatrician's office for a well-child visit. His mother reports that he is being "bullied and teased" at school because he has stooled in his underwear almost daily for the last 3 months. The family reports that he was toilet trained at 2 years of age without difficulty, but over the previous 18 months has developed intermittent episodes of soiling himself while stating that "I didn't know I had to go." His development is normal for age. When evaluated alone he denies any abuse or inappropriate touching. On physical examination he has a temperature of 37°C (98.5°F), a heart rate of 100 beats per minute, a respiratory rate of 19 breaths per minute, and a blood pressure of 102/60 mm Hg. His abdomen is soft and without hepatosplenomegaly. The left lower quadrant seems to be a bit "full" but not tender. Anal sphincter tone appears a bit lax, and a small amount of stool is noted at the os and in the rectal vault. The plain radiograph of his abdomen is shown. Which of the following is the most appropriate initial management?

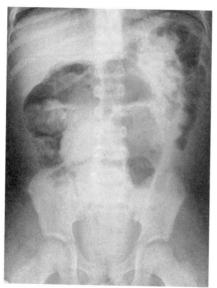

(Used with permission from Susan John, MD.)

a. Barium enema and rectal biopsy
b. Family counseling
c. Timeout when he stools in his underwear
d. Clear the fecal impaction and begin several months of stool softener use
e. Daily enemas for 4 weeks

14. A 2-year-old child is seen in the pediatrician's office as a new patient for a well-child visit. The family is concerned that the child has "bowlegs" that has worsened over the previous 6 months. They report that she was the product of a term, uneventful pregnancy. She takes no medications, has had no serious illnesses or injuries, and her vaccines are current. On physical examination her vital signs are normal. The weight is at the 95th percentile, the length at the 50th percentile, and the head circumference at the 50th percentile. The lower extremities have significant bowing with internal tibial torsion. A radiograph of her lower leg is shown in the photograph. Which of the following is the most likely diagnosis?

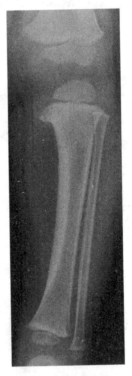

(Used with permission from Susan John, MD.)

a. Osgood-Schlatter disease
b. Physiologic genu varum
c. Slipped capital femoral epiphysis
d. Legg-Calvé-Perthes disease
e. Blount disease

15. A 2-year-old child is seen by the pediatric nurse practitioner. The mother reports that the child has had two episodes of a brief, shrill cry followed by a prolonged expiration. She reports the child became cyanotic, had a few generalized clonic jerks, an apneic episode, and a few moments of what seemed like unconsciousness. After about 3 or 4 seconds the child awakened and had no residual effects. The first episode occurred after the mother refused to give the child some juice, and the second occurred when the mother took away her favorite doll to put her to bed. The child was the product of a normal pregnancy, the growth and development have been normal, and the family history is positive for hypertension in the maternal grandmother. On physical examination she has a temperature of 37°C (98.5°F), a heart rate of 100 beats per minute, and a respiratory rate of 24 breaths per minute. She is awake, alert, and is happily running around the room showing off her favorite doll. Cranial nerves are normal, and no focal neurologic findings are noted. Which of the following is the most appropriate next step in management?

a. Order an EEG
b. Obtain a urine drug screen
c. Begin a trial of methylphenidate
d. Refer to a psychologist for developmental testing
e. Provide reassurance to the family

16. A 10-year-old child is seen in the pediatrician's office for new-onset bed-wetting. He denies dysuria, fever, vomiting, headache, change in behavior, or new stressors in his life. He has had no serious illnesses, takes no medications, and is doing well in school. On physical examination the temperature is 37°C (98.5°F), heart rate is 95 beats per minute, respiratory rate is 18 breaths per minute, and blood pressure is 120/80 mm Hg. Height is 140 cm (55 in), the length is at 50th percentile, and weight is 49 kg (109 lb) which is greater than 97th percentile. BMI is 26.6 kg/m^2. The mucous membranes are moist and without lesions. Skin around the neck is hyperpigmented and velvety in texture. The chest is clear. Heart has a normal S1 and S2 without murmur. His abdomen is soft and without hepatosplenomegaly. Genitourinary examination shows normal uncircumcised male genitalia. Which of the following laboratory findings confirm the correct cause of his symptoms?

a. Fasting plasma glucose of 135 mg/dL
b. Random plasma glucose of 170 mg/dL
c. Two-hour plasma glucose during glucose tolerance test of 165 mg/dL
d. Urine culture by clean catch demonstrating less than 1000 colonies of *Staphylococcus epidermidis*
e. Urine microscopy demonstrating three to five epithelial cells and two WBCs per high-power field

17. A 2-month-old infant in the office for a well-child visit is noted to have an erupted left central mandibular incisor; the mother notes it was there at birth. It is firmly in place and doesn't seem to interfere with the baby's bottle feeding. Correct statements regarding this natal tooth include:

a. The tooth is likely to be supernumerary, or extra.
b. The tooth should be removed.
c. The tooth is indicative of a genetic condition.
d. The tooth should be left in place.
e. The tooth is more likely to become discolored.

18. A 14-day-old neonate is seen in the pediatrician's office for hospital follow-up. The baby was delivered vaginally at term to a 23-year-old primigravida woman. The mother and the baby were discharged after an uneventful 48-hour hospital stay. The baby is breast-feeding well, is voiding and stooling well, and is above birth weight. The physical examination is significant for a "rash" on the face (Photograph). Which of the following is the most likely diagnosis?

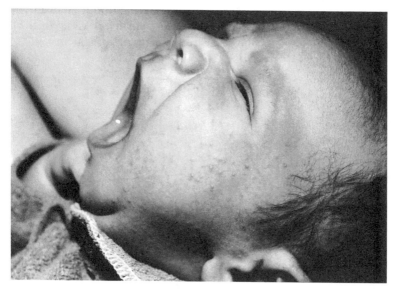

(Used with permission from Adelaide Hebert, MD.)

a. Herpes simplex infection
b. Neonatal acne
c. Milia
d. Seborrheic dermatitis
e. Eczema

19. A 2-year-old child and his 3-month-old sibling are seen in the emergency center for a rash. The mother reports the 2-year old (Photograph A) has had a 4-day history of the rash limited to the feet and ankles. She states the child is constantly scratching the rash. The 3-month-old sibling (Photograph B) has had a similar rash, also of 4-days' duration, involving the head and neck. The mother denies that either child has had fever, vomiting, travel, or change in environments. On physical examination the 2-year old has an erythematous papular eruption on the feet and ankles with evidence of excoriation. The 3-month old is cranky with a similar erythematous papular eruption on the head, neck, and in the axilla. Which of the following is the most appropriate treatment for this condition?

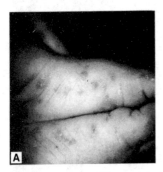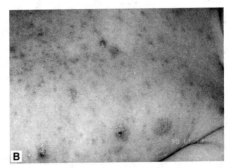

(Used with permission from Adelaide Hebert, MD.)

a. Coal-tar soap
b. Permethrin
c. Hydrocortisone cream
d. Emollients
e. Topical antifungal cream

20. An 8-hour-old neonate in the normal newborn nursery develops tachypnea and increased work of breathing. He was born at term by vaginal delivery in the triage area to a 22-year-old primigravida. The mother had limited prenatal care but reports no complications. The infant's Apgar scores were 9 and 9 at 1 and 5 minutes, respectively. Resuscitation was routine. He passed stool and urine in the delivery room. He was placed on the breast within the first hour and latched well. Maternal laboratory data from an ED visit at 6 months' gestation show her to be blood type AB+, screen negative, rubella immune, and HIV negative. On physical examination the temperature is 35.4°C (95.8°F), heart rate is 180 beats per minute, respiratory rate is 80 breaths per minute, blood pressure is 70/40 mm Hg, and oxygen saturation is 89%. The nose has nasal flaring. The chest has subcostal and intercostal retractions, grunting, and rales. Laboratory data show:

Hemoglobin: 13 g/dL
Hematocrit: 39%
WBC: 1000/mm^3
Segmented neutrophils: 30%
Band forms: 50%
Lymphocytes: 20%
Platelet count: 20,000/mm^3

The chest radiograph shows diffuse, bilateral granular infiltrates. Which of the following is the most likely diagnosis?

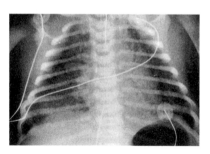

(Used with permission from Susan John, MD.)

a. Congenital syphilis
b. Diaphragmatic hernia
c. Group B streptococcal pneumonia
d. Transient tachypnea of the newborn
e. Chlamydial pneumonia

21. A 16-year-old boy is seen in the pediatrician's office for pain in his knees. He reports that the pain began about 2 months ago at the start of basketball season and seems to be worsening. He denies fever, vomiting, weakness, weight loss, or bruising. He is sexually active with three lifetime partners and reports inconsistent condom use. He denies alcohol or other drug use. On physical examination the temperature is 37°C (98.5°F), heart rate is 74 beats per minute, respiratory rate is 16 breaths per minute, and blood pressure is 110/64 mm Hg. Height and weight are 90th percentile. His joint examination is normal. The area immediately below both knees is tender with swollen and prominent tibial tubercles noted. Which of the following is the most likely diagnosis?

a. Osgood-Schlatter disease
b. Popliteal cyst
c. Slipped capital femoral epiphysis
d. Legg-Calvé-Perthes disease
e. Gonococcal arthritis

22. A 1-year-old child is seen by the pediatric nurse practitioner for a well-child examination. The family has no concerns other than a slight URI for the previous 2 days. The infant has been growing and developing normally. On physical examination vital signs are normal. Growth parameters are at the 50th percentile for age. The examination is normal other than a slightly congested nose and the finding pictured. Which of the following is the most appropriate next step in management?

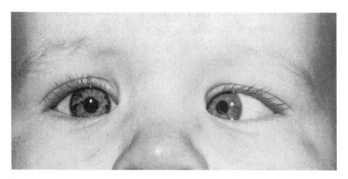

(Used with permission from Kathryn Musgrove, MD.)

a. Patch the eye with the greater refractive error.
b. Patch the eye that deviates.
c. Reevaluate the infant when the URI is resolved.
d. Reassure the mother that he will outgrow it.
e. Refer immediately to ophthalmology.

23. A 7-year-old boy is seen in the emergency room for fever and facial swelling. The mother reports that he was healthy until about 2 days prior when the area surrounding his left eye became red and swollen. He denies insect bites and trauma to the area. On physical examination the temperature is 38.5°C (101.1°F), heart rate is 110 beats per minute, respiratory rate is 22 breaths per minute, and blood pressure is 100/69 mm Hg. The left eye has marked swelling that affects the upper and lower lids. The eye is proptotic and with limited range of motion. The sclera on the affected side is hyperemic. Other mucous membranes are moist and without lesions. Which of the following is the most appropriate next step in management?

a. Parental reassurance and close follow-up
b. CBC, blood culture, IM ceftriaxone, and follow-up with primary care provider in 24 hours
c. Ocular antibiotic drops for 7-10 days
d. Oral antibiotics for 7-10 days
e. Admit and start IV antibiotics

24. A 2-year-old girl is seen in the ED with fever and refusal to walk. Her father reports that she was in good health until about 24 hours prior when she developed irritability, low-grade fever, and a limp. When she awoke in the morning (4 hours prior to the ED visit) her temperature was 38.5°C (101.1°F) and she refused to bear weight on the leg. He reports no previous serious illnesses or hospitalizations, normal diet and development, and vaccines that are current. On physical examination the temperature is 39.2°C (102.5°F), heart rate is 110 beats per minute, and respiratory rate is 20 breaths per minute. On examination, the child refuses to walk and has significant pain upon external rotation of the right leg is noted. Laboratory data show:

Hemoglobin: 13.5 g/dL
Hematocrit: 41%
WBC: 22,000/mm^3
    Segmented neutrophils: 80%
    Band forms: 10%
    Lymphocytes: 10%
Platelet count: 175,000/mm^3

Which of the following is the most likely diagnosis?

a. Legg-Calvé-Perthes disease
b. Leukemia
c. Osteomyelitis
d. Septic arthritis of the hip
e. Transient synovitis

25. A 7-month-old white boy was admitted 4 days ago to the pediatric unit by a general practitioner for failure to thrive. A pediatric consultation is requested after the infant demonstrates inadequate weight gain while in the hospital despite appropriate nutrition. The caregivers at the bedside report the infant has had poor weight gain for the previous 3 months, with occasional URIs but no serious illnesses. He takes daily vitamins. The dietary history suggests that he has been given appropriate infant formula and solid food. The social history reveals the biologic mother to be incarcerated in the state penitentiary and the infant to be in custody of the maternal grandmother. On physical examination the temperature is 37°C (98.5°F), heart rate is 120 beats per minute, and respiratory rate is 24 breaths per minute. Weight is less than the 5th percentile (50th percentile for a 4-month old), the length at the 5th percentile, and the head circumference 25th percentile. He is a happy, alert infant in no distress and with a strong suck. The mucous membranes are moist with some white plaques on the cheeks. The chest is clear. Heart has a normal S1 and S2 without murmur. His abdomen is soft and with hepatomegaly. He has submandibular, posterior auricular, and inguinal adenopathy. Which of the following is the most appropriate next step?

a. Increase caloric intake
b. Order HIV polymerase chain reaction (PCR)
c. Draw blood cultures and start empiric antibiotics
d. Perform a sweat chloride test
e. Send stool for fecal fat

26. A 5-year-old boy is seen in the emergency center for an itchy rash. His mother reports that "the rash has been present his whole life." He states that as an infant the rash involved his face, but as he has gotten older the rash seems to be especially intense in the flexural areas of elbows and knees. She states the rash is worse in the winter months. She reports no serious illnesses or hospitalization, and his vaccines are current. His development has been normal. On physical examination the child is awake, alert, and is scratching intensely at the red, weepy, maculopapular rash (Photographs A and B). Which of the following is the most appropriate treatment of this condition?

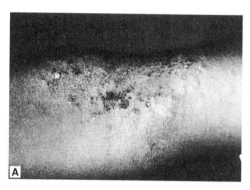

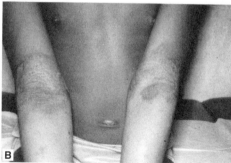

(Used with permission from Adelaide Hebert, MD.)

a. Coal-tar soaps and shampoo
b. Topical antifungal cream
c. Ultraviolet light therapy
d. Moisturizers and topical steroids
e. Topical antibiotics

27. A 14-year-old boy is seen in the emergency room having just been rescued from an avalanche that was caused by a barking Chihuahua. He complains that his feet hurt. Emergency medical services personnel report that when they extricated him from the snowbank his feet were whitish-yellow and numb. He had no loss of consciousness and no obvious injuries. On physical examination the temperature is 35.6°C (96°F), heart rate is 90 beats per minute, and respiratory rate is 18 breaths per minute. He is awake, alert, and oriented. His feet are cool, blotchy in color and painful to touch. Which of the following is the most likely diagnosis?

a. Frostnip
b. Frostbite
c. Chilblain
d. Cold panniculitis
e. Trench foot

28. A 2-month-old infant and her 18-month-old sibling are seen by the pediatrician for well-child visits. The mother reports that the 2-month-old infant has been healthy, but notes that the 18-month-old child has had an intensely itchy scalp for about 4 days. On physical examination the 2-month old is normal. The 18-month old is alert, happy, and is scratching her scalp, especially in the occipital region. The occipital scalp is somewhat weepy, boggy, and red. Numerous tiny lesions are noted at the base of the hair shafts (Photograph). The posterior auricular and suboccipital lymph nodes are slightly swollen but not tender. Which of the following is the most appropriate treatment for them?

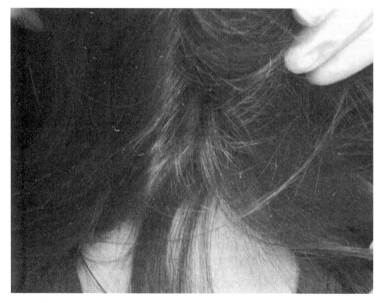

(Used with permission from Adelaide Hebert, MD.)

a. Topical ivermectin for the 18-month old and observation for the 2-month old
b. Oral griseofulvin for both
c. Topical antibiotic ointment for both
d. Oral ivermectin for both
e. Topical 1% lindane for the 2-month-old infant and topical ivermectin for the 18-month-old child

29. A 3-year-old boy is seen by the pediatrician for a 3-week history of vomiting. The family reports that he has had intermittent episodes of vomiting, has become more irritable, listless, and is now anorectic. They have not measured his temperature but report that he "feels warm." He has had no serious illnesses in the past and takes no medications. He sat at 6 months and walked at 12 months. He babbled by 4 months, said "dada" by 10 months, said two syllable words at 24 months, and until the previous 3 weeks was able to put together two- to three-word sentences. He now is able to say single words only. They deny travel, sick contacts, and medications or drugs in the home. Which of the following is the most likely diagnosis?

a. Expanding epidural hematoma
b. Herpes simplex virus (HSV) encephalitis
c. Tuberculous meningitis
d. Food allergy
e. Bacterial meningitis

30. A 4-year-old child is seen by the pediatrician for a well-child visit. The family reports no new problems. The past medical history is significant for multiple episodes of otitis media, some with perforation. The last ear infection was about 3 months ago; it was not associated with perforation. Growth and development (including language) has been normal. On physical examination he is awake, alert, and happy. On otoscopic examination a discrete, whitish polyp extends through the left tympanic membrane. Which of the following is the most likely diagnosis?

a. Cholesteatoma
b. Tympanosclerosis
c. Acute otitis media with perforation and drainage
d. Dislocation of the malleus from its insertion in the tympanic membrane
e. Excessive cerumen production

31. An 8-month-old infant is seen in the ED for diarrhea. The family reports that the child has had a 2-day history of nonbloody diarrhea and poor fluid intake. Triage vital signs show heart rate of 180 beats per minute, respiratory rate of 30 breaths per minute, and blood pressure of 60/40 mm Hg. On physical examination he has poor skin turgor, 5-second capillary refill, and cool extremities. Which of the following fluids is most appropriate first step in the management of this condition?

a. Dextrose 5% in ¼ normal saline (D_5 ¼ NS)
b. Dextrose 5% in ½ normal saline (D_5 ½ NS)
c. Normal saline
d. Whole blood
e. Dextrose 10% in water ($D_{10}W$)

32. A 2-month-old infant is seen by the pediatrician for routine care. The family reports that he was a term, vaginal delivery with discharge at about 48 hours of age. He has had no illnesses since birth. His diet consists of exclusive breast milk. Medications include daily multivitamins that contain vitamin D and iron. On physical examination the vital signs are normal. Weight, length, and head circumference are at the 75th percentile for age. He is awake and alert. The chest is clear. Heart has a normal S1 and S2 without murmur. His abdomen is soft, nontender, and without hepatosplenomegaly. The umbilical cord is firmly attached. Which of the following is the most likely mechanism for these findings?

a. Muscular defect of the abdominal wall
b. Inherited condition of abnormal neutrophil recruitment
c. Immunoglobulin deficiency
d. Repeated trauma to the umbilicus
e. Persistence of a congenital structure

33. A 4-year-old girl is seen by the pediatric nurse practitioner for vaginal itching and irritation. The mother states that the child is toilet trained, has not complained of frequency or urgency, nor has she noted any blood in her urine. She denies fever and abdominal pain. The child has had an occasional URI but no serious illness. She takes no medications. The home consists of the mother and father, one dog, and one bird. The mother does not work outside the home. On physical examination the vital signs are normal. The child is happy, alert, and in no distress. The chest is clear. Heart has a normal S1 and S2 without murmur. Her abdomen is soft, nontender, and without hepatosplenomegaly. The perineum has some erythema of the vulvar area, and no evidence of trauma, foul odor, or discharge. Which of the following is the most appropriate next course of action?

a. Refer to pediatric gynecology for a vaginal examination under anesthesia for a possible foreign body.
b. Counsel mother to stop giving the girl bubble baths, have the girl wear only cotton underwear, and improve hygiene.
c. Refer to social services for suspected physical or sexual abuse.
d. Send urine nucleic acid amplification test (NAAT) for *N. gonorrhoeae* and *Chlamydia*.
e. Treat with an antifungal cream for suspected yeast infection.

34. A 2-month-old infant is seen by the pediatrician for well-child care. The family is concerned that the back of the infant's head is flat. Delivery was vaginal, at term, and without pregnancy complications to a 30-year-old gravida 5 mother. On physical examination the weight and length are 45th percentile and the head is 50th percentile. The anterior fontanel is about 1.25 by 2 cm and the posterior fontanel is about 0.5 cm. Suture line ridges and splitting are absent. Facial features are normal. The posterior occiput is flat. The infant smiles spontaneously, tracks past the midline, and brings her hands to her mouth. Cranial nerves and deep tendon reflexes are normal. When placed prone she lifts her head from the table. Which of the following is the most appropriate initial step in management?

a. Neurosurgical evaluation
b. CT scan of the head with attention to bone windows
c. Increase prone position when awake
d. Refer for cranial remolding orthosis (helmet)
e. Place infant prone when asleep

35. A 14-year-old African American boy is seen in the medical clinic of a ski resort. He was reportedly on a Boy Scout-sponsored hiking expedition during winter break when he became tired, clumsy, and began to hallucinate. His father reports he has been generally healthy, taking methylphenidate during the school year for his attention-deficit/hyperactivity disorder (ADHD). On physical examination the temperature is 34.7°C (94°F), heart rate is 45 beats per minute, and respiratory rate is 12 breaths per minute. He is awake and somewhat interactive. He stares at the door stating "the wolves are coming in." The chest is clear. Heart has a normal S1 and S2 without murmur. His abdomen is soft, nontender, and without hepatosplenomegaly. The extremities are cool. Cranial nerves are intact, deep tendon reflexes are normal, and no focal neurologic abnormalities are noted. Which of the following is the most likely diagnosis?

a. Sickle cell trait with acute stroke
b. Drug ingestion
c. Altitude sickness
d. Malingering
e. Hypothermia

36. A 5-year-old boy is seen in the emergency room for a dog bite. The family reports that the child was attempting to dress the neighbor's immunized Chihuahua as a superhero when the unfortunate altercation occurred. They applied pressure and the small amount of bleeding stopped prior to arrival to the emergency room. The child has been in good health, takes no medications, and is current on his immunizations. On physical examination the child is alert, awake, and is in no distress. The right forearm has several less than 0.5-cm irregularly shaped superficial lacerations with a small amount of dried blood on the surface. The arm and hand have good movement and strength. Sensation and perfusion are normal. Which of the following is the most appropriate next step in management?

a. Copious irrigation and antimicrobial prophylaxis
b. Tetanus booster immunization and tetanus toxoid in the wound
c. Copious irrigation
d. Primary rabies vaccination for the child
e. Destruction of the dog and examination of brain tissue for rabies

37. A 16-year-old girl is seen in the ED with vomiting, diaphoresis, and malaise. The friends that brought her to the ED report that she was in the bathroom at a local theater crying, reportedly having had a fight with her boyfriend earlier in the day. She told her friends that she took a handful of pills about 12 hours earlier. Her past medical history is negative. On physical examination the temperature is 37°C (98.5°F), heart rate is 118 beats per minute, respiratory rate is 24 breaths per minute, and blood pressure is 90/50 mm Hg. She is awake, pale, and diaphoretic. The abdomen is soft, tender in the right upper quadrant, bowel sounds active, and without hepatosplenomegaly.

Hemoglobin: 13.5 g/dL
Hematocrit: 41%
WBC: 8000/mm^3
   Segmented neutrophils: 40%
   Band forms: 3%
   Lymphocytes: 57%
Platelet count: 175,000/mm^3
Aspartate aminotransferase (AST): 1500 IU/L
Alanine aminotransferase (ALT): 1600 IU/L
Urine drug screen negative

Administration of which of the following is the most appropriate next step in management?

a. Deferoxamine
b. Naloxone (Narcan)
c. N-acetylcysteine (Mucomyst)
d. Crotalidae Polyvalent Immune Fab (CroFab)
e. Dimercaptosuccinic acid (DMSA, succimer)

38. As a city public health officer, you have been charged with the task of screening high-risk children for lead poisoning. Which of the following is the best screen for this purpose?

a. Careful physical examination of each infant and child
b. Erythrocyte protoporphyrin levels (EP, FEP, or ZPP)
c. CBC and blood smear
d. Blood lead level
e. Environmental history

39. A 15-year-old boy is seen in the ED with confusion and combativeness. He is accompanied by his high school football coach who reports he was at afternoon practice with his other team members when he complained of headache and nausea. He was given some water and returned to practice. A short time later he became confused and combative on the field. His past medical history is positive for a broken clavicle and an episode of concussion about 12 months ago. He takes no medications, and is not known to smoke, drink alcohol, or take other drugs. On physical examination the temperature is 41°C (105.8°F), heart rate is 130 beats per minute, respiratory rate is 24 breaths per minute, and blood pressure is 110/80 mm Hg. He is awake, dizzy, and sweating profusely. Which of the following is the most appropriate next step?

a. Provide oral rehydration solutions
b. Administer acetaminophen rectally
c. Obtain CT scan of the head
d. Initiate whole body cold water immersion
e. Obtain a urine drug screen

40. A neonate is seen in the normal newborn nursery by the pediatric nurse practitioner. The delivery was vaginal and at term to a 33-year-old woman whose pregnancy was uncomplicated. The physical examination is normal. At 48 hours of age the baby has been eating well, has voided and stooled; weight has dropped by 5% to 3300 g. Which of the following is the most appropriate advice for this family for their infant's sleep?

a. Supine position in a crib or bassinet
b. Prone position in a crib or bassinet
c. Seated position in a car seat
d. Trendelenburg position in a crib or bassinet
e. Use an infant hammock

41. A 14-year-old boy is seen in the physicians' office for a laceration on his hand. The mother reports that he was at school when he became agitated and punched a wall. His past medical history reveals a diagnosis of mild autism and obsessive compulsive disorder for which he takes fluoxetine (Prozac). He does poorly in special education classes at the local school. On physical examination the temperature is 37°C (98.5°F), heart rate is 74 beats per minute, respiratory rate 16 breaths per minute, and blood pressure of 110/64 mm Hg. Height and weight are 35th percentile, and the head circumference is 95th percentile. He has a long and thin face. The ears are large and protruding. The mucous membranes are moist and without lesions; the palate is arched and high. The chest is clear and with mild pectus excavatum. Heart has a normal S1 and S2 with a click over the mitral valve area. His phallus is normal in size and shape, and testes are enlarged. Which of the following is the most likely diagnosis?

a. Trisomy 21
b. Trisomy 18
c. Trisomy 13
d. Fragile X syndrome
e. Williams syndrome

42. A 5-month-old infant is brought by EMS to the ED for seizure. The EMS personnel report that they were told he was in his normal state of health when he had a generalized tonic-clonic seizure lasting about 30 minutes that stopped upon their administration of lorazepam. The family is not yet present for an interview. On physical examination the temperature is 37°C (98.5°F), heart rate is 100 beats per minute, respiratory rate is 18 breaths per minute, and blood pressure is 90/50 mm Hg. Height and weight are less than the 25th percentile, and head circumference is 50th percentile. He is sleepy but arousable. Head is normocephalic with fingertip-sized anterior fontanelle. Eyes and ears are normal size, shape, and position. The mucous membranes are moist and without lesions. The chest is clear. Heart has a normal S1 and S2. The abdomen is soft, nontender, and without hepatosplenomegaly. Which of the following historical bits of information gathered from the mother is most likely to lead to the correct diagnosis in this patient?

a. He has had congestion but no fever for the previous 3 days.
b. He smiles responsively, sits with some assistance, babbles and coos, and holds his own bottles; his siblings aged 5 and 8 are in regular classes at school.
c. The mother recently lost her job and has been diluting his formula to make it last longer.
d. The household contains two dogs and one cat at home; none have been vaccinated.
e. The mother previously worked as an attorney in an energy-trading firm.

Questions 43 to 48

Many rashes and skin lesions can be found first in the newborn period. For each of the descriptions listed below, select the most likely diagnosis. Each lettered option may be used once, more than once, or not at all.

a. Sebaceous nevus
b. Salmon patch
c. Neonatal acne
d. Pustular melanosis
e. Erythema toxicum
f. Seborrheic dermatitis
g. Milia

43. A 1-week-old neonate's mother reports that the newborn has a transient rash that appears all over the body. The rash consists of discrete splotchy areas of erythema up to about 2 cm and with a central clear pustule. Microscopic examination of the liquid in the pustule reveals eosinophils.

44. An adolescent boy reports a splotchy red rash on the nape of his neck, discovered by his teammates when he had his head shaved for football season. The rash is about 3-5 cm in size and is reported by his teammates to become more prominent with exercise or emotion. His mother notes that he has had the rash since infancy, but that it became invisible as hair grew. He had a similar rash on his eyelids that resolved in the newborn period.

45. A 3-day-old African American neonate is seen in the pediatrician's office for a "staph infection." On physical examination the pustules are about 3 mm in size, are filled with a milky fluid, are easily wiped away and reveal an underlying small hyperpigmented macule.

46. A 1-day-old boy is seen in the normal newborn nursery. The delivery was vaginal after an uneventful term pregnancy. On physical examination the vital signs are normal. The scalp reveals a 0.5-cm oval lesion on the right occiput. The yellowish lesion is slightly raised, hairless, and is "orange-peel" in texture.

47. A 2-day-old girl is seen in the pediatrician's office. The mother reports that the infant has numerous very small raised white dots around her chin and on the nose. On physical examination the vital signs are normal. The nose and chin have numerous pinpoint-sized white lesions without surrounding erythema. The lesions are not easily removed.

48. A 2-week-old neonate is seen by the pediatrician. The father reports no issues other than "dandruff." On physical examination the newborn has many yellowish, waxy flakes of skin on the scalp. Scrapping of the firmly adherent skin lesions also results in dislodgment of hair. A similar eruption is noted on the eyebrows.

Questions 49 to 53

For each otherwise normal child presented, choose the nocturnal disturbance most consistent with the history. Each lettered option may be used once, more than once, or not at all.

a. Night terrors
b. Nightmares
c. Learned behavior
d. Obstructive sleep apnea
e. Somniloquy
f. Temporal lobe seizures
g. Allergic rhinitis
h. Simple snoring

49. A 3-year-old boy awakens nightly at about 2:00 AM screaming incoherently. His parents report that when they check on him he is agitated, seems awake but unresponsive, and goes back to sleep within a few minutes. He has no memory of the episodes in the morning.

50. A 15-month-old toddler awakes nightly with crying. The parents report they give her a nighttime bottle, rock and sing to her to help her go back to sleep.

51. A 5-year-old girl is heard over the baby monitor to be crying out during her sleep. The parents report that when they check on her, she is sleeping comfortably and is in no apparent distress.

52. A 10-year-old boy is seen for a refill of his methylphenidate. The family reports he is healthy other than loud snoring and has new-onset nocturnal enuresis. On physical examination the weight is at the 95th percentile and he has "kissing" tonsils.

53. A 5-year-old child refuses to sleep in his bed, claiming there are monsters in his closet and that he has bad dreams. The parents report that they allow him to sleep with them in their bed to avoid the otherwise inevitable screaming fit. When sleeping with them, the parents note that the child sleeps soundly, waking only at sunrise.

Questions 54 to 56

For each numbered patient presentation, select the one lettered immunization most likely required. Each lettered heading may be selected once, more than once, or not at all.

a. Measles vaccine alone
b. Measles-mumps-rubella (MMR) and varicella vaccine
c. Meningococcal, human papilloma virus (HPV), and tetanus toxoid, reduced diphtheria toxoid and acellular pertussis (Tdap) vaccines
d. Diphtheria and tetanus toxoids, acellular pertussis, inactivated poliovirus, *Haemophilus influenzae* type b conjugate, and rotavirus vaccines
e. Pneumococcal 23-valent vaccine
f. Immunizations contraindicated

54. An 11-year-old boy is seen by the pediatrician for a well-child evaluation. He has been in good health and reports no illness. He reports that he is helping to care for his older brother's twin, 3-week-old daughters. His physical examination is normal.

55. A 6-month-old girl is seen by the pediatric nurse practitioner for a well-child examination. The father reports that the infant has had a runny nose and cough for the previous 3 days. He reports a temperature of 38.1°C (100.6°F) for 1 day, but no vomiting, diarrhea, or change in diet. The physical examination is pertinent only for a slight nasal and eye discharge.

56. A 2-year-old child is seen by the pediatrician for well-child care. The past medical history is significant for sickle cell disease (SSD). Medications include daily folate and penicillin. The physical examination is normal.

Questions 57 and 58

For each numbered item (patient presentation), select the one lettered heading (most likely missed immunization opportunity) most closely associated with it. Each lettered heading may be selected once, more than once, or not at all.

a. MMR
b. Varicella
c. Meningococcal
d. HPV
e. Tetanus toxoid, reduced diphtheria toxoid and acellular pertussis (Tdap)
f. Pneumococcal 23 valent

57. A 3-year-old boy is seen by the pediatrician for well-child visit. He has been healthy according to his mother, but she reports that for the last several weeks his voice has become hoarse.

58. A 4-year-old previously healthy but unimmunized child is admitted to the pediatric intensive care unit with sepsis. The family reports that she developed a fever and a pruritic rash with crops of blisters on erythematous bases all over her body 2-3 days prior. Over the preceding 48 hours one area of lesions near her posterior left knee has spread to include the entire left thigh. The thigh is bright red, exquisitely tender, and very swollen.

Questions 59 and 60

For each disorder mentioned later, select the dietary deficiency that is likely to be responsible. Each lettered option may be used once, more than once, or not at all.

a. Folate deficiency
b. Thiamine deficiency
c. Niacin deficiency
d. Vitamin D deficiency
e. Vitamin C deficiency
f. Vitamin B_{12} deficiency
g. Vitamin B_6 deficiency
h. Biotin deficiency
i. Riboflavin deficiency

59. A 9-month-old boy is seen by the health worker in a refugee camp. He has a history of pallor, irritability, and poor weight gain. He is from a war-torn area of the world and has been fed only cow's milk since birth. On physical examination his arms and legs have extreme pain and tenderness with movement. His preferred position of comfort is "frog leg" (semiflexion of the hips and knees).

60. A 14-year-old child is seen by the pediatrician. She has a history of ulcerative colitis, poor appetite, abdominal pain, diarrhea, rash, and irritability. On physical examination the tongue is erythematous and smooth with loss of papillae. Skin has acute areas that are red with large blisters, especially in areas of sun exposure. In older areas the rash is dusky and brown in color. The muscles are weak, and the gait is abnormal.

Questions 61 to 64

Match each clinical presentation with the most likely syndrome. Each lettered option may be used once, more than once, or not at all.

a. Trisomy 13
b. Cri du chat syndrome
c. Angelman syndrome
d. VATER
e. Cornelia de Lange syndrome

61. An infant is noted in the normal newborn nursery to have unusual facies. He was born at 36 weeks' gestation to a 32-year-old woman whose pregnancy was complicated by intrauterine growth restriction. On physical examination his weight and head circumference are at the 5th percentile and the length at the 25th percentile. The cry is high-pitched and the infant is hypertonic. The eyebrows are confluent and the eyelashes long and curly. He has low-set and posteriorly rotated ears and a high-arched palate. The neck is short. Testes are high in the canal. The limbs are short with oligodactyly on upper extremities.

62. A 17-year-old boy is seen by the pediatrician for his annual visit. His past medical history is significant for a seizure disorder for which he takes phenytoin; his last generalized tonic-clonic seizure was 2 months prior. On physical examination he has an unusual gait, microcephaly, blond hair, pale blue eyes, and a large mouth with tongue protrusion. He is developmentally delayed and has unprovoked bursts of laughter.

63. A 6-week-old boy is seen in the pediatrician's office for routine visit. He was born at term to a 29-year-old woman whose pregnancy was complicated by intrauterine growth retardation. At birth he was noted to be small for gestation age. He had feeding problems that required his initial hospital stay to be 10 days, and he has gained weight slowly over the first 6 weeks of life. On physical examination the weight and head circumference are less than the 5th percentile. The cry is high-pitched. The face is rounded with full cheeks, the eyes have hypertelorism, strabismus, and epicanthal folds. The mouth has micrognathia. The ears are low-set.

64. A neonatologist is called to the delivery room to evaluate a newborn that has unusually short arms. The pregnancy was at term to a 23-year-old woman whose pregnancy was complicated by poor prenatal care that revealed on an early ultrasound left renal agenesis. The newborn is transported to the transition nursery in the neonatal intensive care nursery where he is noted to choke on feeds. On physical examination he has shortened arms and anal atresia. Further evaluation demonstrates vertebral defects on plain chest radiograph and a large ventricular septal defect on echocardiogram.

Questions 65 to 68

For each patient seen in a pediatric clinic, select the age most closely associated with the description. Each lettered heading may be selected once, more than once, or not at all.

a. 1-month old
b. 2-month old
c. 4-month old
d. 6-month old
e. 9-month old
f. 12-month old
g. 15-month old
h. 18-month old
i. 24-month old
j. 36-month old
k. 48-month old
l. 72-month old

65. A boy can regard the examiner's face, follow to midline, lift his head from the examining table, smile spontaneously, and respond to a bell. He does not regard his own hand, follow past the midline an object presented before his face, nor lift his head to a 45° angle off the examining table.

66. A girl is able to put on a t-shirt but requires a bit of help dressing otherwise. She can copy a circle well but has difficulty in copying a square. Her speech is understandable and she knows four colors. She balances on each foot for 2 seconds but is unable to hold the stance for 5 seconds.

67. A girl walks well holding on to furniture but is slightly wobbly when walking alone. She uses a neat pincer grasp to pick up a pellet, and she can release a cube into a cup after the act has been demonstrated to her. She tries to build a tower of two cubes with variable success.

68. A boy follows his father imitating his housework, uses a spoon but spills some, and is able to help take off some clothes for baths. He can build a tower of two cubes, can dump raisin from a bottle after the act has been demonstrated to him, and has three words other than mama and dada. He walks well and is variably successful in attempts to walk backward.

Questions 69 to 73

For the most likely toxic substance involved in each case, select the appropriate treatment. Each lettered option may be used once, more than once, or not at all.

a. Atropine and pralidoxime (2-PAM)
b. *N*-acetylcysteine (Mucomyst)
c. Dimercaptosuccinic acid (DMSA, succimer)
d. Naloxone (Narcan)
e. Sodium bicarbonate
f. Naloxone (Narcan) and atropine

69. A previously healthy and developmentally normal 2-year-old girl is seen in the ED for vomiting and altered mental status. The family reports that over the previous 2 weeks she began to have a poor appetite, periods of lethargy with naps at unusual times, and when awake is more irritable than normal. She no longer sleeps well at night. Social history reveals they recently moved to a home that is undergoing extensive renovation but is closer to the father's downtown work location. On physical examination the child has acute encephalopathy, ataxia, and variable consciousness.

70. A 30-month-old boy is seen in the emergency center for lethargy. The family reports that they were helping a relative move into a new apartment when the toddler was found to be playing with the contents of his 67-year-old great aunt's purse. At triage the temperature is 37°C (98.5°F), heart rate is 40 beats per minute, respiratory rate is 12 breaths per minute, and blood pressure is 80/40 mm Hg. He is lethargic. Eyes show miosis. The chest is clear. Heart has a normal S1 and S2 without murmur. The abdomen is soft and nontender. While in the ED his respiratory rate drops further, he becomes apneic, and requires intubation.

71. A newborn is seen in the delivery room by the neonatologist for minimal respiratory effort. The pregnancy was term and complicated by positive maternal group B *Streptococcus* (GBS). Rupture of membranes occurred 14 hours prior to delivery. Medications included 3 doses of penicillin during labor and pain medication just prior to the vaginal delivery. On physical examination the newborn is somewhat pale, has poor tone, poor respiratory effort, and a heart rate of 110 beats per minute.

72. A 4-year-old girl is seen in the ED for an ingestion of an unknown substance. The family reports that she was found at her grandfather's house consuming a bottleful of small, chewable pills. While enroute they reported several episodes of vomiting. At triage the temperature is 39.2°C (102.5°F), heart rate is 120 beats per minute, respiratory rate is 28 breaths per minute, and blood pressure is 100/55 mm Hg. She is disoriented and complains of a bell is ringing in her ears. The pupils are equally round and reactive. Laboratory data reveal:

Arterial blood gas
  pH: 7.0
  $PaCO_2$: 34 mm Hg
  PaO_2: 100 mm Hg
  HCO_3: 12 mEq/L
  BE: –15 mmol/L

73. A 14-year-old boy is seen in the ED after having a generalized, 2 minute long tonic-clonic seizure. His father reports that they were working in the yard when the boy complained of abdominal pain, weakness, and felt like his muscles were twitching. His father noted that the boy began to drool, urinated and soiled himself, and then collapsed before the seizure began. At triage the temperature is 37°C (98.5°F), heart rate is 130 beats per minute, respiratory rate is 22 breaths per minute, and blood pressure is 120/85 mm Hg. He is awake, alert, and restless. The eyes have profuse drainage and the pupils are pinpoint. Mucous membranes reveal copious drainage and no lesions. Chest has some wheezes. The abdomen has mild tenderness and increased bowel sounds.

Questions 74 to 78

Each patient in the following vignettes has a parasitic disease. Match the patient's condition with the correct first-line treatment. Each lettered option may be used once, more than once, or not at all.

a. Metronidazole
b. Albendazole
c. Amoxicillin
d. Trimethoprim/sulfamethoxazole
e. Sodium stibogluconate
f. Chloroquine
g. Praziquantel

74. An 18-year-old girl is seen by the student health center doctor for dyspareunia and dysuria. On physical examination she has a frothy gray malodorous vaginal discharge.

75. A 7-year-old boy is seen by the pediatrician for fever, headache, and drowsiness. He is just back from a mission trip with his family to Haiti. On physical examination he has splenomegaly and pallor.

76. A 4-year-old girl is seen by the pediatric nurse practitioner for diarrhea. The mother reports that the child developed 3 days prior foul-smelling flatulence, nonbloody but greasy diarrhea, abdominal cramping, and generalized weakness. She reports no travel; the child spends 3 days a week in a Mother's Day Out program. On physical examination the child is alert, active, and in no distress. The mucous membranes are moist and without lesion. The abdomen is distended, nontender, and with active bowel sounds.

77. A 2-year-old boy is seen in the ED for diarrhea. The mother reports that he has had 11 days of nonbloody diarrhea, fatigue, abdominal cramping, and weight loss. The child attends day care, and the mother reports many other children had "bad raspberries" and are demonstrating similar symptoms. At triage the temperature is 38.6°C (101.5°F), heart rate is 102 beats per minute, respiratory rate is 18 breaths per minute, and blood pressure of 90/55 mm Hg. He is wake, alert, and in no distress. Mucous membranes are moist without lesions. Chest is clear. The abdomen is soft, nontender, distended and without organomegaly.

78. A 16-year-old boy is seen in the ED for syncope. His father reports that he was assisting in repairs on their Alaskan king crab fishing boat when he became dizzy when standing and then fainted. The father reports no previous serious illnesses and denies his son smokes, drinks alcohol, or ingests other drugs. On physical examination the temperature is 37°C (98.5°F), heart rate is 130 beats per minute, respiratory rate is 18 breaths per minute, and blood pressure is 90/55 mm Hg. He is awake, alert, and in no distress while lying down but becomes dizzy when sitting up. Mucous membranes are pale, moist, and without lesions. Mouth has a beefy red, swollen tongue with loss of papillae, especially at the edges. Chest is clear. The abdomen is soft, nontender, and without organomegaly. Laboratory data reveal:

Hemoglobin: 8.8 g/dL
Hematocrit: 24.2%
Mean corpuscular volume (MCV): 135 fL
WBC: 8500/mm^3
   Segmented neutrophils: 49%
   Band forms: 0%
   Lymphocytes: 51%
Many macrocytes and hypersegmented neutrophils are noted on smear.
Platelet count: 127,000/mm^3

Questions 79 to 83

The normal development of the fetus can be adversely affected by exposure to a number of environmental factors, including infectious agents, physical agents, chemical agents, and maternal metabolic and genetic agents. Match each maternal history of teratogen exposure with the most likely clinical presentation in the infant. Each lettered option may be used once, more than once, or not at all.

a. Small palpebral fissures, ptosis, midfacial hypoplasia, smooth philtrum
b. Hypoplasia of distal phalanges, small nails
c. Bilateral microtia or anotia, congenital heart disease, central nervous system (CNS) abnormalities
d. Spina bifida
e. Ebstein anomaly
f. Renal dysgenesis, oligohydramnios
g. Cataracts
h. Hemangiomatosis

79. A 15-year-old girl is seen by the pediatrician for severe acne. She has failed treatments of topical benzoyl peroxide, topical antibiotics, and is started on an oral preparation of retinoic acid. She has unexpectedly become pregnant, receives no prenatal care, and delivers a male infant at 37 weeks' gestation.

80. A 32-year-old woman delivers a term infant vaginally. She has received no prenatal care, and reports a diet low in green vegetables and enriched grain products.

81. A 33-year-old woman has a long-standing history of hypertension treated with angiotensin-converting enzyme (ACE) inhibitors. She delivers a term infant vaginally after having received no prenatal care.

82. A 17-year-old primiparous mother delivers a 36-week gestation infant. Her pregnancy was complicated by a first trimester fever associated with "3-day" measles.

83. A 23-year-old pregnant woman with manic-depressive disorder has had poor prenatal care. Her psychiatric condition was well-maintained with lithium. She delivers a term female infant.

Questions 84 to 87

Match each common skin condition with the most appropriate therapy. Each lettered option may be used once, more than once, or not at all.

a. Mild cleansing cream, topical moisturizers, and topical steroids
b. Ivermectin
c. Oral antihistamines alone
d. Reassurance only
e. Permethrin 5% cream
f. Topical steroids or a selenium sulfide-containing product
g. Topical antifungal agents
h. Isotretinoin

84. An 18-year-old boy is seen by the pediatrician for a pruritic lesion on his foot. He reports that he just returned from spring break from a coastal town in Central America where the intensely pruritic rash had begun to develop. On physical examination the lesion on his foot is raised, red, serpiginous, and has a few associated bullae.

85. A 6-week-old boy is seen by the pediatric nurse practitioner for a rash on his scalp. The mother reports that the rash developed at about 3 or 4 weeks of age and has progressed. She initially tried emollients with little effect. On physical examination the scalp has scaly, yellow patches with associated hair loss.

86. A 4-year-old child is seen in the pediatrician's office for a well-child visit. The family reports her to be in good health without recent illnesses. Her father reports that he and his daughter developed a splotchy hyperpigmented rash 2 days prior after the family attended a backyard pool party where all enjoyed hotdogs, hamburgers, and fajitas. The children enjoyed limeade and the adults partook of margaritas. He reports his rash on his chest, while the rash on his daughter is around her mouth. On physical examination the child is healthy other than a slight sunburn and some hyperpigmentation around her face and on her hands.

87. A 4-month-old boy is seen by the pediatrician for a rash. The mother reports the pruritic rash began about a month earlier on his cheeks, arms, and upper chest. She denies fever, new soaps or lotions, or medications. Family history reveals his 10-year-old sister with a similar rash at approximately the same age which is now confined to her antecubital and popliteal fossa; her rash worsens in winter months. On physical examination the infant has a dry, scaly maculopapular eruption on the face, arms, and upper chest with evidence of excoriation.

Questions 88 to 90

Match each clinical finding with the most likely cause. Each lettered option may be used once, more than once, or not at all.

a. Patent ductus arteriosus
b. Severe anemia
c. Heart block
d. VSD
e. Arteriovenous malformation
f. Coarctation of the aorta

88. A 6-month-old infant is seen by the pediatrician for a well-child visit. He was born vaginally at term after an uncomplicated pregnancy to a 23-year-old mother. He is exclusively breast-fed and takes daily vitamins containing iron, vitamin D, and fluoride. On physical examination weight, length, and head circumference are at the 75th percentile for age. He is awake, alert, and in no distress. The chest is clear. Heart has a harsh blowing holosystolic murmur at the left lower sternal border that radiates over the precordium. His abdomen is soft, nontender, and without hepatosplenomegaly.

89. A 900-g neonate born at 28 weeks' gestation and currently in the neonatal intensive care nursery has developed a continuous machinery-like murmur at the second left intercostal space that radiates well to the anterior lung fields but not to the back.

90. A 1-day-old neonate is seen by the nurse practitioner in the normal newborn nursery. He was delivered vaginally at term to a 22-year-old woman whose pregnancy was complicated by active systemic lupus erythematosus (SLE).

Questions 91 to 96

The Committee on Nutrition of the American Academy of Pediatrics has concluded that children on a normal diet generally do not need vitamin supplements. There are, however, some clinical situations in which special needs do occur. Match each situation with the appropriate supplement. Each lettered option may be used once, more than once, or not at all.

a. All fat-soluble vitamins
b. Pyridoxine
c. Vitamin A
d. Vitamin C
e. Vitamin D
f. Vitamin K
g. Folate
h. Niacin

91. A 14-year-old boy is seen by the neurologist in follow-up for seizures. He was diagnosed with seizures 3 years prior and has been treated successfully having had no seizures in 24 months. His physical examination is unchanged from the previous year. Laboratory data reveal:

Hemoglobin: 10.2 g/dL
Hematocrit: 31.2%
MCV: 135 fL
WBC: 8500/mm³
   Segmented neutrophils: 49%
   Band forms: 0%
   Lymphocytes: 51%
Numerous macrocytes and a few hypersegmented neutrophils are noted on smear.
Platelet count: 127,000/mm³
Phenytoin level: 15 μg/mL

92. A developing country has an epidemic characterized by high fever associated with malaise, fever, and anorexia. Almost all affected patients develop cough, conjunctivitis, and coryza and many have been noted to have a bluish-gray area on the buccal mucosa opposite the second molars. This prodrome is typically followed 2-4 days later by a confluent rash.

93. A 2-year-old child is seen by the pediatrician for failure to thrive. The family reports the child to have large, foul-smelling stools that float in the toilet. The history is positive for delayed passage of stool at birth.

94. A term infant is seen at 3 days by the pediatric nurse practitioner for early follow-up. The pregnancy was complicated by gestational diabetes and hypertension. The neonate is being exclusively breast-fed. The newborn stools several times per day and has eight wet diapers per day. The current weight is down about 3% from birth weight. Physical examination is normal other than mild jaundice and milia.

95. A 6-month-old infant is seen by the pediatric hospitalist on the inpatient unit of the local children's hospital. The infant was admitted from the emergency room after having been seen for a fever of 39.2°C (102.5°F). On physical examination the temperature is now 37°C (98.5°F), heart rate is 135 beats per minute, respiratory rate is 18 breaths per minute, and blood pressure is 90/55 mm Hg. He is awake, alert, and in no distress. Mucous membranes are pale, moist, and without lesions. Chest is clear. Heart has a 2/6 systolic ejection murmur at the left lower sternal border. Pulses and perfusion are normal. The abdomen is soft, nontender, and the spleen is felt 3 cm below the left costal margin. Laboratory data reveal:

Hemoglobin: 8.8 g/dL
Hematocrit: 24.2%
WBC: 9500/mm^3
 Segmented neutrophils: 70%
 Band forms: 1%
 Lymphocytes: 29%
Many target cells, elongated cells, and sickle erythrocytes noted on smear
Platelet count: 159,000/mm^3
ESR: 12 mm/h
Reticulocyte count: 9%

96. A 1-hour-old neonate and his mother are receiving routine care in the postanesthesia care unit. The neonate was born at 41 weeks' gestation by scheduled cesarean section. The pregnancy was complicated by advanced maternal age and gestational diabetes that was controlled with diet. At birth the newborn was vigorous, was placed skin to skin on the mothers' chest, and then to the breast for feeding at 10 minutes of life. The newborn has since voided and stooled. The physical examination is normal.

Questions 97 to 101

Match each clinical condition with the most appropriate diagnostic laboratory test. Each lettered option may be used once, more than once, or not at all.

a. ESR
b. Serum immunoglobulin levels
c. Dihydrorhodamine 123 (DHR) oxidation test
d. CH50 assay
e. CBC demonstrating Howell-Jolly bodies
f. Platelet count
g. Intradermal skin test using *Candida albicans*

97. A hospitalized 1-year-old boy is seen by the pediatric surgeon for a hepatic abscess identified on ultrasound. He has been admitted three times previously with abscess formation on his legs or buttocks requiring incision and drainage.

98. A 5-month-old infant is admitted by the emergency room attending to the local children's hospital pediatric intensive care unit for respiratory distress. The infant was diagnosed with varicella 3 days prior, and per the family the lesions have spread and cover the infant's entire body. Past medical history is significant for a history of severe atopic dermatitis and frequent epistaxis, the last occurring 3 months prior and required nasal packing in the ED.

99. A 3-year-old boy is seen by the pediatrician for follow-up of osteomyelitis of the femur due to *S aureus*. Past medical history reveals normal birth, growth, and development through the first 4 or 5 months of age with repeated episodes of sinusitis and otitis media thereafter. Family history reveals a maternal uncle with similar infectious problems; that uncle died at the age of 3 years from a "lung infection." On physical examination vital signs are normal. Mucous membranes are moist and without lesions; tonsillar tissue is not seen. Chest is clear. Heart has normal S1 and S2 without murmur. The abdomen is soft, nontender, and without hepatosplenomegaly. Lymph nodes are not found in the axilla, groin, or head and neck regions.

100. A 3-year-old boy is seen by the pediatrician in consultation from the local general practitioner for "frequent infections." The family reports him to be a term, vaginal delivery with a 2-week newborn nursery course complicated by "low calcium" and "seizures." Current medications include daily over-the-counter multivitamins and prescription calcium supplementation. On physical examination vital signs are normal. Ears are small, low-set, and posteriorly rotated. Eyes are widely spaced and down-slanting. The nose is upturned. The jaw is small. Heart has a loud systolic murmur.

101. A 2-year-old girl was admitted 24 hours prior to the local children's hospital for fever, thrombocytopenia, and hypotension. Her family reports she was in good health until about 12 hours prior to admission when she developed irritability, poor feeding, and fever. A sepsis evaluation was done in the ED and broad-spectrum antibiotics were initiated. The child's past history is positive for two previous episodes of *Neisseria meningitidis* septicemia. Current blood cultures are positive for *Streptococcus pneumoniae.*

General Pediatrics

Answers

1. The answer is e. (*Hay et al, pp 819-820. Kliegman et al, pp 844, 3014-3015. Rudolph et al, p 2233.*) Bell palsy is an acute, unilateral facial nerve palsy that begins about 2 weeks after a viral infection. Although the exact pathophysiology is unknown, reactivation of herpes simplex or varicella-zoster virus seems to be the most common cause; demyelination through an autoimmune process or allergic inflammation may also play a part in some cases. On the affected side, the upper and lower face are typically paretic, the mouth droops, and the patient cannot close the eye. Treatment consists of maintaining moisture to the affected eye (especially at night) to prevent keratitis. Complete, spontaneous resolution occurs in about 85% of cases, 10% of cases have mild residual disease, and about 5% of cases do not resolve. Occasionally infants will have facial nerve palsy at birth; this is usually related to compression from forceps and spontaneously resolves over several weeks. As this is a compression neuropathy, it should not be called congenital Bell palsy.

When evaluating a facial weakness, special care must be taken to evaluate the movement of the forehead. A peripheral facial neuropathy like Bell palsy will cause upper and lower facial weakness on the affected side. However, a central facial palsy will spare the forehead due to bilateral innervation.

Guillain-Barré syndrome is classically described as a demyelinating neuropathy that causes ascending weakness and diminished reflexes. Symptoms of paresthesia (occasionally pain) classically start in the hands or feet and then move centrally before affecting facial, respiratory, or other central structures.

The most common form of botulism in the United States is "infant botulism," classically described as resulting from the ingestion of honey but more often the source is unknown. Other forms of botulism occur as "food-borne" or "wound." In older patients with food-borne or wound botulism the first symptoms are cranial nerve findings of diplopia and blurred vision, dry mouth, and then descending weakness and paralysis. Infant botulism typically presents in the 2- to 4-month-old infant as constipation, poor gag reflex, and then descending weakness and paralysis.

Ischemic stroke typically is an abrupt onset of neurologic symptoms that might include a combination of visual defects, blurred vision, ataxia, aphasia, and change in consciousness. Hemorrhagic stroke may also have the symptoms of nausea, vomiting, and headache. Isolated facial droop would be unusual for either.

A brainstem tumor likely would present with a combination of cranial nerve deficits (sixth and seventh nerves common), long track signs (hyper-reflexia, clonus, muscle spasticity, bladder abnormalities), truncal or limb ataxia, nystagmus, and papilledema.

2. The answer is b. (*Hay et al, pp 830-831, 871. Kliegman et al, pp 3281-3283. Rudolph et al, pp 855-856.*) Slipped capital femoral epiphysis is a disease of unknown etiology and occurs typically in adolescents; the disorder is most common among obese boys with delayed skeletal maturation or in thin, tall adolescents having recently undergone a growth spurt. The onset of this disorder is frequently gradual; pain referred to the knee in 20% of cases can mask the hip pathology.

Legg-Calvé-Perthes disease is avascular necrosis or idiopathic osteonecrosis of the femoral head; the cause of this disorder is unknown. Boys between the ages of 2 and 12 years are most frequently affected (incidence in boys is four- to fivefold greater than in girls), with a mean of 6-7 years old. Presenting symptoms include a limp and pain in the anterior thigh, groin, or knee, although classic symptoms include a painless limp.

Septic arthritis requires urgent intervention to preserve joint mobility. Joint aspiration is diagnostic and can be helpful in treatment. Opening the joint space may be required in a septic hip to assist in draining purulent material. These children need treatment for 4-6 weeks.

Transient synovitis is a disorder of unknown etiology, affecting children usually from 2 to 6 years of age. These children usually present with a painful limp. This is a diagnosis of exclusion; septic hip and osteomyelitis must be ruled out. The WBC count and ESR may be normal or slightly elevated. Early aspiration of the joint space may assist in diagnosis. Transient synovitis is a self-limited disorder.

Osteomyelitis usually presents with focal bone tenderness and fever. Early evaluation is best done through nuclear medicine studies or MRI, as plain film bony changes usually take a week or so before becoming evident.

3. The answer is e. (*Hay et al, pp 844-845. Kliegman et al, p 1175. Rudolph et al, pp 1620-1630.*) Transient synovitis is a disorder of unknown etiology, affecting children usually from 2 to 6 years of age. These children usually present with a painful limp. The WBC count and ESR may be normal or slightly elevated. This is a diagnosis of exclusion; septic hip and osteomyelitis must be ruled out. Early aspiration of the joint space may assist in diagnosis. Transient synovitis is a self-limited disorder.

Legg-Calvé-Perthes disease is avascular necrosis or idiopathic osteonecrosis of the femoral head and occurs when the blood supply to the femoral head is interrupted. The cause of blood flow disruption is often not known. Boys between the ages of 2 and 12 years are most frequently affected (incidence in boys is four- to fivefold greater than in girls), with a mean of 6-7 years old. Presenting symptoms include a limp and pain in the anterior thigh, groin, or knee, although classic symptoms include a painless limp. Laboratory data are typically normal.

A septic joint can occur as a direct inoculation into the joint space or as a hematogenous spread of bacteria into the epiphysis (osteomyelitis) with subsequent seeding of the joint space. Septic arthritis of the hip requires urgent intervention to preserve joint mobility. Joint aspiration is diagnostic and can be helpful in treatment. Opening the joint space may be required in a septic hip to assist in draining purulent material. These children need treatment for 4-6 weeks. Osteomyelitis usually presents with focal bone tenderness and fever prior to joint involvement. Early evaluation is best done through nuclear medicine studies or MRI, as plain film bony changes usually take a week or so before becoming evident. In both cases, an elevated WBC and a significant elevation of ESR and C-reactive protein would be expected.

Leukemia can present with orthopedic findings of bone pain, limping, and swollen joints. Associated findings of anemia (pallor, fatigue, weakness), thrombocytopenia (bruising, petechiae, bleeding), generalized lymphadenopathy, and hepatosplenomegaly would be anticipated. Laboratory data would demonstrate evidence of bone marrow replacement with leukemic cells including anemia, thrombocytopenia, elevated or reduced WBCs, and demonstration of immature cells on peripheral smear.

4. The answer is a. (*Hay et al, pp 889-892. Kliegman et al, pp 1160-1170. Rudolph et al, pp 800-806.*) Oligoarticular JIA asymmetrically involves large joints, especially the knee, and often has no other symptoms. A major morbidity of oligoarticular JIA is chronic uveitis, resulting in blindness. About 20% of girls who have the oligoarticular form of JIA have iridocyclitis (anterior uveitis) as their only significant systemic manifestation. Because this eye disorder can require treatment with local or systemic steroids and develop without signs or symptoms, it is recommended that all children with this form of arthritis have frequent slit-lamp eye examinations.

The other choices listed in the question do not have characteristic eye findings, nor are eye findings expected.

Slipped capital femoral epiphysis is a disease of unknown etiology and occurs typically in adolescents; the disorder is most common among obese boys with delayed skeletal maturation or in thin, tall adolescents having recently enjoyed a growth spurt. The onset of this disorder is frequently gradual; pain referred to the knee in 20% of cases can mask the hip pathology. Laboratory data are typically normal.

Henoch-Schönlein purpura (HSP or anaphylactoid purpura) is a generalized, acute vasculitis of unknown etiology involving small blood vessels. The skin lesion is classically described as palpable purpura of the lower extremities and buttocks. It is often accompanied by arthritis, usually of the large joints, and by gastrointestinal symptoms. Colicky abdominal pain, vomiting, and melena are common. Renal involvement occurs in a significant number of patients and is potentially the most serious manifestation of the disease. Although most children with this complication recover, a few will develop chronic nephritis. Laboratory studies are not diagnostic. The platelet count, serum complement, and IgA levels can be normal or elevated. Coagulation studies and platelets are normal.

Legg-Calvé-Perthes disease is avascular necrosis or idiopathic osteonecrosis of the femoral head and occurs when the blood supply to the femoral head is interrupted. The cause of blood flow disruption is often not known. Boys between the ages of 2 and 12 years are most frequently affected (incidence in boys is four- to fivefold greater than in girls), with a mean of 6-7 years old. Presenting symptoms include a limp and pain in the anterior thigh, groin, or knee, although classic symptoms include a painless limp. Laboratory data are typically normal.

Osgood-Schlatter disease is repeated microfracture of the tibial tubercle at the insertion of the patellar tendon. This is an overuse injury typically seen in adolescents, and presents with swelling and knee pain localized to the tubercle.

5. The answer is b. (*Hay et al, pp 408-409, 1258. Kliegman et al, pp 3206-3207. Rudolph et al, p 1093.*) Also known as Ritter disease, staphylococcal scalded skin disease is seen most commonly in children less than 5 years of age. The rash is preceded by fever, irritability, and erythroderma (widespread erythema with extraordinary tenderness of the skin). Circumoral erythema; crusting of the eyes, mouth, and nose; and blisters on the skin are frequently present in areas of friction, such as intertriginous areas. Intraoral mucosal surfaces are not affected. Peeling of the epidermis in response to mild shearing forces (Nikolsky sign) leaves the patient susceptible to problems similar to those of a burn injury, including infection and fluid and electrolyte imbalance. Cultures of the bullae are negative, but the source site or blood often may be positive. Treatment includes antibiotics (to cover resistant *S aureus*) and localized skin care. Outcome is typically good and scaring unusual, unless a secondary infection develops.

Epidermolysis bullosa is a group of inherited conditions of the skin associated with blister formation due to trauma. Often a family history of similar lesions will be obtained. On physical examination common areas of trauma in pediatrics include the upper extremities (fingers, hands, and elbows), the legs (feet and toes) and in the diaper area of infants.

Erythema multiforme is a type IV hypersensitivity reaction to infections, medications, or other unknown triggers. Erythema multiforme minor is classically described as a localized skin eruption with no or minimal mucosal involvement in a "target" or "iris" shaped lesion. Erythema multiforme major (Stevens-Johnson syndrome) is a life-threatening condition that often begins on face or trunk as purpuric macules that then also involve the mucosa. A prior drug ingestion is often noted with this condition. Nikolsky sign is not an expected feature.

The findings of a classic drug eruption vary, but classically consist of widespread eruptions of papules, pustules, hives, or blisters after ingestion of a medication. Pruritus may be seen. A severe reaction might also include mucous membrane involvement and Nikolsky sign.

Scarlet fever is caused by erythrogenic toxin-producing group A β-hemolytic streptococci. It consists of an acute febrile illness with a scarlatiniform (sandpaper-like) rash, erythema of the mucous membranes that produces an injected pharynx and strawberry tongue, cervical lymphadenopathy, and desquamation of skin on the hands and feet 7-10 days later. Nikolsky sign is not an expected feature.

6. The answer is d. The advertisement includes the findings of a meta-analysis of four studies deemed by the company to be of "high quality"; the methodology used to choose these articles for analysis (and the reasons other studies were not chosen for analysis) is not described and potentially biases the conclusions. For example, if dozens of other high-quality studies were available that had opposite findings from those described but had been excluded from the analysis, the results would be dramatically affected.

The 75% relative risk reduction of colic suggests that as compared to the baseline rate of colic in the cow's milk group, 75% fewer infants fed this advertised product would experience colic. Importantly, the rate of colic among infants fed a cow's milk product is not stated. Thus, if the baseline rate of colic among infants fed intact cow's milk protein was 5%, 5 out of 100 children would have colic. A 75% relative reduction would reduce this incidence from 5 in 100 children to about 2 in 100 children. The "relative risk reduction" is often used in advertising as it is a large, eye-catching number. This reduction may or may not be "clinically" important if the baseline rate of the disease or condition is low.

While general references to breast milk are made in the advertisement, no outcome data presented suggest that the digestive health, gastrointestinal function or other conditions of infants fed this product match those of infants fed breast milk. Similarly, despite the inclusion of the words "just like mom" in the product name, no clinical data support the contention that this product's overall benefit is truly as good as breast milk.

No conclusion regarding the use of this product for a child whose family history is positive for allergies can be drawn. The small print suggests that this product has not been studied for this benefit.

7. The answer is c. (*Hay et al, pp 1258-1259. Kliegman et al, pp 2263-2269. Rudolph et al, p 1854.*) The child in the question has endocarditis as confirmed by the vegetations on the mitral valve. The American Heart Association updates the guidelines for the use of prophylactic antibiotics regularly. Among those patients currently recommended to receive prophylactic antibiotic treatment are patients for whom any heart infection would result in the highest incidence of adverse outcome: previous history of endocarditis, prosthetic valve or material for repair, heart transplant patients, and severe or partially repaired congenital heart defects (2017 AHA guideline revision). Activity is not usually limited unless there is extensive destruction of heart muscle or the conducting system leading to failure. Minimizing salt intake is generally a good idea, but not any more so in an individual who has endocarditis. Bed rest should be instituted only in the case of heart failure. Family members are not typically at risk.

8. The answer is b. (*Hay et al, p 330. Kliegman et al, pp 3447-3450. Rudolph et al, pp 446, 863.*) Human bites can pose a significant problem. They can become infected with oropharyngeal bacteria, including *S aureus, Streptococcus viridans, Eikenella corrodens*, and anaerobes. A patient with an infected human bite of the hand (fever, poor feeding, reduced activity, and red, indurated and tender hand) requires hospitalization for appropriate drainage procedures, Gram stain and culture of the exudate, vigorous cleaning, debridement, and appropriate antibiotics. The infected wound should be left open and allowed to heal by secondary intention (healing by granulation tissue rather than closure with sutures). Empiric antibiotic therapy for an infected bite should be penicillinase-resistant; amoxicillin-clavulanate orally, or ticarcillin-clavulanate or ampicillin-sulbactam IV are good choices. Antibiotic prophylaxis for noninfected bite wounds remains controversial, but some experts recommend prophylaxis for all significant human bites.

9. The answer is b. (*Hay et al, p 416. Kliegman et al, pp 3163-3164. Rudolph et al, p 1262.*) Pityriasis rosea is a benign condition that usually presents with a herald patch, a single round or oval lesion appearing anywhere on the body. Usually about 5 to 10 days after the appearance of the herald patch, a more diffuse rash involving the upper extremities and trunk appears. These lesions are oval or round, slightly raised, and pink to brown in color. The lesion is covered in a fine scale with some central clearing possible. The rash can appear in a Christmas tree pattern on the back, identified by the aligning of the long axis of the lesions with the cutaneous cleavage lines. The rash lasts 2-12 weeks and can be pruritic. This rash is commonly mistaken for tinea corporis, and the consideration of secondary syphilis is important. Treatment is usually unnecessary but can consist of topical emollients and oral antihistamines, as needed. More uncommonly, topical steroids can be helpful if the itching is severe.

Lichen planus is rare in children. It is intensely pruritic, and additional lesions can be induced with scratching. The lesion is commonly found on the flexor surfaces of the wrists, forearms, inner thighs, and occasionally on the oral mucosa.

Seborrheic dermatitis can begin anytime during life; it frequently presents as cradle cap in the newborn period. This rash is commonly greasy, scaly, and erythematous and, in smaller children, involves the face, neck, axilla, and diaper area. In older children, the rash can be localized to the scalp and intertriginous areas. Pruritus can be marked.

Contact dermatitis is characterized by redness, weeping, and oozing of the affected skin. The pattern of distribution can be helpful in identification of the offending agent. The rash can be pruritic; removal of the causative agent and use of topical emollients or steroids is curative.

Psoriasis consists of red papules that coalesce to form plaques with sharp edges. A thick, silvery scale develops on the surface and leaves a drop of blood upon its removal (Auspitz sign). Additional lesions develop on scratching older lesions. Commonly affected sites include scalp, knees, elbows, umbilicus, and genitalia.

10. The answer is b. (*Hay et al, pp 1043-1045. Kliegman et al, pp 2589-2590. Rudolph et al, pp 179, 1746.*) The infant in the question is a happy, chubby, normally developed boy. Many boys, especially those who are overweight, have an inconspicuous penis; when skin and fat lateral to the penis shaft are retracted, a normally sized and shaped penis is revealed. If, after performing this maneuver, the penis is found to be more than 2.5 standard deviations below the mean in size for age, and especially if other abnormal physical examination findings are noted, then further evaluation such as those listed in the question would be initiated.

11. The answer is a. (*Hay et al, pp 938-939. Kliegman et al, pp 1216-1218. Rudolph et al, pp 810-812.*) The clinical presentation described supports the diagnosis of anaphylactoid purpura (also known as Henoch-Schönlein purpura, or HSP), a generalized, acute vasculitis of unknown cause involving small blood vessels. In this condition, the skin lesion, which is classic in character (palpable purpura) and distribution, is often accompanied by arthritis and arthralgias, usually of the lower extremity joints, and by gastrointestinal symptoms. Colicky abdominal pain, vomiting, and melena are common. Renal involvement occurs in a significant number of patients and is potentially the most serious manifestation of the disease; early findings include a few red blood cells and protein in the urine. Although most children with this complication recover, a few will develop chronic nephritis; for this reason, children with HSP must be monitored for renal disease for 1-2 years after the episode. Laboratory studies are not diagnostic. The platelet count, serum complement, and IgA levels can be normal or elevated. Coagulation studies and platelets are normal.

Meningococcal (bacterial) infection and leukemia (infiltrate of skin by blasts) should be in the differential diagnosis, as both can cause purpura, but in a well-appearing child with normal vital signs and normal blood counts as presented they are unlikely. Child abuse (inflicted injury) and hemophilia (coagulation disorder) will typically result in bruises, not petechiae.

12. The answer is e. (*Hay et al, pp 213-221. Kliegman et al, pp 236-244. Rudolph et al, pp 139-140.*) The radiograph showing a fracture (or a radiograph showing multiple fractures in various stages of healing) indicates trauma. This information should be reported to the medical examiner and appropriate social agencies, including the police, so that an investigation can be started and other children in the home or under the care of the same babysitter can be protected. Although an autopsy (and death-scene investigation) should be done in every such case, medical examiners sometimes diagnose SIDS without an autopsy, particularly if the parents object to one, unless further information is provided by the emergency room staff, as in this case. For none of the other conditions (except osteogenesis imperfecta [OI]) would bone injuries at various levels of healing be expected. OI would be expected to present with symptoms of a broken bone and not with death at 4 months of age. The bone findings of scurvy are classically described as causing a "ground glass osteopenia" while those in congenital syphilis classically are described as periostitis of long bones and osteochondritis of the wrists, elbows, ankles, and knees.

Physical abuse should always be considered when the child's injuries do not align with the history, and the child's developmental status plays a major role in this assessment. For example, lower extremity bruising on this 4-month old would not be expected, but would be completely normal in an active 2-year old who periodically falls while running. Inconsistency in the caregiver's story should also raise the concern of abuse.

13. The answer is d. (*Hay et al, pp 76-77, 644-645. Kliegman et al, pp 1807-1808. Rudolph et al, pp 1386-1389.*) *Encopresis* is defined as the passage of feces in inappropriate locations after bowel control would be expected (usually older than 4 years). Encopresis is seen both with chronic constipation and overflow incontinence (retentive encopresis), and without constipation (non-retentive encopresis). Retentive encopresis is more common, and is the source of this child's problem. A leakage of liquid stool around a large fecal impaction can result in fecal soiling. The radiograph demonstrates a dilated, stool-filled colon consistent with retentive encopresis. Treatment involves clearing the fecal mass, maintaining soft stools for 3-6 months with mineral oil or stool softeners, and behavioral modification. Most children will outgrow this condition. Timeout would be ineffective, because these children usually have dysfunctional anal sphincters and little control over the problem; they do not know they are soiling their clothes until it is too late. Daily enemas could potentially be harmful. A rectal biopsy would help diagnose Hirschsprung disease, but this condition typically presents in the newborn period with delayed stooling, or more rarely in the older child with constipation and abdominal distention but without encopresis.

14. The answer is e. (*Hay et al, p 828. Kliegman et al, pp 3261-3263. Rudolph et al, p 844.*) Genu varum (bowlegs) is a common finding in infants and toddlers younger than 2 years of age. Improvement occurs spontaneously with time, and most children have straight legs by the time they are 2 years old. A few children with bowlegs, however, continue to progress and worsen, and in some cases the bowing is unilateral. This is termed Blount disease (or idiopathic tibia vara) and is characterized by an abnormality in the medial aspect of the proximal tibial epiphysis. Radiographically there is a prominent step abnormality with beaking and calcification at the proximal tibial epiphysis. Aggressive treatment is essential, as the disease can be rapidly progressive and lead to permanent growth disturbances. Bracing can be effective up to the age of 3; later correction may require surgery. Blount disease can occur in several forms: infantile (ages 1-3 years; more common in African American children and is associated with obesity as in this case), juvenile (ages 4-10 years), and adolescent (age 11 years and older). Clinically, the findings are the same; in the adolescent group, radiograph findings of metaphyseal beaking are less prominent than in the earlier age groups.

Legg-Calvé-Perthes disease is avascular necrosis of the femoral head, caused by an interruption of the blood supply by a currently unknown cause. The onset is usually between 2 and 12 years of age and classically presents with a painless limp, although mild pain of the thigh is common. Repeated microfracture of the tibial tubercle at the insertion of the patellar tendon is called Osgood-Schlatter disease. This is an overuse injury, and presents with swelling and knee pain localized to the tibial tubercle. Improvement occurs with rest. Slipped capital femoral epiphysis (SCFE) typically occurs in overweight adolescents, and presents with a limp. Radiographically, the capital femoral epiphysis is separated from the neck of the femur and remains in the acetabulum as the rest of the femur moves anteriorly.

15. The answer is e. (*Hay et al, pp 83-85. Kliegman et al, pp 175, 2858. Rudolph et al, pp 2222-2223.*) The child in this question most likely has breath-holding spells; two forms exist. Cyanotic spells consist of the symptoms outlined and are predictable upon upsetting or scolding the child. They are rare before 6 months of age, peak at about 2 years of age, and resolve by about 5 years of age. Avoidance of reinforcing this behavior is the treatment of choice. Pallid breath-holding spells are less common and are usually caused by a painful experience (such as a fall). With these events, the child will stop breathing, lose consciousness, become pale and hypotonic, and may have a brief tonic episode. Although the family may be concerned that these "tonic episodes" are seizures, the temporal relationship with an inciting event makes this diagnosis highly unlikely and an EEG is not warranted. These pallid events, too, resolve spontaneously. Again, avoidance of reinforcing behavior is indicated. Assuring the family that this is a benign condition is important.

The child's development appears to be normal as she is interactive with the family and the examiner; developmental testing for such things as autism or other forms of pervasive developmental delay is not indicated.

The trial of methylphenidate suggests a diagnosis of ADHD. The diagnosis is made by fulfilling a series of criteria that include among other criteria a child's attention and activity being disruptive in two settings such as home and school or work, and the condition being present for at least 6 months. A 2-year old can rarely meet those initial requirements.

16. The answer is a. (*Hay et al, pp 1055-1056. Kliegman et al, pp 2760-2763. Rudolph et al, p 2104.*) The case description is of a hypertensive obese patient (> 97th percentile for weight) with physical examination findings of acanthosis nigricans. The criteria for diagnosis of diabetes mellitus, as established by the Expert Committee on the Diagnosis and Classification of Diabetes Mellitus (sponsored by the American Diabetes Association), include a fasting glucose level ≥ 126 mg/dL or symptoms of diabetes mellitus plus a random plasma glucose ≥ 200 mg/dL. Although an oral glucose tolerance test is not typically used in children, a level above 200 mg/dL 2 hours after a load helps confirm the diagnosis. Acanthosis nigricans in children usually suggests insulin resistance, but is not, in and of itself, diagnostic, nor are symptoms alone diagnostic. Previous standards suggested a fasting glucose between 100 and 125 mg/dL or a 2-hour glucose during an oral glucose tolerance test between 140 and 200 mg/dL indicated impaired glucose tolerance. The bed-wetting in the question can be explained by increased liquid consumption due to the hyperosmolar state caused by hyperglycemia. The two urine specimen findings are probably normal. The clean catch urine does not contain enough bacteria to suggest urinary tract infection; the bacterium is a normal skin contamination. Additionally, microscopy demonstrated several epithelia cells in the clean catch urine suggesting contamination.

17. The answer is d. (*Hay et al, p 470. Kliegman et al, p 1769. Rudolph, et al, p 178.*) A *natal* tooth is present at birth, while a *neonatal* tooth erupts in the first 30 days of life. The incidence of natal tooth is estimated to be

1:3000 live births, with a female predominance. About 95% of natal teeth are primary incisors; only 5% are supernumerary, or extra, teeth. If the tooth is loose, it is usually removed to prevent accidental aspiration. If, however, it is firmly in its socket, the tooth is generally left in place. As a natal tooth is typically the primary tooth, early removal will leave a gap until the secondary teeth erupt between 5 and 7 years of age.

A natal tooth in the proper location rarely suggests a genetic anomaly, while a single midline central incisor is more typically related to a genetic condition. Conditions associated with natal teeth include chondroectodermal dysplasia (Ellis-van Creveld syndrome) and oculo-mandibulo-dyscephaly with hypotrichosis (Hallermann-Streiff syndrome). Natal teeth do not discolor at a higher rate than other teeth.

18. The answer is b. (*Hay et al, p 401. Kliegman et al, p 3234. Rudolph et al, pp 1287-1288.*) The clinical description and the pictured neonate represent a classic case of neonatal acne, which peaks at 2-4 weeks of age. The condition results from maternal hormone transmission. It resolves in a few weeks to months, and occasionally is severe enough to require treatment with agents such as topical tretinoin or benzoyl peroxide.

Neonatal herpes infection can occur in 14-day-old neonates, but the clinical scenario is of a healthy child; children with neonatal herpes are usually ill. Milia are benign, tiny white keratin plugs on the nose, cheeks, or chin. Seborrheic dermatitis is a weepy rash that can be found on the face or on the scalp (cradle cap); it is not usually found at 14 days of age but rather later in infancy. Eczema commonly occurs on the face of children in the early years of life (later occurring in the more "adult" pattern of extremities), but would be unusual in a 14-day-old neonate.

19. The answer is b. (*Hay et al, pp 1371-1372. Kliegman et al, pp 3224-3226. Rudolph et al, pp 1301-1302.*) Scabies is caused by the mite *Sarcoptes scabiei* var. *hominis*. Most older children and adults present with intensely pruritic and threadlike burrows in the interdigital areas, groin, elbows, and ankles; the palms, soles, face, and head are spared. Infants, however, usually present with bullae and pustules, and the areas spared in adults are often involved in infants. The clinical manifestations closely resemble those of atopic dermatitis, which is treated with emollients and hydrocortisone cream. Gamma benzene hexachloride (lindane) can cause neurotoxicity through percutaneous absorption, especially in small infants and those with abnormal skin (impetigo, etc), and is, therefore, not recommended in children as first-line therapy for scabies. An excellent alternative—5% permethrin cream (Elimite)—is safer and is more often recommended. Coaltar soaps often are used to treat psoriasis. Antifungal creams commonly are utilized to treat tinea corporis, cruris, or pedis.

20. The answer is c. (*Hay et al, pp 1250-1253. Kliegman et al, pp 1337-1341. Rudolph et al, pp 1097-1099.*) The clinical scenario is of an essentially normal newborn who rapidly becomes ill with hypothermia, tachycardia, tachypnea, hypotension, and respiratory distress. The rapid onset of the symptoms, the low WBC count with left shift and thrombocytopenia, along with the chest x-ray findings of diffuse, bilateral granular infiltrates are typical of a patient with GBS pneumonia. Appropriate management for the child with GBS sepsis would include rapid recognition of symptoms, cardiorespiratory support, and prompt institution of antibiotics. Despite these measures, mortality from this infection is not uncommon. The other infectious causes listed do not present so early, and the noninfectious causes listed do not cause elevations in the band count. GBS disease in the newborn is decreasing in incidence with better prevention strategies in the perinatal period; early screening in pregnancy and treatment with antibiotics just prior to delivery to eliminate GBS colonization markedly decreases the risk to the neonate.

Congenital syphilis can cause pneumonia, but it is diagnosed at birth along with other features including hepatosplenomegaly, jaundice, rashes, hemolytic anemia, and others. Diaphragmatic hernia presents with early respiratory distress, but the diagnosis is confirmed clinically with bowel sounds heard in the chest and a radiograph that has loops of bowel located above the normal placement of the diaphragm. Transient tachypnea of the newborn (TTN) causes an increase in respiratory rate and occasionally a supplemental oxygen requirement; the history is often positive for a scheduled cesarean delivery, and the radiograph shows retained fluid in the fissures. TTN does not cause temperature instability nor an abnormal CBC. Chlamydial pneumonia is not a condition that occurs in an 8-hour-old neonate; it is generally a mild pneumonia that can develop in an exposed infant at several weeks of life.

21. The answer is a. (*Hay et al, p 874. Kliegman et al, pp 3271-3272. Rudolph et al, p 852.*) This history is typical of Osgood-Schlatter disease. Microfractures in the area of the insertion of the patellar tendon into the tibial tubercle are common in athletic adolescents. Swelling, tenderness, and an increase in size of the tibial tuberosity are found. Radiographs can be used to rule out other conditions. Treatment consists of rest.

Legg-Calvé-Perthes disease is avascular necrosis of the femoral head. This condition usually produces mild or intermittent pain in the anterior thigh but can also present as a painless limp. Gonococcal arthritis, although common in this age range, is uncommon in this anatomic site. More significant systemic signs and symptoms, including chills, fever, migratory polyarthralgia, and rash are commonly seen. Slipped capital femoral epiphysis is usually seen in a younger, more obese child (mean age between 12-14 years) or in a thinner, older child who has just undergone a rapid growth spurt. Pain upon movement of the hip is typical, and surgical stabilization of the slip is required.

Popliteal (Baker) cysts are found on the posterior aspect of the knee. Observation is usually all that is necessary, as they typically resolve over several years. Surgical excision is indicated if the cyst progressively enlarges or if there are unacceptable symptoms associated with the cyst.

22. The answer is e. (*Hay et al, pp 462-463. Kliegman et al, pp 3026-3031. Rudolph et al, pp 2293-2298.*) To prevent monocular blindness and to ensure the development of normal binocular vision, early recognition and treatment of strabismus are essential. Infants can be screened for strabismus by observing the location of a light reflection in the pupils when the patient fixes on a light source. Normally, it should be in the center or just nasal of the center in each pupil. Persistence of a transient or fixed deviation of an eye beyond 4 months of age requires referral to an ophthalmologist. Another method of testing for strabismus is the "cover" or "cover-uncover" test, using the principle that children with strabismus will use the "good" eye for fixation. By covering the good eye, the other eye will deviate. The aim of treatment is to prevent loss of central vision from foveal suppression of a confusing image in the deviating eye. This is accomplished by surgery, eyeglasses, or patching of the normal eye. The prognosis for normal vision if the diagnosis is delayed beyond 6 years of age is guarded. Routine vision and strabismus screening are essential at age 3-4 years. A mild URI should not create strabismus.

23. The answer is e. (*Hay et al, pp 458-459. Kliegman et al, pp 3063-3064. Rudolph et al, p 1293.*) The description is of a child with orbital cellulitis, an infection and inflammation of the tissues around the orbit. While some cases arise from direct infection through trauma, most pediatric orbital cellulitis is a direct extension from nearby sites such as the paranasal sinuses. It is a potentially vision-threatening infection, and as such necessitates hospital admission and IV antibiotics. Imaging with a CT or MRI is performed to determine the extent of the infection, and surgical drainage of orbital or subperiosteal abscesses is required in some cases. Complications include cavernous sinus thrombosis, meningitis, brain abscess, and vision loss from increased intraorbital pressure with retinal artery occlusion. Common causative organisms include MRSA, *Streptococcus* species, and *Haemophilus* species.

Orbital cellulitis typically results in a febrile, ill-appearing child with proptosis and restriction of eye movement, whereas periorbital (or preseptal) cellulitis has a lower fever, the children do not look so ill, and there is no proptosis or restriction in eye movements. While orbital cellulitis is usually managed as an inpatient with IV antibiotics and ophthalmologic consultation, periorbital cellulitis in an era where vaccines have eliminated *H influenzae* type b as a cause can usually be managed as an outpatient with oral antibiotics and close follow-up.

24. The answer is d. (*Hay et al, pp 843-844. Kliegman et al, pp 3327-3330. Rudolph et al, pp 2141, 854-856, 934-938.*) The clinical picture is of a febrile, irritable child with extreme pain with manipulation of one hip. The CBC shows elevated WBC with left shift. Septic arthritis requires urgent intervention to preserve joint mobility. Joint aspiration is diagnostic and can be helpful in treatment. Opening the joint space may be required in a septic hip to assist in draining purulent material. The joint tap will reveal cloudy fluid containing a predominance of polymorphonuclear leukocytes. Organisms are readily seen on Gram stain examination, and cultures of joint fluid and blood are usually positive. Radiography reveals a widened joint space. Finding pus in the joint indicates the need for immediate surgical drainage and prompt institution of IV antibiotic therapy to avoid serious damage to the joint and permanent loss of function. The most common organism found to cause septic arthritis is *S aureus*. Since immunization against *H influenzae* type b has become an established practice, invasive disease such as septic arthritis caused by this organism is rarely seen. In sexually active adolescents, *Neisseria gonorrhoeae* is a common cause of septic arthritis. Treatment is typically for 4-6 weeks.

Legg-Calvé-Perthes disease is avascular necrosis or idiopathic osteonecrosis of the femoral head; the cause of this disorder is unknown. Boys between the ages of 2 and 12 years are most frequently affected (incidence in boys is four- to fivefold greater than in girls), with a mean of 6-7 years old. Presenting symptoms include a limp and pain in the anterior thigh, groin, or knee, although classic symptoms include a painless limp.

Leukemia can present with orthopedic findings of bone pain, limping, and swollen joints. Associated findings of anemia (pallor, fatigue, and weakness), thrombocytopenia (bruising, petechial, and bleeding), generalized lymphadenopathy, and hepatosplenomegaly would be anticipated. Laboratory data would demonstrate evidence of bone marrow replacement with leukemic cells including anemia, thrombocytopenia, elevated or reduced white blood, and immature cells on peripheral smear.

Osteomyelitis usually presents with focal bone tenderness and fever. Early evaluation is best done through nuclear medicine studies or MRI, as plain film bony changes usually take a week or so before becoming evident. The most common pathogen is *S aureus*, estimated to cause about two-thirds of all pediatric cases. Other less common organisms include group A *Streptococcus* (*S pyogenes*), *S pneumoniae*, and *Kingella kingae*. *Escherichia coli* can be seen in neonatal osteomyelitis. While *H influenzae* type b previously was a frequent cause of osteomyelitis, universal immunization has significantly diminished infection with this organism.

Transient synovitis is a disorder of unknown etiology, affecting children usually from 2 to 6 years of age. These children usually present with a painful limp. This is a diagnosis of exclusion; septic hip and osteomyelitis must be ruled out. The WBC count and ESR may be normal or slightly elevated. Early aspiration of the joint space may assist in diagnosis. Transient synovitis is a self-limited disorder.

25. The answer is b. (*Hay et al, pp 1233-1245. Kliegman et al, pp 1650-1654. Rudolph et al, p 1165.*) This infant in the vignette is presenting with failure to thrive (FTT), especially in weight gain, and the differential diagnosis of this problem is extensive. While any of the answers provided may have a place in an FTT evaluation, the best single recommendation in this case would be to evaluate for HIV. In this case, the biologic mother was in jail for unknown reasons (possibly for prostitution, drugs, or other high-risk activities); the risk for congenital HIV is higher. In addition, the presenting symptoms (lymphadenopathy, hepatomegaly, and persistent oral candidiasis) are most consistent with HIV. An HIV ELISA may still reflect maternal antibody at this age; thus, an antigen test like the HIV PCR is preferred.

Increasing caloric count would be appropriate for the child with simple caloric deficiency; this child has demonstrated failure to gain weight despite adequate nutrition. Blood cultures and antibiotics are appropriate for a febrile child where treatable infections are suspected. Sweat chloride testing (cystic fibrosis) would be appropriate initial testing if the child had had delayed stooling at birth (meconium ileus), a history of large stools (malabsorption), or evidence of fat-absorbable vitamin deficiency (rash, anemia). Fecal fat content (malabsorption) would be appropriate initial testing for the child with diarrhea and failure to thrive. Sweat chloride testing and fecal fat measurement might be appropriate subsequent diagnostic considerations if the HIV testing proves to be negative.

26. The answer is d. (*Hay et al, pp 412-415. Kliegman et al, pp 1116-1121. Rudolph et al, pp 1257-1260.*) Eczema is a chronic dermatitis that occurs in a population with a strong personal or family history of atopy. The skin presents initially as an erythematous, papulovesicular, weeping eruption, which progresses over time to a scaly, lichenified dermatitis. From about 3 months to about 2 years of age, the rash is prominent on the cheeks, wrists, scalp, postauricular areas, and the extensor surfaces of the arms and legs. In a child 2-12 years of age, mainly the flexural folds of the arms and legs and the neck are involved. Pruritus is a predominant feature, and scratching leads to excoriation, secondary infection, and lichenification of the skin. The rash has a chronic and relapsing course, and treatment is determined by the major clinical features. Cutaneous irritants (bathing in hot water, scrubbing vigorously with soap, wearing wool or synthetic clothing) should be avoided, and maximal skin hydration with emollients is essential. Topical moisturizers and steroids are the mainstays of therapy for atopic dermatitis; topical calcineurin inhibitors (tacrolimus and pimecrolimus) are second-line therapy. The use of antihistamines can provide additional relief from pruritus. Tar preparations and sun exposure (while avoiding excessive sweating and sunburn) can help in some cases, but have been less effective than topical steroids. Tar and light treatments are more commonly used to manage psoriasis. Similarly, topical antibiotics are added as temporary treatment of eczema when a bacterial superinfection is suspected. Topical antifungal creams are appropriate for tinea corporis, cruris or pedis.

27. The answer is b. (*Kliegman et al, p 577. Rudolph et al, pp 1264, 1316.*) Frostbite is the condition in which tissue is frozen and destroyed. Initial stinging is replaced by aching and culminates in numb areas. Rapid rewarming is the mainstay of treatment; thrombolysis may help in certain cases. Once rewarmed, the area becomes red, blotchy, and painful. Early surgical consultation is recommended, as there are frequently areas of necrotic tissue that require debridement, and amputation may be required in severe cases.

Frostnip is manifest by small, firm, white, cold patches of skin in exposed areas; treatment is rewarming the areas before they become numb. Chilblains are small, ulcerated lesions on exposed areas such as the ears and fingers. Lesions may last 1-2 weeks. Cold panniculitis is destruction of fat cells caused by exposure to cold weather or a cold object (such as a Popsicle); it is usually a benign condition that self-resolves. Trench foot, also known as immersion foot, occurs with prolonged exposure to cold (but not freezing) temperatures and moisture. The foot will become cold, numb, pale, edematous, and clammy. A prolonged autonomic disturbance after this condition can persist for years. Gangrene may develop.

28. The answer is a. (*Hay et al, p 412. Kliegman et al, pp 3226-3227. Rudolph et al, p 1302.*) The photo and history are consistent with head lice (*Pediculosis capitis*). In the past, head lice treatment was simple, as over-the-counter pediculicides (Rid, Nix) were effective. Recent data suggest increased resistance to these products making treatment more complicated. In many areas with high-resistance patterns, a second-line therapy may be required. Of the choices presented, topical ivermectin for the 18-month-old sibling (approved for children > 6 months of age) and observation of the 2-month-old infant (less likely to get the disease) is the best option. Lindane is contraindicated for young children due to its potential of neurotoxicity. Oral griseofulvin would be appropriate for the treatment of tinea capitis, topical antibiotics for the treatment of impetigo or other superficial bacterial infection, and oral ivermectin for helminths (worm) infection.

29. The answer is c. (*Hay et al, pp 1293-1296. Kliegman et al, pp 1452-1453. Rudolph et al, p 1052.*) Of the options, tuberculous (TB) meningitis is most likely to linger for 3 weeks with regression of normal milestones. TB meningitis as outlined in this case is most commonly seen between 6 months and 4 years of life. The first stage lasts 1-2 weeks and includes nonspecific symptoms like those in the vignette. The second stage begins abruptly with seizures, lethargy, hypertonicity, hydrocephalus, and focal neurologic signs. The third stage includes coma, hypertension, posturing, decompensation, and death. Unfortunately, this life-threatening illness often will go unrecognized, or the patient will be initially diagnosed with a viral illness.

The other infectious causes listed (HSV encephalitis or bacterial meningitis) may have overall similar signs and symptoms but lead to rapid deterioration. HSV typically presents with fever, headache, lethargy, altered consciousness, and seizure. CSF shows a lymphocytic pleocytosis with an elevated protein. Bacterial meningitis typically presents with a few days of fever and progresses with CNS symptoms including headache, lethargy and irritability; typical organisms include *S pneumoniae* and *N meningitidis.*

An epidural hematoma is an acute event, typically with rapid deterioration. A food allergy does not typically cause the CNS manifestations described.

While many patients with nonspecific complaints have trivial diseases that resolve spontaneously, the patient presented here has a 3-week history of progressive symptoms and developmental regression. Diagnoses that cause a slowly progressive course should be considered foremost.

30. The answer is a. (*Hay et al, p 486. Kliegman et al, p 3098. Rudolph et al, pp 1314-1315.*) A cholesteatoma may be congenital or acquired. It is a small epithelium-lined sac containing debris. Acquired cholesteatoma can present in children with recurrent otitis media, or in the face of a chronically draining ear. The mass can grow aggressively, leading to CNS complications like facial nerve damage, hearing loss, and intracranial extension. Referral to an otolaryngologist is required; a CT scan of the temporal bones can define the extent of the growth.

Tympanosclerosis, or scarring on the surface of the tympanic membrane is a sequela of frequent otitis media. Acute otitis media with perforation and drainage would present with a hole in the tympanic membrane and with (often) purulent drainage. Dislocation of the malleus from its insertion in the tympanic membrane can occur, but would not produce a mass extending through the tympanic membrane. Excessive cerumen production would result in waxy build-up that is removable with irrigation.

31. The answer is c. (*Hay et al, pp 719-725. Kliegman et al, pp 388-391. Rudolph et al, pp 1643-1647.*) The patient has severe dehydration as outlined in the case by tachycardia, hypotension, and skin findings. The dehydration can be estimated to be in the 10%-15% range and requires rapid expansion of the vascular space to prevent organ failure and eventual death. Assuming this patient is in shock, it is vital to restore circulatory volume quickly, thereby improving tissue perfusion and shifting anaerobic toward aerobic metabolism. Isotonic intravenous (IV) fluids appropriate for rapid bolus infusion include Ringer's lactate and normal saline, although Ringer's lactate contains potassium and thus should not be used in oliguric or anuric patients. Albumin, plasma, and blood offer no significant advantages over the cheaper and more available crystalloid. An initial fluid bolus should be 20 mL/kg; this may be repeated if the patient has an inadequate response to the first bolus.

The hypotonic dextrose fluids listed are various forms of maintenance fluids and should never be used for rapid volume replacement. A rapid infusion of hypotonic fluid causes a brisk drop in serum sodium with a concomitant reduction in serum osmolality, leading to significant fluid shifts out of the vasculature and into cells. This fluid shift results in cerebral edema and death. Blood can be used for resuscitating hypovolemia due to rapid blood loss.

32. The answer is b. (*Hay et al, p 924. Kliegman et al, pp 1040-1044. Rudolph et al, pp 1593-1594.*) The umbilical cord typically separates from a newborn 10-14 days after birth, although some will remain for 3-4 weeks. An intact cord after 1 month of age is considered "delayed separation." Leukocyte adhesion deficiency type 1 (LAD-1) has been described with delayed cord separation. These children are at risk for overwhelming bacterial infection. A CBC usually shows a marked leukocytosis, and diagnosis is made by measuring surface CD11b using flow cytometry. Most patients with LAD-1 have normal antibody production.

A complete lack of abdominal wall musculature development would point toward Prune Belly syndrome, but a partial defect hints at an omphalocele, an abdominal wall opening with intestine or liver protruding into the base of the umbilical cord, covered by peritoneum but not by skin. It should be readily recognizable at birth. Umbilical granulomas can occur with repeated trauma of the umbilical area and form after the cord has separated; they are easily treated with application of silver nitrate. Depending on the specific immunoglobulin deficiency, expected findings would include a variety of recurrent, unusual, or especially severe infections. A persistent urachus is a remnant of a congenital structure that will produce ongoing clear or yellow fluid from the umbilicus.

33. The answer is b. (*Kliegman et al, pp 2607-2613.*) A nonspecific vulvovaginitis is common in this age group, often caused by chemical irritants such as bubble baths or by poor hygiene. Parents should be counseled to use only cotton underwear for young children, stop bubble baths (or at least splash fresh, clean water in the vaginal area at the end of a bath), and reemphasize wiping front to back after urination or bowel movements. Vaginal foreign bodies in young girls are usually either toilet paper or stool, and are accompanied by a foul odor and discharge that is sometimes bloody. Removal of vaginal foreign bodies is frequently done under general anesthesia in the operating room. While child sexual abuse is always a possibility, there is no verbal or physical evidence that this is a problem in this child. Gonorrhea and chlamydia would go along with abuse and are usually accompanied by a mild discharge in the prepubertal child.

34. The answer is c. (*Kliegman et al, pp 2819-2823. Rudolph et al, pp 710-711.*) The patient in the case has a normal physical and developmental examination with the exception of a flat posterior occiput which is caused by her being placed in the supine position for prolonged periods of time. While "back to sleep" is recommended, that is placing children supine (on their backs) and not in the prone position when they are put to sleep to help reduce the incidence of SIDS, "tummy time" when they are awake likely will prevent the flattening (posterior plagiocephaly) described. If the infant were found to have an abnormally shaped head with evidence of craniosynostosis (abnormally shaped head in the anterior-posterior direction with ridging over the suture lines, developmental delay, small head circumference) then imaging and neurosurgical evaluation would be indicated. An orthosis (in the form of a helmet) may be required if the molding does not resolve with conservative maneuvers.

35. The answer is e. (*Hay et al, pp 326-327. Kliegman et al, pp 577-579. Rudolph et al, pp 1264, 1316.*) The patient in the scenario has hypothermia, bradycardia, and confusion. Hypothermia can develop in any cold weather exposure. As the core temperature drops, the individual becomes lethargic, tired, uncoordinated, apathetic, mentally confused, irritable, and bradycardic. Removal from the cold and rewarming him will return his condition to baseline.

Patients with sickle cell trait who are exposed to high altitude and hypoxia are at risk (albeit relatively low) to the complications of sickling. Thus, all of the complications of sickle cell disease (SSD) are possible, including stroke. The patient with SSD-associated stroke present with sudden onset of focal neurologic signs, especially hemiparesis. Drug ingestions are always possible, but none would typically cause low temperatures. Altitude sickness symptoms typically are seen in the first 24 hours after ascent to a high altitude and include headache (usually throbbing and frontal), anorexia, nausea, vomiting, weakness, lightheadedness, and dizziness. While adolescents are known to occasionally be malingerers, physical findings of low temperature and bradycardia are not expected.

36. The answer is c. (*Hay et al, pp 329-331. Kliegman et al, pp 3447-3450. Rudolph et al, pp 445-446.*) Mammalian bites should be promptly and thoroughly scrubbed with soap and water and debrided. The decision to suture depends on the location, age, and nature of the wound. Antibiotic prophylaxis is extremely controversial. Most experts suggest a short course of antibiotics should be started for cat, human, or monkey bites. Only 4% of dog bites become infected (and therefore do not necessarily need antibiotic prophylaxis), compared with 35% of cat bites, and 50% of monkey bites (which require antibiotics in most cases). Cat bites are usually deep punctures. Human bites almost invariably become infected.

The etiologies of these infections are polymicrobial. *Pasteurella multocida* is a common organism in infected cat and dog bites. Infected human bites tend to have positive cultures for *S viridans*, *S aureus*, and *E corrodens*. Treatment with amoxicillin-clavulanate orally or ampicillin-sulbactam IV is recommended. Antibiotic prophylaxis is recommended for any bite sustained by an infant, a diabetic, or an immunocompromised patient because of the higher risk of infection in these persons. Since the child is fully immunized, tetanus boosters are not required. Similarly, as the dog was provoked and was fully immunized, rabies should not be a concern.

37. The answer is c. (*Hay et al, pp 337-339. Kliegman et al, pp 456-457. Rudolph et al, pp 458-459.*) The patient in the case has an unknown ingestion with vomiting, diaphoresis, and malaise, along with vital sign findings of mild tachycardia and hypotension. Laboratory data suggest a normal CBC with elevation of liver enzymes with a negative drug screen. The picture is most likely reflective of acetaminophen ingestion. The appropriate next steps in addition to supportive care include measurement of serum acetaminophen levels and administration of *N*-acetylcysteine.

Deferoxamine is used to treat iron overdose. Symptoms classically are described as including GI symptoms of nausea, hematemesis, abdominal pain, and diarrhea. Ultimately hypovolemia due to vomiting and diarrhea ensue. A "honeymoon" period is classically described in which supportive care results in the patient seemingly returning to baseline but often followed 18-24 hours later with profound acidosis and liver failure.

Naloxone is a medication used in a number of situations, but the most common use is for opioid ingestion. The clinical triad associated with opioid ingestion includes CNS depression, respiratory depression, and pupillary miosis.

CroFab typically is used as an antidote after an envenomation from the North American Crotalinae subfamily of venomous snakes which includes rattlesnakes, copperheads and water moccasins. Clinical findings after the bite are varied but might include pain and swelling at the bite site, a metallic taste in the mouth, respiratory difficulty or chest pain, nausea and vomiting, and generalized weakness.

Dimercaptosuccinic acid is used for heavy metal exposures such as lead or arsenic poisoning. Lead toxicity typically is a chronic condition with findings of microcytic anemia, constipation or abdominal pain, and alteration in mental status such as inattention, hyperactivity, or learning difficulty. Acute arsenic poisoning causes tachycardia, hypotension, and altered mental status or seizures.

38. The answer is d. (*Hay et al, pp 231-232. Kliegman et al, pp 3433-3434. Rudolph et al, p 45.*) There is no accepted "safe" blood lead level in children. Impaired cognitive function can occur at blood lead levels previously thought to be safe; the toxic concentration of lead in whole blood was revised downward in 1991 from 25 to 10 μg/dL, and currently the CDC recommends that public health actions are initiated at levels of ≥ 5 μg/dL. The blood erythrocyte protoporphyrin concentration is not elevated in such low-level poisoning, rendering this test useless as a screening test. The definitive screen, then, is the blood lead level, preferably via venous sampling which avoids the risk of environmental contamination with lead that is more likely with finger sticks. Most lead poisoning is clinically inapparent. A careful history will help identify sources of lead in the environment. However, neither the history nor the anemia that accompanies severe lead poisoning is an appropriate means of screening for lead poisoning. In most areas, lead screening recommendations are made by the state or local health department, based on local risk factors (e.g., number of older houses potentially containing lead-based paint).

39. The answer is d. (*Hay et al, p 326. Kliegman et al, pp 3354-3355. Rudolph et al, pp 470-472.*) Hyperthermia with dry, hot skin and mental status changes characterizes classic heat stroke, typically seen in the elderly with a gradual onset. Young athletes exerting themselves in a hot environment may develop acute heat stroke with signs and symptoms of hyperthermia and mental status changes; the difference, however, is that the athletes may continue to sweat profusely, thus the presence of sweat should not be used to eliminate heat stroke from the differential. Heat stroke is a medical emergency. These otherwise healthy athletes should be rapidly rehydrated with IV fluids, undergo aggressive cooling (cold water immersion, cool mist fans, removal of clothing), and perhaps oxygen, laboratory evaluation, and ICU admission. Heat stroke can have a high mortality; prevention is certainly the best option, but prompt recognition is essential. Oral rehydration therapy might have been preventive if instituted before symptoms of heat stroke were manifest, but once the syndrome has started IV fluids are indicated. Acetaminophen and other antipyretic administration have no role in the treatment of heat stroke. Without evidence of trauma to the head, CT scanning is not indicated. While drug ingestion is always possible, the clinical scenario presented is not consistent of any typical drugs of abuse.

40. The answer is a. (*Hay et al, pp 558-560. Kliegman et al, pp 2005-2006. Rudolph et al, pp 710-711.*) About 3500 infants die in the United States each year suddenly and unexpectedly. Extensive research in infants clearly demonstrates the prone (facedown) sleeping position to be a risk factor for SIDS. A higher risk of SIDS in the prone position has been noted when the infant sleeps on a soft, porous mattress or in an overheated room, is swaddled, or has recently been ill. The American Academy of Pediatrics recommends that healthy infants be positioned on their back when being put down for sleep. While the rate of SIDS has declined in areas where the change from prone to supine (face up) sleeping positions has been implemented, the rate of positional plagiocephaly (the flattening of the occiput that occurs when infants are always on their back) has increased. Infants should spend some time in the prone position (tummy time) while they are awake to avoid this condition.

41. The answer is d. (*Hay et al, pp 95-96. Kliegman et al, pp 622-623. Rudolph et al, pp 742-747.*) The physical features associated with the fragile X syndrome become more obvious after puberty, many of which are outlined in the case. They include macrocephaly, a long face, large ears, prominent jaw, high-arched palate, evidence of mitral valve prolapse, macroorchidism, pectus excavatum, hypotonia, repetitive speech, gaze avoidance, and hand flapping. Even in the absence of physical findings, boys of all ages with developmental delay, autism, and abnormal temperament of unknown cause probably should be tested for the fragile X syndrome. The genetics of the fragile X syndrome are unique. Most males who carry the fragile X mutation are mentally impaired and show the clinical phenotype; however, 20% of males who inherit the genetic mutation are normal in intelligence and physical appearance. They are also cytogenetically normal in that the fragile site on their X chromosome is not seen by the karyotyping method. These normal transmitting males (NTMs) transmit the fragile X mental retardation (*FMR-1*) gene to all of their daughters and often have severely affected grandchildren. It is thought that a premutation carried by these NTMs must go through oogenesis in their daughters to become a full mutation. Daughters of NTMs are usually normal but are obligate carriers of the *FMR-1* gene. Daughters who inherit the gene from the mother are mentally retarded about one-third of the time. Because both males and females can be affected, the fragile X syndrome is best described as a dominant X-linked disorder with reduced penetrance in females. Direct DNA analysis is available for diagnosis of phenotypically affected persons as well as suspected carriers of fragile X; it has supplanted cytogenetic testing for the fragile site on the X chromosome. The DNA test can also be used for prenatal testing.

Trisomy 21 (Down syndrome) has a wide variety of features including hypotonia, epicanthal folds, transpalmar crease, cardiac lesions (VSD or atrioventricular [AV] canal), mental retardation, and a propensity for leukemia. Trisomy 18 (Edwards syndrome) features include small for gestational age, micrognathia, low-set ears, a variety of cardiac defects, small palpebral fissures, microcephaly, cleft lip/palate, and rocker bottom feet. Trisomy 13 (Patau syndrome) features include microcephaly, cutis aplasia of the scalp, a variety of cardiac defects, holoprosencephaly, cleft lip/palate, and coloboma. Williams syndrome features include short stature, blue irides, a variety of cardiac abnormalities involving the pulmonary vessels, hypercalcemia in infancy, and a friendly and outgoing personality.

42. The answer is c. (*Hay et al, pp 721-722. Kliegman et al, pp 353-356. Rudolph et al, pp 1680-1681.*) The differential diagnosis of seizure activity is extensive, and a detailed history and physical examination is essential. While knowing the occupation of the mother and the developmental status of the infant and his siblings are important, the most helpful historical detail for acute management of this patient is the dilution of the formula, especially in light of the history of poor growth (weight and length < 25th percentile with preservation of head size). Over time, inappropriate dilution can cause hyponatremia and water intoxication, leading to seizure activity. Slow correction of the sodium is curative. The technique used to correct the patient's hyponatremia depends on the etiology. In this case, the infant likely has chronic hyponatremia from poor intake. If the infant continues to seize, 3% sodium chloride may be used to rapidly increase serum sodium and, theoretically, decrease cerebral edema. Otherwise, starting the infant on a regular formula and eliminating excess water will correct the deficiency over time.

43 to 48. The answers are 43-e, 44-b, 45-d, 46-a, 47-g, 48-f. (*Hay et al, pp 401-404. Kliegman et al, pp 3116-3118, 3132-3133. Rudolph et al, pp 1253-1257, 1260, 1285-1286.*) Erythema toxicum is a benign, self-limited condition of unknown etiology. It is found in about 50% of term newborns. The lesions are 2-3 cm erythematous macules; some have a central yellow-white pustule. Examination of the fluid from these lesions demonstrates eosinophils. This rash waxes and wanes over the first days to weeks of life. No therapy is indicated.

Salmon patches (also known as nevus simplex or nevus flammeus) are flat vascular lesions that occur in the listed regions and appear more prominent during crying. The lesions on the face fade over the first few years of life. Lesions found over the nuchal and occipital areas often persist. No therapy is indicated.

Pustular melanosis is another benign, self-limited disease of unknown etiology of the newborn period. It is more common in African Americans than in whites. These lesions are usually found at birth and consist of 2- to 10-mm pustules that result in a hyperpigmented lesion encircled by a collarette of scale upon rupture of the pustule. The pustular stage of these lesions occurs during the first few days of life, with the hyperpigmented stage lasting for weeks to months. No therapy is indicated.

Sebaceous nevi (nevus of Jadassohn) are small, sharply edged lesions that occur most commonly on the head and neck of infants. These lesions are yellow-orange in color and are slightly elevated. They usually are hairless. Malignant degeneration is possible, most commonly after adolescence.

Milia are fine, yellowish white, 1- to 2-mm firm raised lesions scattered over the face of the neonate. They are cysts that contain keratinized material. Commonly, these lesions resolve spontaneously without therapy. Epithelial cysts on the palate are called Epstein pearls. Milia should be distinguished from sebaceous gland hyperplasia, which manifests as smooth white to yellow papules, usually found on the infant's nose; as maternal androgen levels drop, the hyperplasia resolves.

Seborrheic dermatitis can begin anytime during life and frequently presents as cradle cap in the newborn period. This rash is commonly greasy, scaly, and erythematous and in smaller children involves the face, neck, axilla, and diaper area. In older children, the rash can be localized to the scalp and intertriginous areas. Pruritus can be marked.

49 to 53. **The answers are 49-a, 50-c, 51-e, 52-d, 53-c.** (*Hay et al, pp 80-83, 554-555. Kliegman et al, pp 111-123. Rudolph et al, pp 1944-1948.*) Sleep disturbances are fairly common in childhood. Many children resist going to bed, and parents frequently give in just to get the child to sleep by allowing the child to sleep in the parents' bed or allowing them to stay up late. Unfortunately, children learn remarkably well how to get what they want, and the parents' concessions only make the problem worse. Learned behavior (behavioral insomnia, dyssomnia) is the root of many sleep disturbances in young children.

Other types of sleep disturbance in children fall into the category of sleep disruptions, such as nightmares and night terrors.

A nightmare is a scary or disturbing dream that usually awakens the child and causes agitation about the content of the dream. Nightmares occur during rapid eye movement (REM) sleep. Many children and adults have an occasional nightmare; recurrent or frequent nightmares, however, may be indicative of an ongoing stress in the child's life.

Night terrors (pavor nocturnus) are non-REM phenomena seen less commonly than nightmares, occurring in 1%-6% of all children. The child will be described as apparently awake but unresponsive; they can have evidence of autonomic arousal such as tachycardia, sweating, and tachypnea, and appear frightened and agitated. Attempts at calming the child are usually not effective, and the child will eventually go back to sleep. Although usually seen in early childhood, night terrors can sometimes continue through adolescence.

Somnambulism, or sleepwalking, occurs in 15% of children and is described as recurrent episodes of rising from bed and walking around. The child is typically hard to arouse and will have amnesia after the event. This usually happens in the first third of the sleep cycle, during stage 4 non-REM sleep. Somniloquy, or sleeptalking, can occur at any sleep stage and is seen in all ages.

Obstructive sleep apnea is seen more commonly in obese children or in children who have recently gained significant weight. The family may report loud snoring or other abnormal sleep breathing patterns. These children may have new-onset nocturnal enuresis, difficulty in morning awakening, daytime sleepiness, or hyperactivity/behavior problems. On physical examination the child may have evidence of enlarged and "kissing tonsils" or excessive adenoidal tissue. Contributing factors include children with micrognathia, short neck, and significant allergic rhinitis.

Temporal lobe seizures have features of aura, memory impairment, special sensory phenomena (olfactory or gustatory aura), auditory or visual hallucinations, a feeling of déjà vu, anxiety and autonomic changes (piloerection, nausea). Physical findings include lip smacking or chewing, stereotyped manual movements, and occasionally generalization to tonic-clonic activity.

Allergic rhinitis presents with rhinorrhea, nasal congestion, sneezing, and itching eyes and palate. Physical examination findings include clear discharge; dark, puffy, lower eyelids (allergic shiners); lines under the lower eyelids (Dennie-Morgan); transverse crease at lower third of nose (allergic crease) secondary to nose rubbing (allergic salute); papillary hypertrophy of tarsal conjunctivae; watery ocular discharge; enlarged, pale-blue nasal turbinates; and cobblestoning of the posterior pharynx.

Simple snoring is a commonly seen vibratory noise heard on a sleeping child during inspiration. Oxygen desaturation, hypercapnia, and sleep disruption are not seen. Polysomnography, if done, is normal.

54 to 56. The answers are 54-c, 55-d, 56-e. (*Hay et al, pp 259-261, 266-268. Kliegman et al, pp 1246, 1348, 1381-1382, 1546-1548. Rudolph et al, p 985.*) Measles vaccination alone (rather than in the form of the MMR combination) is not part of the routine immunization schedule. It typically is indicated only during a measles outbreak.

MMR and varicella are typically given at the 12- to 15-month-old visit and again at the 4- to 6-year-old visit.

Meningococcal, HPV, and tetanus toxoid, reduced diphtheria toxoid and acellular pertussis (Tdap) are commonly initiated at about 11 years of age. A second dose of meningococcal vaccine is given at about 16 years of age. A second dose of HPV is given 1-2 months after the first and a third dose given 6 months after the first.

Diphtheria and tetanus toxoids, acellular pertussis, inactivated poliovirus, *H influenzae* type b conjugate vaccine, and rotavirus vaccines (alone or in combination) are the primary series of childhood vaccines which are started at about 2 months of age, repeated at 4 months of age, and completed at 6 months of age.

Pneumococcal 13-valent conjugate vaccine is routinely given at the 2-, 4-, and 6-month visits with a booster at the 12- to 15-month-old visit. The 23-valent vaccine is not a routine vaccine given to all children but rather is reserved for the high-risk population of children including SSD, immune deficiencies, congenital heart disease, etc.

Few true contraindications to vaccines exist, but many misconceptions about contraindications circulate widely. The one contraindication for all vaccines is a prior history of a severe allergic reaction to a component of the vaccine. For the DTaP, another contraindication is the occurrence of encephalopathy (such as coma, altered level of consciousness, or prolonged seizures) within 7 days of administration of the previous dose. Minor illnesses; current antibiotic therapy; history of local reaction (such as erythema or swelling) after previous immunizations; family history of seizures, SIDS, or adverse events due to DTaP; and stable, nonprogressive neurologic conditions (e.g., cerebral palsy, controlled seizure disorder, or developmental delay) are not contraindications.

57 and 58. The answers are **57-d, 58-b.** (*Hay et al, pp 1206-1208, 1368-1370. Kliegman et al, pp 1579-1586, 1621. Rudolph et al, p 985.*) A woman who fails to receive the HPV vaccine is at risk for developing venereal warts and later cervical cancer. A child born to a woman who has active HPV infection may develop colonization of mucous membranes, often presenting as a "hoarse cry" when the congenitally-acquired lesions are located on the vocal folds. Failure to receive the varicella vaccine places a child at risk of developing chicken pox, which begins as vesicles on a red base that later crust and eventually resolve. Infection by methicillin-resistant staphylococcus during the early portion of this condition can lead to localized infection, regional spread, and possibly sepsis.

59 and 60. The answers are **59-e, 60-c.** (*Hay et al, pp 289-293. Kliegman et al, pp 321-341. Rudolph et al, p 92.*) Vitamin C deficiency classically causes "scurvy," a condition in the small child consisting of pallor, irritability, and poor weight gain. Later findings progress to include extreme pain and tenderness in the arms and the legs. A characteristic posture of semiflexion of the hips and knees in the "frog leg" position is due to extreme subperiosteal pain. Petechiae and ecchymosis may also be seen. Milk is a poor source of vitamin C.

Niacin deficiency causes pellagra, a condition that begins with lassitude, weakness, and digestive disturbances. Ultimately the classic triad of "dermatitis, diarrhea, and dementia" develops. The first stage of the skin findings includes redness and blebs or blisters that exfoliate leaving large areas of denuded epithelium similar to sunburn. About one-third of patients with niacin deficiency develop oral mucous membrane involvement including edema, furrowing, erosions, ulcers, and atrophy of the tongue.

Vitamin B_6, or pyridoxine, deficiency occurs in patients with low levels of this vitamin in their diet, because of a vitamin B_6-dependent syndrome whereby enzyme structure problems result in poor absorption, or as a result of vitamin inhibition due to drug ingestion including isoniazid, penicillamine, corticosteroids, and anticonvulsants. Seizures, peripheral neuritis, dermatitis, and microcytic anemia are commonly seen evidence of deficiency.

Folate deficiency can occur from a number of etiologies including poor intake or absorption, in high-demand diseases such as sickle cell, and in inborn errors of metabolism. It can also be seen in conjunction with a variety of medication uses including high-dose nonsteroidal anti-inflammatory drugs (NSAIDs), methotrexate, and phenytoin. Deficiency results in megaloblastic anemia, glossitis, pharyngeal ulcers, and impaired immunity.

Deficiencies of the other vitamins listed include: vitamin B_{12} (cobalamin) and neurologic symptoms including weakness, failure to thrive, irritability, fatigue, sensory defect, delayed or loss of milestones, seizures, neuropsychiatric changes, and megaloblastic anemia; riboflavin deficiency and cheilosis, glossitis, a variety of ocular problems (keratitis, conjunctivitis, and corneal vascularization), and seborrheic dermatitis; thiamine and beriberi; vitamin D and rickets, and; biotin and dermatitis/seborrhea.

61 to 64. The answers are 61-e, 62-c, 63-b, 64-d. (*Hay et al, pp 1107, 1109, 1112-1113, 1115, 1120. Kliegman et al, pp 602-603, 615-616, 2165, 2813. Rudolph et al, pp 694-695, 702, 703.*) Features of Cornelia de Lange include intrauterine growth retardation, prematurity, low-pitched cry, early hypertonicity, and feeding difficulty. Physical examination findings include short stature, microcephaly, confluent eyebrows, long curly eyelashes, poorly developed orbital arches, hirsutism, limb defects (micromelia most common), VSD, and undescended testes. All have intellectual disability.

Angelman syndrome is also called "happy puppet syndrome" because of the unusual gait and the unprovoked outbursts of laughter. In most cases, it is caused by an interstitial deletion of chromosome 15q11-13; the deleted material always comes from the maternal side (the same deleted segment from the paternal side results in Prader-Willi). Other features include developmental delay, seizures, microcephaly, speech impairment, hyperactivity, a fascination with water, and poor sleeping.

The distinctive, catlike cry associated with cri du chat syndrome is likely caused by abnormal laryngeal development; it tends to resolve with time. Intrauterine growth retardation, early failure to thrive with poor suck and swallow, round face with full cheeks, hypertelorism, micrognathia, low-set ears, and single palmar crease are commonly seen. Profound intellectual disability, self-injurious behavior, hypersensitivity to sound, and repetitive behaviors are commonly seen. Deletion of the short arm of chromosome 5 is the etiology. About 85% of cases are paternal in origin.

VATER (or VACTERL) is an association of commonly seen findings of unknown etiology. The patients affected have **v**ertebral defect, **a**nal atresia, **c**ardiac defects, **t**racheo**e**sophageal fistula, **r**enal/**r**adial defect (or both), and **l**imb abnormalities. Intelligence is normal.

Trisomy 13 occurs in about 1:5000-12,000 live births. In most cases, all or a majority of the extra chromosome 13 is present. Failure to thrive, seizures, cleft lip and palate, microphthalmia, cutis aplasia of the scalp, congenital heart disease, and severe intellectual disability are seen. Advanced maternal age is commonly noted. Translocation can be a cause, thus imparting approximately 10% risk of recurrence and the need for parental testing. The survival of these infants is poor with less than 5% survival after 6 months of age.

65 to 68. The answers are **65-a, 66-k, 67-f, 68-h**. (*Hay et al, pp 67-74. Kliegman et al, pp 66-67. Rudolph et al, p 2141.*) In general, motor development occurs in a cephalocaudal and central-to-peripheral direction; truncal control precedes arm control, which precedes finger dexterity. Thus, a 1-month old can regard his parent's face, follow to midline, lift his head from the examining table, smile spontaneously, and respond to a bell.

A 2-month old can smile, fix and follow, coo when smiled at or talked to, and hold his head in a prone position.

A 4-month old is expected to follow a moving toy from side to side and also in the vertical plane. He can roll and reach for an object.

At 6-6½ months of age, infants will be able to sit alone, leaning forward to support themselves with arms extended, in the so-called tripod position. They can reach for an object by changing the orientation of the torso. They can purposefully roll from a prone to a supine as well as from a supine to a prone position.

A 9-month old can turn to his name and bear weight.

By 12 months a child can walk well holding on to furniture but is slightly wobbly when walking alone; can use a neat pincer grasp to pick up a pellet, and can release a cube into a cup after it has been demonstrated to her. Building a tower of two cubes is variably successful.

A 15-month old can walk steadily and scribble with a pen. He has several single words and can point at an object. He assists in dressing and uses a spoon to feed, albeit with much spilling.

An 18-month old should be able to climb, throw a ball, walk up and down stairs with assistance, and walk backward with variable success. Naming body parts and using two-word phrases is seen. He has now learned to build towers of blocks, remove some clothing, and can play with others.

A 24-month old is able to climb up and down stairs one step at a time, kick a ball, use pronouns, and three-word phrases.

Four- and 5-year-old children should be able to copy a square and a cross; children younger than this age have difficulty with this task. By 4 years of age, their language should be fully understandable by the examiner. Children begin to name four colors, define five words, and know three adjectives. A 4-year-old child can stand on each leg for 2 seconds, and by 5 years of age that skill can be maintained for at least 5 seconds. A 4-year-old child may require some help with some clothing, but by 5 years of age, they are able to dress themselves independently, skip, and ask questions about word meaning.

69 to 73. The answers are 69-c, 70-f, 71-d, 72-e, 73-a. (*Hay et al, pp 337-361. Kliegman et al, pp 450-467. Rudolph et al, pp 67, 458, 461, 464-465, 469.*) The findings of chronic lead exposure include those listed in the question including a history of vomiting, altered mental status, poor appetite, lethargy, and irritability. Physical examination findings include evidence of acute encephalopathy, ataxia, and variable levels of consciousness. The most important aspect of the management of lead poisoning is the identification and withdrawal of the source of the lead. Patients with symptomatic lead poisoning or extremely high lead levels in the blood (> 70 μg/dL) should be treated with both dimercaprol and calcium EDTA. With milder poisoning, intravenous or intramuscular calcium EDTA or, more commonly, oral dimercaptosuccinic acid can be used.

Clonidine is used for adults for hypertension and in some children for attention-deficit/hyperactivity or tic disorders. Accidental ingestion findings in the first hour include lethargy, miosis, bradycardia, and hypotension. Later respiratory depression progressing to apnea requiring mechanical ventilation is seen. Treatment includes aggressive PICU support and naloxone (which has variable effect) and atropine.

Morphine and other narcotics used in the labor and delivery process produce their major toxic effect by suppression of ventilation. Ventilatory support can be necessary initially, but naloxone is a specific antidote and can be very rapidly effective. The effect of naloxone can wear off more quickly than the effects of the drug for which it was given, so careful observation and repeated doses may be necessary.

Salicylate poisoning produces the demonstrated blood gas findings including metabolic acidosis and respiratory alkalosis (although this latter feature is often missed in young children), hyperglycemia or hypoglycemia, paradoxical aciduria, dehydration, and lethargy. Excretion of salicylates in the urine can be markedly enhanced by the administration of acetazolamide and IV sodium bicarbonate. Hemodialysis can also be used.

Organophosphate insecticides are absorbed from all sites and act by inhibiting cholinesterases, thereby leading to the accumulation of high levels of acetylcholine. This affects the parasympathetic nervous system, muscle, and the CNS. Treatment of a patient contaminated with organophosphate insecticide will include thorough washing of the pesticide from the skin, inducing emesis or performing gastric lavage, supporting ventilation, and administering atropine followed by pralidoxime (2-PAM).

N-acetylcysteine (NAC) is an effective treatment for acetaminophen poisoning and acts as a glutathione substitute by binding directly to *N*-acetyl-*p*-benzoquinone imine, the cytotoxic metabolite of acetaminophen. Ideally it should be given within 8 hours of ingestion; after 36 hours it is probably ineffective.

74 to 78. **The answers are 74-a, 75-f, 76-a, 77-d, 78-g.** (*Hay et al, pp 1312-1316, 1321-1324, 1364-1365. Kliegman et al, pp 1692-1694, 1697-1698, 1713-1718, 1750, 1874. Rudolph et al, pp 925, 1203-1204, 1216, 1219-1220, 1227-1234.*) *Trichomonas vaginalis* causes trichomoniasis, a common sexually transmitted disease characterized by dyspareunia, dysuria, and a frothy malodorous vaginal discharge. First-line treatment is with metronidazole or tinidazole, although tinidazole is contraindicated in pregnancy.

Malaria presents with high spiking paroxysms of fever accompanied by headaches, myalgia, back pain with splenomegaly, and pallor on examination. Malaria in Central America tends to be chloroquine-sensitive, but it would be prudent to consult with an up-to-date resource as resistance patterns change over time.

Giardia does not always present in a typical fashion, but the symptoms in order of reported frequency include diarrhea, weakness, abdominal distension, flatulence, abdominal cramps, and foul-smelling, greasy stools. Tinidazole is first-line treatment; metronidazole is frequently used off-label as well. Albendazole is a secondary option, as it is less effective than tinidazole and metronidazole.

Cyclospora cayetanensis can cause fever, abdominal bloating, low-grade fever, prolonged diarrhea, and weight loss. Exposure through contaminated foods is the source; symptoms begin after about a 7-day incubation period. Diagnosis is confirmed by identifying oocysts in the stool. Trimethoprim/sulfamethoxazole is the treatment of choice; ciprofloxacin is an alternative.

Diphyllobothrium latum is the longest tapeworm affecting humans. It is frequently asymptomatic, but can present with anemia as the worm will use vitamin B_{12} for its own growth. Thus, the patient may present with the signs and symptoms of anemia as noted by the question and the CBC findings of megaloblastic anemia as listed due to B_{12} deficiency. Praziquantel is currently the treatment of choice.

79 to 83.   The answers are 79-c, 80-d, 81-f, 82-g, 83-e. (*Hay et al, pp 31, 56, 1105, 1122. Kliegman et al, pp 812-814, 818, 1550-1551. Rudolph et al, pp 734-737, 739.*) The use of lithium early in pregnancy has been associated with Ebstein anomaly, a congenital heart abnormality consisting of displacement of the tricuspid valve into the right ventricle with partial attachment of the valve to the right ventricular wall instead of the tricuspid annulus. ACE inhibitor antihypertensives have been associated with renal dysgenesis, oligohydramnios, and skull ossification defects. Isotretinoin is a very effective medication for nodular cystic acne, but if taken when a woman is pregnant commonly results in teratogenic effects including hydrocephalus, CNS defects, microtia/anotia, small or missing thymus, conotruncal heart defect, micrognathia, and even fetal death.

Ensuring adequate folate supplementation before and during pregnancy is associated with a reduction in the incidence of neural tube defects.

The congenital rubella syndrome, now rare in the United States, can result in infants born with cataracts and mental retardation. Two-thirds of infants with congenital rubella infection have permanent sensorineural hearing loss. Half have congenital heart disease; patent ductus arteriosus and pulmonary artery stenosis are most common, with other lesions such as valvular stenosis and VSD reported. The "classic" clinical finding is a petechial and purpuric rash; the baby is described as appearing like a blueberry muffin.

84 to 87.   The answers are 84-b, 85-f, 86-d, 87-a. (*Hay et al, pp 412-414, 1327. Kliegman et al, pp 1116-1121, 1736, 3154-3157. Rudolph et al,* *pp 1122-1123, 1194-1195, 1257-1259.*) Cutaneous larva migrans (also known as creeping eruption) is caused primarily by *Ancylostoma braziliense*, a dog and cat hookworm. After exposure (such as walking barefoot on a beach and stepping where an infected dog has recently been), the larvae penetrate the skin at the epidermal-dermal junction and migrate at about 1-2 cm a day. The result is an intensely pruritic lesion as described in the vignette. Left untreated the larvae die over a period of weeks to months, but treatment with anthelminthic medications hastens resolution of symptoms.

Seborrheic dermatitis is a common condition in newborn infants, arising in the first weeks after delivery. The description is as in the vignette. Chronic seborrheic dermatitis, particularly if it is associated with failure to thrive, can be a manifestation of Langerhans cell histiocytosis (formerly called histiocytosis X). Treatment for common seborrheic dermatitis consists of antiseborrheic shampoos; topical corticosteroids may be used for inflamed lesions.

Photosensitive or photoallergic reactions are seen when the offending agent is found on the skin and the patient is exposed to sunlight. In the vignette, lime juice (a common offender along with lemon juice) is found in the limeade and in the margaritas. The distribution on the face and chest of the child would be expected, as might spilling on the chest of her father. Medications that can cause a photoallergic eruption include tetracycline and griseofulvin.

Atopic dermatitis, an immediate hypersensitivity reaction to common environmental irritants, has a prevalence of 2%-3% in children. Inflammatory patches and weeping, crusted plaques on the neck, face, groin, and extensor surfaces characterize the infantile form. In older children, dermatitis of the flexural areas is common. Soaps and hot water are common irritants. Therapy is based on avoidance of irritants, adequate hydration of the skin, and use of topical steroids, as well as treatment of infected lesions.

88 to 90.   The answers are 88-d, 89-a, 90-c. (*Hay et al, pp 40-41, 575-577. Kliegman et al, pp 1180-1181, 2194-2198. Rudolph et al, pp 1279, 1805-1806, 1807-1810.*) VSD is the most common congenital cardiac malformation. Although small lesions result in insignificant left-to-right shunts, the murmur associated with them can be significantly louder as a result of turbulent blood flow. Larger lesions result in significant left-to-right shunting of blood and can result in dyspnea, poor growth, and heart failure, usually during early infancy.

The ductus arteriosus usually closes spontaneously shortly after delivery in a term infant in response to change from placental support to the relatively higher oxygen concentration in room air. In preterm infants, however, the smooth muscle in the wall of the ductus is not so responsive to increased oxygen. Although the PDA can be helpful in the very few patients with cyanotic congenital heart disease, it can lead to complications for most premature infants. The ductus may be closed with indomethacin, with a coil during cardiac catheterization, or with a surgically placed clip.

Neonatal lupus can be responsible for a variety of problems in the newborn. Mothers with antibodies to Ro/SSA and some with antibodies to La/SSB can deliver infants with rashes, thrombocytopenia, and congenital heart block, among the more common problems. Whereas the other symptoms usually resolve during the first months of life, the congenital heart block can be irreversible and can result in heart failure, need for early pacemakers, and an increased incidence of early death.

91 to 96.   The answers are 91-g 92-c, 93-a, 94-e, 95-g, 96-f. (*Hay et al, pp 284-294. Kliegman et al, pp 274-280. Rudolph et al, pp 105, 593, 1055, 1172, 1574-1576, 1984.*)

Children maintained on anticonvulsants such as phenytoin can develop low folate levels that can be associated with megaloblastic anemia as noted in the question (anemia with elevation in MCV and a smear replete with macrocytes and some hypersegmented neutrophils). Folic acid supplementation may be indicated.

The World Health Organization (WHO) recommends that, in communities where vitamin A deficiency is prevalent, it should be given to all children with measles, the classic symptoms (including Koplik spots on the oral mucosa) are described in the question. Compliance with this recommendation has resulted in a definite reduction in measles-related morbidity and mortality. In the United States, vitamin A supplements should be considered for use in measles patients with immunodeficiency, impaired intestinal absorption, and malnutrition. Recent immigrants from areas with a high mortality from measles and who show ophthalmologic evidence of vitamin A deficiency (blindness, Bitot spots, or xerophthalmia) should also be included in that group.

Fat malabsorption occurs: (1) in the absence of pancreatic enzymes, as in cystic fibrosis as described by the signs and symptoms in the question; (2) as a result of failure of micellar solubilization by bile salts, as in chronic liver disease; and (3) with a problematic mucosal uptake, as in celiac sprue. For people with these conditions, attention must be paid to the provision of fat-soluble vitamins A, D, E, and K.

Both human and cow's milk are low in vitamin D content. Cow's milk and infant formulas are fortified with this vitamin. The AAP issued a recommendation in November 2008 that all breast-fed infants receive supplementation with vitamin D beginning in the first few days of life, based on studies suggesting a significant role for vitamin D in immunity as well as disease prevention.

Patients with hemolytic anemia have an ongoing compensatory erythropoiesis. To supply the increased need of rapidly dividing RBC precursors for folate, supplementation is necessary. The child in the question admitted for fever due to increased risk of sepsis has evidence of SSD: pallor, splenomegaly, systolic ejection murmur (due to anemia), as well as CBC findings of anemia and sickled cells on smear.

In newborns, a lack of free vitamin K in the mother and the absence of bacterial intestinal flora that synthesizes vitamin K result in a transient deficiency in vitamin K–dependent factors (II, VII, IX, X). Milk is a poor source of vitamin K. Vitamin K administered shortly after birth prevents hemorrhagic disease of the newborn.

97 to 101. The answers are 97-c, 98-f, 99-b, 100-g, 101-e. (*Hay et al, pp 997-1001. Kliegman et al, pp 999-1006. Rudolph et al, pp 757-758, 761-762, 1588, 1594-1596, 2089.*) The bulk of immunodeficiencies can be ruled out with little cost. The dihydrorhodamine (DHR) flow cytometry test will help identify phagocytic-cell defects such as chronic granulomatous disease (resulting in the liver abscess in the child in question). An older test for CGD is the nitroblue tetrazolium (NBT) test.

Wiskott-Aldrich syndrome must be considered in a patient with severe eczema and unusual infections, and is a strong possibility with this history if the platelet count (frequent nosebleeds) is low (but is unlikely if the platelet count is normal). Other findings include eosinophilia and elevated IgE. B-cell defects are likely to result in low immunoglobulin A, G, and M levels, lack of adenopathy, and result in multiple infections such as that described in the 3-year old with otitis media and sinusitis. An intradermal skin test using *Candida albicans* will result in no response in the patient with T-cell deficiencies, such as in the question of the dysmorphic child who has many of the features of DiGeorge syndrome. Asplenia results in Howell-Jolly bodies and also an increased risk for encapsulated organisms such as pneumococcus or meningococcus; a CBC with a peripheral smear can rule out this disease. Should any of these tests prove to be positive, more extensive, invasive, and expensive testing can be undertaken.

The Newborn Infant

Questions

102. A 2-day-old infant is rooming in with his mother on the mother-baby unit. He was born vaginally at 38 weeks' gestation to a 33-year-old woman with limited prenatal care. On physical examination, weight, height, and head circumference of the infant are less than the 10th percentile. He is somewhat irritable with good tone and cry. In addition to the findings shown (Photograph) he has strabismus and abnormal palmer creases. On auscultation he has a harsh 2/6 holosystolic murmur. Which of the following is the most likely mechanism for this condition?

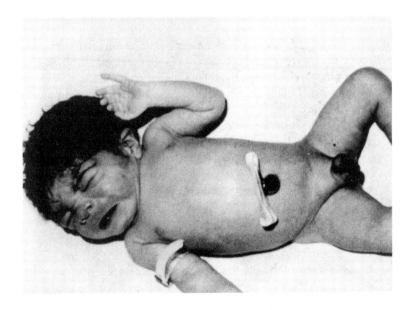

a. Exposure *in utero* to phenytoin
b. Translocation of chromosome 21 genetic material
c. Pathogenetic mutation of the COL4A5 genes on the X chromosome
d. Exposure *in utero* to ethanol
e. Exposure *in utero* to maternal hyperglycemia

103. A 3-day-old neonate is seen by the pediatrician for early follow-up after birth. The boy was born vaginally at term to a 31-year-old woman whose pregnancy was complicated by seizures which were well controlled with phenobarbital. The newborn has been bottle-feeding well, and voiding and stooling several times per day. Physical examination shows his vital signs to be normal. His current weight is about 3% lower than birth weight. The skin is jaundiced and with good turgor. Laboratory data show his total bilirubin to be 17.8 mg/dL (direct bilirubin is 0.3 mg/dL). Which of the following factors would be associated with the development of kernicterus?

a. Metabolic alkalosis
b. Increased attachment of bilirubin to binding sites caused by drugs such as sulfisoxazole
c. Hyperalbuminemia
d. Neonatal sepsis
e. Maternal ingestion of phenobarbital during pregnancy

104. A 2-hour-old full-term infant is noted by the nursing staff in the normal newborn nursery to have episodes of cyanosis and apnea. Per nursery protocol an oxygen saturation monitor is placed on him. The staff report that when they attempt to feed him the oxygen saturation level drops into the 60s. When he is stimulated and cries, the oxygen level quickly increases into the 90s. Which of the following is the most important next step to quickly establish the diagnosis?

a. Obtain an echocardiogram.
b. Order an upper GI series.
c. Attempt to pass a 5 French feeding catheter into each nostril.
d. Obtain a hemoglobin electrophoresis.
e. Perform bronchoscopic evaluation.

105. The triage nurse receives a call from a new mother. She reports that she was just diagnosed with varicella at a local urgent care center. She delivered a term infant 7 days prior. The newborn is being breast-fed only. He has been eating, stooling, and urinating without difficulty. The mother reports the newborn's temperature to be 37°C (98.5°F). Which of the following is the most appropriate next step in management?

a. Isolate the neonate from the mother.
b. Hospitalize the neonate in the isolation ward.
c. Administer acyclovir to the newborn.
d. Administer varicella-zoster immunoglobulin to the neonate.
e. Advise the mother to continue regular well-baby care for the newborn.

106. A term infant is born by scheduled cesarean section for breech lie to a 33-year-old woman. Which of the following maternal conditions would preclude her wish to breast-feed the newborn?

a. Upper respiratory tract infection
b. Cracked and bleeding nipples
c. Mastitis
d. Inverted nipples
e. HIV infection

107. A term infant is seen in the delivery room by the neonatologist after an emergency cesarean delivery for severe fetal bradycardia. The mother is a 19-year-old woman who had no prenatal care but denies any problems. On physical examination the newborn has poor respiratory effort, is meconium stained, and receives Apgar scores of 3 at 1 and 5 minutes of life. She is intubated and transported to the neonatal intensive care unit. Which of the following sequelae is likely to develop in this neonate?

a. Sustained rise in pulmonary arterial pressure
b. Hyperactive bowel sounds
c. Microcephaly with micrognathia
d. Cataracts
e. Thrombocytosis

108. A 2-year-old boy is seen by the pediatrician for well-child care. The child is deaf and developmentally delayed. His mother reports that he was born small for gestational age and had a prolonged newborn hospital course which was complicated by hepatosplenomegaly, thrombocytopenia, chorioretinitis, and deafness. Brain imaging showed him to have periventricular calcifications. The child's mother states that she is currently 8 weeks' pregnant. Which of the following is the most appropriate advice to provide?

a. The mother has developed antibodies that will likely protect the fetus from serious disease.
b. The mother's condition from the first pregnancy cannot become reactivated.
c. The newborn likely will develop similar complications.
d. Termination of pregnancy is advised due to the high risk of complications.
e. Upon birth, the newborn should be isolated from the older child.

109. A term infant is born vaginally to a 28-year-old woman whose pregnancy was complicated by gestational diabetes. Delivery was complicated by marginal placental separation. The birth weight was 2900 g (6 lb, 4 oz) and the Apgar scores were 8 and 9 at 1 and 5 minutes, respectively. At 12 hours of age the neonate is seen by the pediatric nurse practitioner. The nursing staff report normal feeding with one void recorded. On physical examination the temperature is 37°C (98.6°F), heart rate is 140 beats per minute, and respiratory rate is 28 breaths per minute. The abdomen is soft with liver edge palpable 1 cm below the costal margin, and spleen tip is palpable. The skin is pink without petechiae or bruises. The extremities are normal. The diaper has a meconium stool that contains a large amount of blood. Laboratory data reveal:

Hemoglobin: 16 g/dL
Hematocrit: 47.2%
WBC: 15,000/mm³
  Segmented neutrophils: 60%
  Band forms: 1%
  Lymphocytes: 39%
Platelets: 185,000/mm³

Which of the following is the most appropriate next step?

a. Perform barium enema
b. Order an Apt-Downey test
c. Place an orogastric tube and lavage the newborn's stomach with normal saline
d. Obtain an upper gastrointestinal series
e. Order a prothrombin time and partial thromboplastin time

110. A pediatrician is evaluating a 2-hour-old neonate. The neonate was delivered vaginally at term to a 19-year-old woman whose pregnancy was complicated by chronic hypertension and seizures. She has a history of herpes simplex virus infections for which she was given oral antiviral agents in the weeks before pregnancy; she had no lesions during the month before delivery. She attends local community college and takes methamphetamine for her long-standing attention deficit disorder. The mother states that she wishes to breast-feed the newborn. Which of the following would be a contraindication?

a. Ibuprofen as needed for pain or fever
b. Labetalol
c. Methamphetamine
d. Carbamazepine
e. Acyclovir

111. A 50-hour-old neonate develops twitching and tremors of the extremities. The neonate was born at term by cesarean section to a 26-year-old primigravida mother with insulin-dependent gestational diabetes. Birth weight was 4500 g (9 lb, 14.5 oz). The newborn's initial glucose at 1 hour of age was 25 mg/dL, but after breast-feeding subsequent glucoses have all been above 60 mg/dL. On physical examination the temperature is 37°C (98.6°F), heart rate is 140 beats per minute, and respiratory rate is 34 breaths per minute. The newborn is diaphoretic and irritable. The extremities twitch and have tremors. The rest of the examination is normal. Which of the following is the most likely cause of this newborn's condition?

a. Hypernatremia
b. Hypocalcemia
c. Hypoglycemia
d. Hyperphosphatemia
e. Hypokalemia

112. A 36-hour-old neonate is seen in the normal newborn nursery by the pediatric nurse practitioner. The neonate was born vaginally at term to a primiparous woman whose pregnancy was uncomplicated. Maternal laboratory testing reveal:

Blood type: O-positive, antibody screen negative
HIV negative
Rubella immune

On physical examination the newborn's temperature is 37°C (98.6°F), heart rate is 140 beats per minute, and respiratory rate is 30 breaths per minute. The newborn is asleep and resting comfortably. The examination is normal, except the skin is jaundiced. Newborn laboratory test results reveal:

Blood type: A-positive
Hematocrit: 55%
Transcutaneous bilirubin (TcB): 12 mg/dL

Which of the following findings would be characteristic of ABO hemolytic disease in this newborn?

a. A normal reticulocyte count
b. A positive direct Coombs test
c. Crescent-shaped RBCs in the blood smear
d. Elevated hemoglobin
e. Petechiae

113. A neonatologist sees a neonate in the level 2 neonatal intensive care nursery for feeding difficulties. The 7-day-old newborn was born at 32 weeks' gestation and had been doing well on increasing nasogastric feedings of breast milk. In the previous 6 hours the nursing staff report emesis of two feedings and decreased activity. On physical examination the temperature is 36.6°C (97.9°F), heart rate is 165 beats per minute, and respiratory rate is 35 breaths per minute. The newborn is awake and appears uncomfortable. Abdomen is tense and distended with decreased bowel sounds. A grossly bloody stool is noted in the diaper. The plain film of his abdomen is shown. Which of the following is the most appropriate next step?

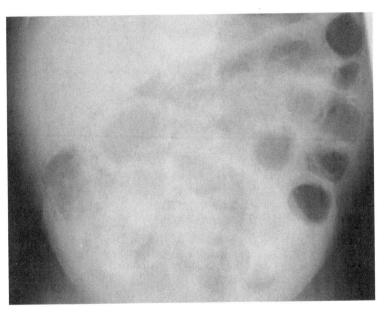

(Used with permission from Susan John, MD.)

a. Obtain a surgical consultation for an emergent exploratory laparotomy.
b. Continue feeding of the newborn, as gastroenteritis is usually self-limited.
c. Culture the stool culture to identify the etiology of the bloody diarrhea and obtain an infectious disease consultation.
d. Stop feeds, begin intravenous fluids, order serial abdominal films, and initiate systemic antibiotics.
e. Remove the nasogastric tube, place a transpyloric tube, and after confirmation via radiograph of tube positioning, switch feeds from nasogastric to nasoduodenal.

114. A neonatologist sees a 1-hour-old neonate for tachypnea. The neonate was born at 32 weeks' gestation to a 21-year-old woman whose pregnancy was uncomplicated until a motor vehicle crash induced her labor. Birth weight was 1600 g (3½ lb). The initial evaluation in the labor and delivery suite was benign, and the newborn was transferred to the level 2 nursery for prematurity. On the current physical examination the temperature is 35°C (95°F), heart rate is 145 beats per minute, and respiratory rate is 80 breaths per minute, oxygen saturation of 98% on room air. The neonate is asleep and appears comfortable. The head is normocephalic with flat fontanel. The chest is clear with good air movement and equal breath sounds. The heart has normal S1 and S2 without murmur. Abdomen is soft, nontender, and without hepatosplenomegaly. The newborn's chest radiograph is shown. Which of the following is the most appropriate next step?

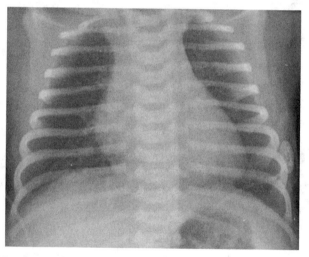

(Used with permission from Susan John, MD.)

a. Obtain a complete blood count and differential.
b. Perform a lumbar puncture.
c. Administer intravenously 5 cc of $D_{50}W$.
d. Place the newborn under a warmer.
e. Administer supplemental oxygen.

115. A 3-day-old neonate, born at 32 weeks' gestation and weighing 1700 g (3 lb, 12 oz), has three episodes of apnea, each lasting 20-25 seconds and occurring after a feeding. During these episodes, the heart rate drops from 140 to 100 beats per minute, and the newborn remains motionless. Between episodes, however, the newborn displays normal activity. On physical examination the newborn is asleep and appears comfortable. The head is normocephalic with a flat anterior fontanel. The chest is clear with good air movement and equal breath sounds. The heart has normal S1 and S2 without murmur. Abdomen is soft, nontender, and without hepatospleno-megaly. Laboratory data show:

Sodium: 135 mEq/L
Potassium: 5.5 mEq/L
Chloride: 105 mEq/L
Bicarbonate: 22 mEq/L
Glucose: 50 mg/dL
Calcium: 8.5 mg/dL

Which of the following is the most likely mechanism for this newborn's apneic periods?

a. An immature respiratory center.
b. Normal periodic breathing.
c. Electrolyte disturbance.
d. Seizures.
e. Underlying pulmonary disease.

116. An 11-day-old term neonate is seen in the pediatrician's office. The neonate was born vaginally at term and weighed 2900 g (6 lb, 4 oz). The mother is a 22-year-old woman whose pregnancy was complicated by HSV-2 positive serology but without active lesions. The newborn breast-fed well and was discharged at 2 days of age after an uneventful newborn course. On physical examination weight is 2800 g (6 lb, 4 oz), temperature is 37°C (98.6°F), heart rate is 135 beats per minute, and respiratory rate is 35 breaths per minute. The newborn is asleep but easily arousable. The physical examination is normal. Laboratory data show the initial newborn metabolic screen to indicate possible galactosemia. Which of the following is the most appropriate next step?

a. Discontinue oral feeds and begin total parenteral nutrition.
b. Supplement her breast-feeding with a multivitamin.
c. Refer to endocrinology for evaluation.
d. Discontinue breast-feeding and initiate soy formula feedings.
e. Obtain an ultrasound of the liver and spleen.

117. A 1-week-old neonate is seen in the pediatrician's office for a shoulder mass. The father reports that he noted the slightly tender mass on his newborn's right anterior shoulder about 2 hours previously. The newborn has been breast-feeding, voiding, and stooling well. Delivery was vaginal with forceps assistance, at term, after an uneventful pregnancy. Birth weight was 3200 g (7 lb, 1 oz). Apgar scores were 9 and 8 at 1 and 5 minutes, respectively. Family history is positive for osteosarcoma in the father at age 15; the father received chemotherapy and a leg amputation at the time. On physical examination weight is 3200 g (7 lb, 1 oz), temperature is 37°C (98.6°F), heart rate 133 beats per minute, and respiratory rate is 32 breaths per minute. The newborn is asleep but easily arousable. The head is normocephalic with flat fontanel. Pupils are equally round and reactive to light; red reflex is normal. The right eye has a small subconjunctival hemorrhage medially. A 2-cm firm, nontender mass at the midpoint of the right clavicle is noted. Which of the following is the most appropriate next step?

a. Obtain a magnetic resonance imaging of the right shoulder.
b. Provide reassurance and supportive care.
c. Arrange for a biopsy of the mass for culture and cytology.
d. Refer child to an orthopedic surgeon.
e. Schedule a skin biopsy to test for osteogenesis imperfecta.

118. A 12-hour-old neonate in the normal newborn nursery is seen by the pediatrician for initial evaluation. The term infant was born vaginally with forceps assistance to a 22-year-old primigravida mother whose pregnancy was complicated by gestational diabetes and obesity. On physical examination weight is 3900 g (8 lb, 9.6 oz), temperature is 37°C (98.6°F), heart rate is 132 beats per minute, and respiratory rate is 32 breaths per minute. The newborn is asleep but easily arousable. The head is elongated with slight bruising on the temporal regions; the fontanel is flat. The left arm is held internally rotated by her side with the forearm extended and pronated. She does not move the left arm spontaneously or during a Moro reflex. Which of the following is the most likely mechanism of injury?

a. Fracture of the left clavicle
b. Fracture of the left humerus
c. Injury to left-sided cervical spine nerves C5 and C6
d. Injury to left-sided cervical spine nerve C8 and thoracic nerve T1
e. Injury to the spinal cord with left hemiparesis

119. A newborn was the product of a benign, term pregnancy and was delivered vaginally. Nursing assessment done 6 hours prior determined the weight to be 2900 g (6 lb, 3 oz), length 48 cm (19 in), and head circumference 36 cm (14.2 in). In the interim period the staff report the newborn has breast-fed, stooled, and voided. On physical examination, temperature is 37°C (98.6°F), heart rate is 180 beats per minute, and respiratory rate is 45 breaths per minute. The newborn is easily arousable and in no distress; he is somewhat pale. Head is nontender with a "squishy" feel over the temporal, frontal, and occipital regions; a fluid wave can be elicited over the scalp. The fontanelles are not easily felt. The head circumference is now 50 cm (20 in). Pupils are equally round and reactive to light; red reflex is normal. The rest of the examination is normal. Which of the following is the most appropriate next step?

a. Transfer to the newborn ICU
b. Observation and parental reassurance
c. CT scan of the skull with bone windows
d. Needle aspiration of the fluid collection
e. Elevation of the head of the crib

120. A 14-hour-old neonate has just had a 2-minute episode of rhythmic tonic-clonic activity of the upper extremities. The neonate was born vaginally at 38 weeks to a 19-year-old primiparous woman. Apgar scores were 1 and 4 at 1 and 5 minutes, respectively. The pregnancy was complicated by preeclampsia in the final trimester of pregnancy that required magnesium sulfate during labor. Physical examination reveals weight 2100 g (4 lb, 10 oz; 5th percentile), length 46 cm (18.5 in; 5th percentile), and head circumference 32 cm (12.5 in; 5th percentile). Temperature is 37°C (98.6°F), heart rate is 150 beats per minute, and respiratory rate is 42 breaths per minute. The newborn is asleep and in no distress. The head is normocephalic with flat fontanels. Pupils are equally round and reactive to light; red reflex is normal. No focal abnormalities are found on neurologic examination. Laboratory data show:

Sodium: 135 mEq/L
Potassium: 5.5 mEq/L
Chloride: 94 mEq/L
Bicarbonate: 22 mEq/L
Glucose: 50 mg/dL
Calcium: 8.7 mg/dL
Magnesium: 2.5 mEq/L
Hemoglobin: 25 g/dL
Hematocrit: 77%
WBC: 15,000/mm³
    Segmented neutrophils: 60%
    Band forms: 1%
    Lymphocytes: 39%
Platelets: 100,000/mm³

Which of the following is the most likely cause of the newborn's condition?

a. Polycythemia
b. Hypoglycemia
c. Hypocalcemia
d. Hypermagnesemia
e. Thrombocytopenia

121. The neonatal resuscitation team is called to the delivery room to assess a lethargic and somewhat limp newborn. The mother is 28-years old with four previous vaginal deliveries. The pregnancy was complicated by obesity and maternal seizure disorder. Fetal monitoring during labor was normal. Labor was rapid, with local anesthesia and intravenous meperidine (Demerol) administered for maternal pain control about 30 minutes prior to delivery. On physical examination the newborn appears to be term and of normal size. He is lethargic, limp, and has a poor respiratory effort. Which of the following is the most appropriate next step?

a. Begin an intravenous infusion of 10% dextrose in water
b. Administer naloxone (Narcan)
c. Administer vitamin K
d. Measure serum electrolytes and magnesium levels
e. Obtain a neurology consultation

122. A newborn is transferred to the neonatal intensive care unit for respiratory distress. He was born at 31 weeks' gestation to a 21-year-old woman whose pregnancy was uncomplicated until about 5 days prior when she developed fever, chills, headache, nausea and vomiting. Rupture of membranes was 6 hours prior to delivery; the fluid was brown. On physical examination height, weight, and head circumference are at the 25th percentile for gestational age. Temperature is 35.9°C (96.6°F), heart rate is 170 beats per minute, and respiratory rate is 72 breaths per minute. The newborn is asleep and pale with audible grunting. The head is normocephalic with flat fontanel. The chest has subcostal and intercostal retractions. Breath sounds are equal. Crackles are heard over both lung fields. Air movement is equal. The heart has normal S1 and S2 without murmur. Capillary refill is about 8 seconds. Abdomen is soft and nontender. Liver edge is about 3 cm below, and the spleen tip is palpable 2 cm below the costal margin. Skin has numerous 2-3 mm pinkish-gray granulomas scattered over the trunk and extremities. Which of the following is the most likely explanation for this newborn's condition?

a. Infection with *Listeria monocytogenes*
b. Aspiration of meconium
c. Deficiency of surfactant
d. Development of pneumothorax
e. Exposure to herpes simplex virus type II

123. A 2-day-old neonate is seen by the pediatrician for eye discharge. The newborn was the product of a term, vaginal home delivery by a midwife. The pregnancy was uncomplicated. The mother reports the newborn has been breast-feeding every 2 hours, stooling two to three times daily, and voids six to eight times daily. On physical examination the eyes are puffy, the eyelids tense, and the conjunctivae red; copious amount of purulent ocular discharge and chemosis is noted (Photograph). Which of the following is the most likely diagnosis?

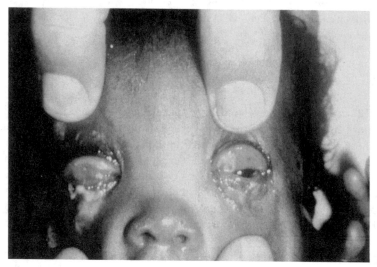

(Used with permission from Kathryn Musgrove, MD.)

a. Dacryocystitis
b. Chemical conjunctivitis
c. Pneumococcal ophthalmia neonatorum
d. Gonococcal ophthalmia neonatorum
e. Chlamydial ophthalmia neonatorum

124. A 28 weeks' gestation neonate admitted to the neonatal intensive care unit develops worsening respiratory distress over a 6-hour period. The newborn weighed 1000 g (2 lb, 3 oz) at birth and had grunting and an increased respiratory rate in the delivery room. On physical examination height, weight, and head circumference are at the 50th percentile for gestational age. Temperature is 37°C (98.6°F), heart rate is 160 beats per minute, and respiratory rate is 68 breaths per minute. Oxygen saturation is 91% while under a 35% oxygen hood and drops to 60% when the hood is removed. The newborn is asleep with audible grunting. The head is normocephalic with flat fontanel. The nose has flaring. The chest has subcostal and intercostal retractions. Breath sounds are equal. Air movement is equal but diminished bilaterally. The heart has normal S1 and S2 without murmur. Which of the following is the most likely mechanism of disease?

a. Decreased lung compliance, reduced lung volume, left-to-right shunt of blood
b. Decreased lung compliance, reduced lung volume, right-to-left shunt of blood
c. Decreased lung compliance, increased lung volume, left-to-right shunt of blood
d. Normal lung compliance, reduced lung volume, left-to-right shunt of blood
e. Normal lung compliance, increased lung volume, right-to-left shunt of blood

125. A 2-hour-old neonate is seen by the pediatrician in the low-risk nursery. The term infant was born by planned cesarean section to a 22-year-old woman whose pregnancy was complicated by past medical history of HSV-2 without recent lesions, HIV infection, and group B streptococcal urinary tract infection at 2 months' gestation. Prenatal medications included oral acyclovir, antiretroviral medications, and three doses of penicillin in the 12 hours prior to delivery. Physical examination show normal vital signs. Growth parameters demonstrate weight, length, and head circumference to be 75th percentile. The head is normocephalic with flat fontanels. Pupils are equally round and reactive to light; red reflex is normal. The chest is clear with good air movement and equal breath sounds. The heart has normal S1 and S2 without murmur. Abdomen is soft, nontender, and without hepatosplenomegaly. Which of the following is the most appropriate next step?

a. Admit the newborn to the neonatal intensive care unit and begin intravenous acyclovir.
b. Obtain an HIV ELISA on the newborn to determine if congenital infection has occurred.
c. Begin a course of oral zidovudine for the newborn.
d. Obtain a neonatal blood culture and begin a course of penicillin G.
e. Administer a dose of intravenous immunoglobulin (IVIG) to the newborn.

126. A pediatrician sees a term 4-hour-old girl in the low-risk nursery for initial evaluation. The neonate was born vaginally to a 23-year-old woman whose pregnancy was complicated by fetal ultrasound findings of nuchal cystic hygroma and horseshoe kidney. On physical examination weight is 2500 g (5 lb, 8 oz). The dorsum of hands and feet shows edema, the nails are hypoplastic, and the digits appear sausage-like in appearance. The hips are dislocated. Which of the following additional findings would be expected to be seen?

a. A liver palpable to 2 cm below the costal margin
b. Tremulous movements and ankle clonus
c. Diminished lower extremity pulses
d. A transient, longitudinal division of the body into a red half and a pale half
e. Softness of the parietal bones at the vertex

127. A pediatrician is advising the local information technology team on the implementation of computerized physician order entry. In the development of the normal newborn admission order set, which of the following vaccines is routinely advised?

a. Rotavirus vaccine
b. Hepatitis B vaccine
c. Combination diphtheria, tetanus, and acellular pertussis vaccine
d. Inactivated polio virus
e. *Haemophilus influenzae* type b vaccine

128. A 1-week-old African American boy is seen by the pediatrician for well-child care. The boy was born vaginally at term to a 22-year-old woman whose pregnancy was complicated by mild gestational diabetes and mild chronic hypertension. Prenatal medications included daily vitamins only. The parents report no problems; the neonate has been exclusively breast-feeding and has been taking daily vitamin D drops. On physical examination the weight is down about 3% from birth; vital signs are normal. The head is normocephalic with flat fontanels. Pupils are equally round and reactive to light; red reflex is normal. The chest is clear with good air movement and equal breath sounds. The heart has normal S1 and S2 without murmur. Abdomen is soft, nontender, and without hepatosplenomegaly. A large, fairly well-defined, gray-blue lesion is noted over the buttocks bilaterally (Photograph). The lesion is not palpable, warm or tender. Which of the following is the most appropriate next step?

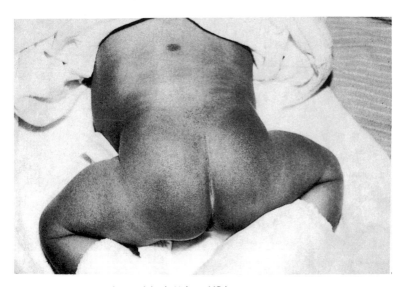

(Used with permission from Adelaide Hebert, MD.)

a. Report the family to child protective services.
b. Provide family reassurance.
c. Obtain soft tissue films of the buttocks.
d. Administer vitamin K intramuscularly.
e. Obtain serum factor VII and XI levels.

129. A newborn is seen by the neonatologist in the delivery room. The neonate was born vaginally at approximately 38 weeks' gestation to a 19-year-old woman who had no prenatal care; she reports no pregnancy complications and took no medications. On initial physical examination the newborn has severe respiratory distress with grunting and subcostal and intercostal retractions. The abdomen is scaphoid. Breath sounds are not heard on the left side of his chest, but are audible on the right. Immediate intubation is successful with little or no improvement in clinical status. Emergency chest x-ray is shown (Photograph A) along with an x-ray 2 hours later (Photograph B). Which of the following is the most likely explanation for this newborn's condition?

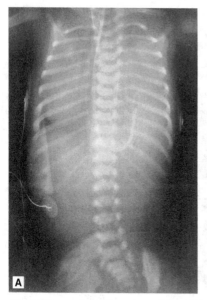 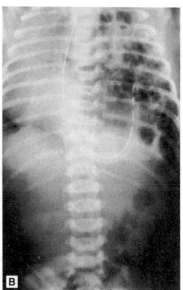

(Used with permission from Susan John, MD.)

a. Pneumonia
b. Congenital pulmonary airway malformation
c. Congenital diaphragmatic hernia
d. Choanal atresia
e. Pneumothorax

130. A 1-hour-old newborn is seen by the pediatric nurse practitioner in the low-risk nursery. The nursing staff report that upon the first breast-feeding she coughed and choked; the feeding seemed to run out of the side of her mouth. On physical examination growth parameters are at the 35th percentile for weight, length, and head circumference. Temperature is 37°C (98.6°F), heart rate is 160 beats per minute, and respiratory rate is 68 breaths per minute. The chest has intercostal retractions and bilateral rales. Abdomen is soft, nontender, distended and without hepatospleno-megaly. Which of the following illustrations of the trachea and esophagus is the most likely mechanism for this clinical presentation?

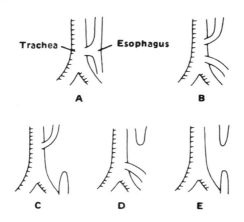

a. Figure A
b. Figure B
c. Figure C
d. Figure D
e. Figure E

131. A pediatric nurse practitioner sees a 1-hour-old neonate in the normal newborn nursery for initial evaluation. The neonate was born vaginally at term to a 21-year-old mother whose pregnancy was complicated by chronic hepatitis B (HBsAg-positive). Which of the following is the most appropriate next step?

a. Screen the newborn for HBsAg.
b. Isolate the newborn with enteric precautions.
c. Screen the mother for hepatitis B "e" antigen (HBeAg).
d. Administer hepatitis B immunoglobulin and hepatitis B vaccine to the newborn.
e. Reassure the family that transplacentally acquired antibody will protect the newborn from infection.

132. A 3-day-old infant is noted to have difficulty feeding, irritability, increased tone, tremors, a high-pitched cry and a temperature of 38.3°C (100.9°F). The infant was born vaginally at 38 weeks (based on an ultrasound just before delivery in the ED) to a 35-year-old mother with no prenatal care. Birth weight was 2200g (4 lb, 13.6 oz), less than 10% for gestational age. The mother denied pregnancy complications, but her history of substance abuse had led Children's Protective Services to take custody of her other children. Withdrawal of which of the following substances is the most likely cause of the infant's symptoms?

a. Marijuana
b. Heroin
c. Cocaine
d. Alcohol
e. Lorazepam

133. A 4-day-old neonate is seen by the pediatrician for "yellow skin." The newborn was delivered vaginally at term to a 28-year-old woman; the hospital course was uneventful with discharge at 48 hours of age. The newborn is fed standard infant formula taking about 2 oz every 3 hours. Stooling and voiding occur with frequency. The parents report the pregnancy was complicated by a life-long maternal history of hypothyroidism managed with thyroid supplementation. On physical examination the weight is 3% lower than birth weight. Vital signs are normal. Laboratory data reveal:

Maternal blood type: O-positive, antibody screen negative
Baby blood type: O-positive, Coombs negative
Total serum bilirubin: 11.8 mg/dL
Direct serum bilirubin: 0.2 mg/dL
Urine bilirubin is positive.
Hemoglobin: 17 g/dL
Hematocrit: 51%
Platelet count: 278,000 mm^3
WBC: 13,000/mm^3
   Segmented neutrophils: 49%
   Band forms: 0%
   Lymphocytes: 51%
No fragments or abnormal cell shapes noted.
Reticulocyte count: 4.5%

Which of the following is the most likely mechanism of disease?

a. Rh or ABO hemolytic disease
b. Physiologic jaundice
c. Sepsis
d. Congenital spherocytic anemia
e. Biliary atresia

134. A 6-hour-old neonate is seen by the pediatrician in the normal newborn nursery for regurgitation of small amounts of mucus and bile-stained fluid. The neonate was born vaginally at term to a 24-year-old woman whose pregnancy was complicated by group B *Streptococcus* infection, and the mother received adequate prophylaxis. Delivery was complicated by use of forceps and a large amount of amniotic fluid. On physical examination growth parameters are at the 75th percentile for weight, length, and head circumference. Temperature is 37°C (98.6°F), heart rate is 140 beats per minute, and respiratory rate is 45 breaths per minute. The chest has equal and unlabored breath sounds. Abdomen is soft, nontender, distended and without hepatosplenomegaly. An abdominal x-ray is obtained (Photograph). Which of the following is the most likely diagnosis?

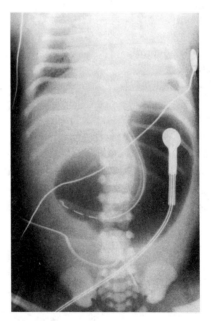

(Used with permission from Susan John, MD.)

a. Gastric duplication
b. Pyloric stenosis
c. Esophageal atresia
d. Duodenal atresia
e. Midgut volvulus

135. A pediatrician sees a 2-week-old neonate in the office for routine care. The parents report the newborn has "colic" and wish to switch to goat's milk from breast milk. Which of the following deficiencies is the main concern for the use of goat's milk as compared to breast or cow's milk?

a. Caloric density
b. Folate concentration
c. Whey composition
d. Casein composition
e. Fat distribution

136. An infant is seen in the low-risk nursery by the pediatrician for initial evaluation. The delivery was vaginally at term to a 31-year-old woman whose pregnancy was uncomplicated. Consultation with plastic and reconstructive surgery as well as the hospital's speech therapist has been initiated (See Photograph). Which of the following statements is appropriate anticipatory guidance for this family?

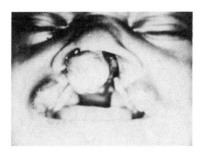

a. Parenteral alimentation is recommended to prevent aspiration.
b. Surgical closure of the palatal defect should be done before 3 months of age.
c. Good anatomic closure will preclude the development of speech defects.
d. Recurrent otitis media and hearing loss are likely complications.
e. The chance that a sibling also would be affected is 1:1000.

137. A 2-week-old neonate is seen in the pediatrician's office with the maternal concern of poor feeding. The mother reports that since birth her bottle-fed newborn sleeps most of the day; she has to awaken her every 4 hours to feed and she will take only 1 oz of formula at a time. She voids about twice a day and passes hard, pellet-like stools every other day. On physical examination growth parameters are at the 50th percentile for weight, length, and 95th percentile for head circumference. Temperature is 35°C (95°F), heart rate 75 beats per minute, and respiratory rate is 35 breaths per minute. The newborn is jaundiced and somewhat difficult to awaken. The head is normocephalic with enlarged, flat anterior and posterior fontanels. Pupils are equally round and reactive to light; red reflex is normal. The chest has equal and unlabored breath sounds. Abdomen is soft, nontender, distended and with a large umbilical hernia. Which of the following is the most likely etiology for these findings?

a. Congenital hypothyroidism
b. Congenital megacolon (Hirschsprung disease)
c. Sepsis
d. Infantile botulism
e. Normal development

138. An infant was born by cesarean section at term to a 24-year-old primigravida mother whose pregnancy was complicated by poor prenatal care. At birth the newborn is noted to have the defect shown. Which of the following statements about this defect is correct?

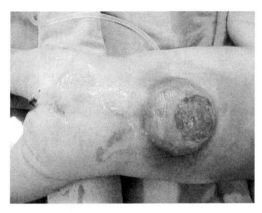

(Used with permission from David I. Sandberg, MD.)

a. The hereditary pattern for this condition is autosomal recessive.
b. The prenatal diagnosis can be made by the detection of very low levels of alpha-fetoprotein in the amniotic fluid.
c. Subsequent pregnancies are not at increased risk compared to the general population.
d. Supplementation of maternal diet with folate leads to a decrease in incidence of this condition.
e. Neither environmental nor social factors have been shown to influence the incidence.

139. A term, 4200 g (9 lb, 4 oz) infant is admitted to the neonatal intensive care unit for respiratory distress. She was delivered via scheduled cesarean section due to cephalopelvic disproportion. The amniotic fluid at the delivery was clear, the newborn cried almost immediately, and the Apgar scores were 9 and 9 at 1 and 5 minutes, respectively. The mother had good prenatal care; the pregnancy was complicated by a history of gestational diabetes which was controlled by diet. At about 15 minutes of life the newborn's respiratory rate increased to 80 breaths per minute, and she began to have intermittent grunting respirations. In the NICU she was noted to have an oxygen saturation of 94%. The initial chest radiograph (Photograph A) and the follow-up chest radiograph performed 24 hours later (Photograph B) are shown. Which of the following is the most likely diagnosis?

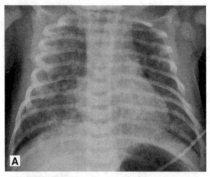

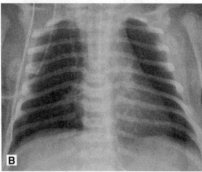

(Used with permission from Susan John, MD.)

a. Diaphragmatic hernia
b. Meconium aspiration
c. Pneumonia
d. Infant respiratory distress syndrome
e. Transient tachypnea of the newborn

140. A 2-week-old neonate is seen by the pediatrician for routine care. The mother reports the newborn to have a constant "runny nose" and rash but to otherwise be healthy taking her infant formula every 2-3 hours. She has been voiding and stooling regularly. The neonate was born vaginally at home by a midwife, reportedly at term, to a 19-year-old woman whose pregnancy was complicated by poor prenatal care. The mother denies smoking or drug use; she did not take prenatal vitamins. On physical examination the growth parameters are at the 35th percentile for weight, length, and head circumference. The temperature is 37°C (98.6°F), heart rate is 135 beats per minute, and respiratory rate is 35 breaths per minute. The newborn is alert and active. Skin is pale and somewhat jaundiced. The head is normocephalic with flat fontanels. Pupils are equally round and reactive to light; red reflex is normal. Nose has copious grayish drainage. The chest has equal and unlabored breath sounds. Abdomen is soft, nontender, and with marked hepatosplenomegaly. Skin is slightly jaundiced with a diffuse, erythematous maculopapular rash (Photographs A and B). Which of the following is the most appropriate next step?

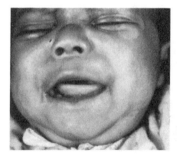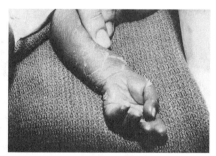

(Used with permission from Adelaide Hebert, MD.)

a. Obtain a computerized tomography of the brain to identify calcifications scattered in the cortex.
b. Take serial measurement of serum glucose and lactate levels.
c. Order serum thyroid function studies.
d. Measure newborn's rapid plasma reagin (RPR).
e. Obtain computerized tomography of the brain to identify periventricular calcifications.

141. An 8-hour-old African American neonate is seen in the normal newborn nursery by the nurse practitioner for initial evaluation. The neonate was born vaginally at term to a 35-year-old woman whose pregnancy was complicated by maternal hypertension. On physical examination the growth parameters are at the 50th percentile for weight, length, and head circumference. Vital signs are normal. Extremities show fifth finger-side (postaxial) abnormalities that appear to have no skeletal duplications and are attached to the rest of the hand by a threadlike soft tissue pedicle (Photograph). The rest of the examination is normal. Which of the following is the most appropriate next step?

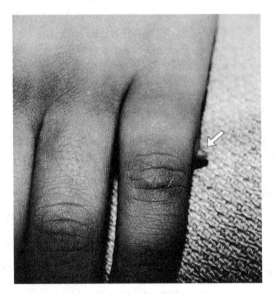

(Used with permission from Adelaide Hebert, MD.)

a. Chromosomal analysis
b. Excision of extra digit
c. Skeletal survey for other skeletal abnormalities
d. Echocardiogram
e. Renal ultrasound

142. An infant born at term after an unremarkable pregnancy is noted to have an exposed glans penis and an incompletely formed foreskin with the urethral meatus noted ventrally at the corona. The other finding most frequently noted with this birth defect is which of the following?

a. Chordee
b. Inguinal hernia
c. Hydrocele
d. Undescended testes
e. Peyronie disease

143. A previously healthy full-term neonate develops on the second day of life several episodes of generalized duskiness and apnea. He was born vaginally at term to a 33-year-old mother whose pregnancy was uncomplicated. The newborn has been rooming in with the parents, has been breastfeeding well, and has stooled and voided. Birth weight, height, and head circumference are at the 50th percentile. Initial physical examination was normal. Which of the following is the most appropriate next step?

a. Obtain newborn blood type and Coombs testing.
b. Order continuous pulse oximetry and an echocardiogram.
c. Arrange for a home apnea monitor.
d. Provide parent reassurance of normalcy of findings.
e. Order serum glucose and insulin levels.

144. Which of the following statements concerning the abstract is correct?

Interaction between Maternal Prepregnancy Body Mass Index and Gestational Weight Gain Shapes Infant Growth

William J. Heerman, MD, MPH; Aihua Bian, MPH; Ayumi Shintani, PhD, MPH; Shari L. Barkin, MD, MSHS

Division of General Pediatrics, Department of Pediatrics (Dr Heerman and Dr Barkin), and Department of Biostatistics (Ms Bian and Dr Shintani), Vanderbilt University Medical Center, Nashville, Tenn
The authors declare that they have no conflict of interest.
Address correspondence to William J. Heerman, MD, 2146 Belcourt Ave, 2nd Floor, Nashville, TN 37212 (e-mail: Bill.Heerman@vanderbilt.edu).

Received for publication February 6, 2014; accepted May 12, 2014.

ABSTRACT

OBJECTIVE: To quantify the combined effect of maternal prepregnancy obesity and maternal gestational weight gain (GWG) on the shape of infant growth throughout the first year of life.

METHODS: A retrospective cohort of mother–child dyads with children born between January 2007 and May 2012 was identified in a linked electronic medical record. Data were abstracted to define the primary exposures of maternal prepregnancy body mass index (BMI) and GWG, and the primary outcome of infant growth trajectory.

RESULTS: We included 499 mother–child dyads. The average maternal age was 28.2 years; 55% of mothers were overweight or obese before pregnancy, and 42% of mothers had excess GWG, as defined by the Institute of Medicine. Maternal prepregnancy BMI ($P < .001$) and the interaction between prepregnancy BMI and maternal GWG ($P = .02$) showed significant association with infant growth trajectory through the first year of life after controlling for breast-feeding and other covariates, while GWG alone did not reach statistical significance ($P = .38$). Among infants of mothers with excess GWG, a prepregnancy BMI of 40 kg/m^2 versus 25 kg/m^2 resulted in a 13.6% (95% confidence interval 5.8, 21.5; $P < .001$) increase in 3-month infant weight/length percentile that persisted at 12 months (8.4%, 95% confidence interval 0.2, 16.5; $P = .04$).

CONCLUSIONS: The combined effect of excess maternal GWG and prepregnancy obesity resulted in higher infant birth weight, rapid weight gain in the first 3 months of life, with a sustained weight elevation throughout the first year of life. These findings highlight the importance of the preconception and prenatal periods for pediatric obesity prevention.

KEYWORDS: infants; mothers; obesity; pediatric; pregnancy; weight gain

ACADEMIC PEDIATRICS: 2014;14:463–470

a. A woman's prepregnancy body mass index was nonpredictive of infant growth in the first year of life.

b. Gestational weight gain alone is associated with higher rates of weight gain in infants during the first year of life.

c. Rapid weight gain of neonates born to obese women will continue throughout childhood and lead to adolescent obesity.

d. Maternal obesity combined with high pregnancy weight gain is associated with more rapid weight gain in infants.

e. A prospective study evaluating the relationship between maternal body mass index and pregnancy weight gain will demonstrate more rapid weight gain in infants during their first year of life.

145. Twin newborns are seen by the pediatrician in the normal newborn nursery for their initial evaluation. The monozygotic diamniotic twins were born by planned cesarean section at 38 weeks' gestation to a 32-year-old woman whose pregnancy was uncomplicated other than twin gestation and preterm labor at 32 weeks' gestation. The first twin weighs 2800 g (6 lb, 3 oz) and has a hematocrit of 70%; the second twin weighs 2100 g (4 lb, 10 oz) and has a hematocrit of 40%. Which of the following statements is correct?

a. The second twin is at risk for developing respiratory distress, cyanosis, and congestive heart failure.
b. The first twin is more likely to have hyperbilirubinemia and seizures.
c. The second twin is at risk for renal vein thrombosis.
d. The second twin probably has hydramnios of the amniotic sac.
e. The first twin is likely to be pale, tachycardic, and hypotensive.

146. A 15-minute-old neonate is seen by the pediatrician in the delivery area for initial evaluation. The delivery was vaginal, reportedly at term, to a 19-year-old G2P1001 woman who received no prenatal care but reports no problems during this pregnancy. She arrived to the emergency room in active labor denying rupture of membranes; the biophysical profile done in the emergency center reveals severe oligohydramnios. Upon close evaluation of this newborn, which of the following is the most likely abnormality to be found?

a. Anencephaly
b. Trisomy 18
c. Renal agenesis
d. Duodenal atresia
e. Tracheoesophageal fistula

147. A newborn becomes markedly jaundiced on the second day of life. He was born vaginally at term to a 17-year-old woman whose pregnancy was complicated by chlamydia that was successfully treated in the first trimester. Birth parameters were at the 50th percentile, and initial examination on the first day of life was notable only for milia, Mongolian spots on the buttocks and a diffuse, faint petechial rash. He has been breast-feeding well, has voided, and has stooled. The current physical examination shows weight to be decreased by 2% and vital signs to be normal. The newborn is asleep and easily awakened. The head is normocephalic with flat fontanels. Pupils are equally round and reactive to light; red reflex is normal. The chest has equal and unlabored breath sounds. Abdomen is soft, nontender, and with hepatosplenomegaly. Skin has a diffuse, generalized purpuric rash and jaundice. Neurologic examination is nonfocal. Which of the following is the most appropriate next step?

a. Order a liver and spleen ultrasound.
b. Isolate the newborn from pregnant hospital personnel.
c. Obtain a urine drug screen on the newborn.
d. Discharge the newborn with the mother with an early follow-up visit in 48 hours.
e. Measure thyroid function studies.

Questions 148 to 151

For each clinical scenario mentioned later, select the most likely congenital condition. Each lettered option may be used once, more than once, or not at all.

a. Toxoplasmosis
b. Syphilis
c. Rubella
d. Cytomegalovirus (CMV)
e. Herpes simplex virus (HSV)

148. A 6-hour-old neonate was born by vaginal delivery to a 32-year-old woman whose pregnancy was complicated by intrauterine growth retardation. The newborn has bilateral cataracts and microphthalmia, hemorrhagic skin lesions scattered throughout the body, and a harsh systolic murmur heard best at the left sternal border and radiating to the lung fields.

149. A 1-week-old neonate is seen in the emergency department with a 3-hour history of fever. The family reports that he has been fussy for the day and has had decreased eating. On physical examination he has tonic-clonic activity isolated to the left hand.

150. A 1-hour-old neonate born by cesarean section to a 24-year-old woman is noted to have an enlarged head. The mother reports limited prenatal care but no known pregnancy problems. Initial evaluation of this newborn demonstrates the head circumference to be more than 95th percentile. Further evaluation demonstrates chorioretinitis, hydrocephalus, intracranial calcifications, and anemia.

151. A 14-hour-old neonate is seen by the pediatrician in the newborn nursery. He was born by vaginal delivery to an 18-year-old woman after a pregnancy notable for scant prenatal care. On initial examination the newborn has microcephaly and hepatosplenomegaly. He develops marked hyperbilirubinemia and requires phototherapy. Further evaluation demonstrates periventricular intracranial calcifications and thrombocytopenia.

Questions 152 to 155

For each clinical scenario presented, select the most likely diagnosis. Each lettered option may be used once, more than once, or not at all.

a. Bronchopulmonary dysplasia
b. Respiratory distress syndrome (hyaline membrane disease [HMD])
c. Pulmonary interstitial emphysema
d. Bronchiolitis
e. Primary pulmonary hypoplasia
f. Pneumothorax
g. Asthma
h. Meconium aspiration
i. Phrenic nerve paralysis
j. Bacterial pneumonia

152. A large-for-gestational-age term neonate is delivered via scheduled cesarean section. At 15 minutes of age he develops tachypnea, grunting, flaring, and retractions. On physical examination he does not move his left arm well. The clavicle and bony structures on the left arm are normal. A chest radiograph shows the left diaphragm to be markedly higher than the right.

153. A 43-weeks' gestation newborn is delivered by a midwife after a prolonged and difficult labor. The newborn is brought to the hospital at 1 hour of life because of rapid breathing. The family notes that the newborn seemed well initially, but then developed increased work of breathing. On physical examination growth parameters of weight, length, and head circumference are at the 50th percentile for gestational age. The newborn is asleep and in moderate respiratory distress. Chest radiograph shows the heart to be pushed to the right side and the left lung field to have loss of lung markings.

154. A baby is born to a 16-year-old mother who has received no prenatal care; the newborn has immediate respiratory distress in the delivery room. The delivery was at about term but uncertain dates via emergent cesarean section for nonreassuring heart tones. No amniotic fluid was noted at the time of the delivery. On physical examination the growth parameters of weight, head circumference, and length are less than 10th percentile for a term infant. The face has a flattened nose, recessed chin, epicanthal folds, and low-set ears. The chest has diminished breath sounds throughout. The extremities, especially the legs, are poorly formed. A chest radiograph reveals a poorly developed chest with little lung tissue.

155. A 9-week-old infant is seen in the emergency center on Thanksgiving Day for cough and cold symptoms. The infant is a former 29-week infant who required mechanical ventilation for 2 weeks, was weaned off respiratory support and oxygen at 3 weeks of age, and was just discharged a week ago. The family reports poor feeding, cough, and congestion for the previous 2 days. Sick contacts include the 2-year-old sibling with upper respiratory symptoms of cough, congestion, and nasal discharge. On physical examination the temperature is 38.8°C (101.9°F), heart rate is 160 beats per minute, respiratory rate is 70 breaths per minute, and pulse oximeter on room air is 85%. The infant is in mild respiratory distress, is irritable but is easily consoled. The mouth is moist. The nose has much clear nasal discharge and nasal flaring. The chest has equal breath sounds, diffuse wheezing, and intercostal and subcostal retractions. A chest radiograph reveals patchy infiltrates and hyperexpansion in both lung fields.

Questions 156 to 159

Most developed countries have a newborn screening program that screens infants for metabolic disease that may not otherwise be identified until later in its course when intervention would be less successful. Select the most appropriate treatment for each disease mentioned below. Each lettered option may be used once, more than once, or not at all.

a. Special infant formula
b. Hormone therapy
c. Vitamin therapy
d. Antibiotic prophylaxis
e. Sunlight

156. Galactosemia

157. Phenylketonuria

158. Biotinidase deficiency

159. Maple syrup urine disease

Questions 160 to 163

For each of the following descriptions of a patient with a congenital anomaly, select the major abnormality with which it is most likely to be associated. Each lettered option may be used once, more than once, or not at all.

a. Deafness
b. Seizures
c. Wilms tumor
d. Congestive heart failure
e. Optic glioma

160. A term infant is born vaginally to a 32-year-old woman after an uneventful pregnancy. She reports taking prenatal vitamins and denies tobacco, alcohol, or other drug exposure. Family history is positive for type 2 diabetes on the paternal side. On physical examination the newborn's left arm and leg are noticeably larger than those on the right. Eyes show aniridia and normal red reflex. Chest has equal, unlabored breath sounds. Abdomen is flat, nontender, and without hepatosplenomegaly.

161. A term infant is born by cesarean section for nonreassuring fetal heart rate to a 23-year-old woman after a pregnancy complicated by maternal hypertension. The family history is positive for hypertension and stroke in the maternal grandfather. On physical examination the head is normocephalic with flat fontanelles. A white forelock is noted over the left frontal scalp. Eyes have fusion of the eyebrows and heterochromic irises. The nasal root is broad with lateral displacement of the medial canthi.

162. A 37-week gestation boy is born by spontaneous vaginal delivery to a 21-year-old mother after an uneventful pregnancy. The newborn is noted in the delivery room to have a large facial lesion. The family history is positive for a 2-year-old sibling with a hemangioma on the left arm that was about 0.5 cm in size at birth, grew to about 1.5 cm over the first year, and has since begun to shrink in size. On physical examination the head is normocephalic with flat fontanelles. A large, flat vascular malformation is noted over the left face and scalp. Pupils are equally round and reactive to light; red reflex is normal. The vascular lesion extends over the left eye. Heart has normal S1 and S2 without murmur. The chest has equal and unlabored breath sounds. Abdomen is soft, nontender, and without hepatosplenomegaly.

163. A 2-week-old neonate is seen by the pediatric resident in continuity clinic for routine care and "rash." The mother reports no new problems since the early follow-up visit at 3 days of age. The newborn is breast-feeding well, voids and stools often, and is taking daily vitamin D drops. Family history is positive for stroke in the baby's maternal great grandmother and the baby's maternal uncle with "hypopigmented skin spots" and a brain tumor. On physical examination pupils are equally round and reactive to light; red reflex is normal. Heart has normal S1 and S2 without murmur. The chest has equal and unlabored breath sounds. Abdomen is soft, nontender, and without hepatosplenomegaly. Skin has six hypopigmented oval macules about 1 cm by 1.5 cm in size over the trunk and extremities.

The Newborn Infant

Answers

102. The answer is d. (*Hay et al, pp 96-97. Kliegman et al, pp 895-896. Rudolph et al, p 738.*) Fetal alcohol syndrome is caused by prenatal exposure to ethanol. Findings include small-for-gestation birth, microcephaly, small palpebral fissures, short nose, smooth philtrum, thin upper lip, ptosis, strabismus, microphthalmia, and central nervous system abnormalities including intellectual disability. Cardiac defects, particularly septal defects, are commonly seen.

Common findings with trisomy 21 include protruding tongue, Brushfield spots, redundant neck skin, developmental delay, brachycephaly, upslanting palpebral fissures, epicanthal folds, flat face, small ears, cardiac abnormalities (especially ventricular septal defect or endocardial cushion defect), palmar creases, and clinodactyly of the fifth digit.

Dilantin exposure causes midface hypoplasia, low nasal bridge, ocular hypertelorism, and accentuated Cupid's bow of the upper lip. Other features include cleft lip and palate, growth retardation, mental deficiency, distal phalangeal hyperplasia, cardiovascular anomalies, and skeletal defects.

Alport syndrome is the most common of the hereditary nephritis conditions, frequently leading to end-stage renal disease. In 85% of patients with Alport syndrome, an X-linked dominant form (pathogenic mutation of the COL4A5 gene on the X chromosome) of inheritance is found; about 15% are autosomal recessive (due to pathogenic mutations of the COL4A3 or 4 genes on chromosome 2). All cause hematuria and progressive nephritis. Other findings include deafness and ocular defects.

Infants of diabetic mothers have an increased chance of congenital heart disease, caudal regression syndrome, and a small left colon. They are large-for-gestational age and frequently have a number of biochemical abnormalities such as hypoglycemia and hypocalcemia.

103. The answer is d. (*Hay et al, p 22. Kliegman et al, pp 876-880. Rudolph et al, pp 229-233.*) The described neonate is essentially normal but with jaundice on examination and hyperbilirubinemia on laboratory data. Significant unconjugated serum bilirubin levels in a full-term newborn can lead to diffusion of bilirubin into brain tissue and to irreversible neuro-logic damage; this condition is called *kernicterus*. Sulfisoxazole and other drugs compete with bilirubin for binding sites on albumin; therefore, the presence of these drugs can cause displacement, not increased affinity, of bilirubin to tissues. Metabolic acidosis also reduces binding of bilirubin, and neonatal sepsis interrupts the blood-brain barrier, thus allowing easier diffusion of bilirubin into the brain. Administration of phenobarbital has been used to induce glucuronyl transferase in newborn and can reduce, rather than exacerbate neonatal jaundice. Other factors that reduce the amount of unconjugated bilirubin bound to albumin (and therefore cause an increase in free unconjugated bilirubin) include hypoalbuminemia and certain compounds (eg, nonesterified fatty acids, which are elevated during cold stress) that compete with bilirubin for albumin-binding sites. Of the answers provided, only sepsis typically results in higher levels of unconju-gated bilirubin. Based on the Bhutani nomogram for hyperbilirubinemia, phototherapy is the next step for this infant.

104. The answer is c. (*Hay et al, p 495. Kliegman et al, p 2007. Rudolph et al, p 1260.*) It is important to make the diagnosis of choanal atresia quickly because it responds to treatment but can be lethal if unrecognized and untreated. Most neonates are obligate nose breathers and cannot breathe adequately through their mouths. Infants with choanal atresia have increased breathing difficulty during feeding, sleeping, and improved res-pirations when crying. A variety of temporizing measures to maintain an open airway have been used, including oropharyngeal airways, positioning, tongue fixation, and endotracheal intubation, but surgical correction with placement of nasal tubes is most effective. The diagnosis can be made by failure to pass a catheter through the nose to the pharynx or by checking for fog developing on a cold metal instrument placed under each naris. About half of patients with choanal atresia will have CHARGE association (**C**oloboma, **H**eart disease, **A**tresia of the choanae, **R**etarded growth and development, **G**enital hypoplasia, and **E**ar abnormalities).

Bronchoscopy would help diagnose lower airway anomalies. An upper GI series would identify esophageal atresia, but these babies will have gagging and choking with feeds, not just desaturation. A newborn with a hemoglobinopathy such as sickle cell or thalassemia would not present as this infant did, so an electrophoresis would not be helpful. An echocardio-gram would be useful if you suspected congenital cyanotic heart disease. The lack of a murmur in a newborn does not rule out pathology; this would be a reasonable next step if the catheter passed through both nares without difficulty.

105. The answer is e. (*Hay et al, p 56. Kliegman et al, p 1581. Rudolph et al, p 1296.*) Per current CDC recommendations, varicella-zoster immunoglobulin (VZIG) should be administered to the newborn immediately after delivery if the mother had the onset of varicella within 5 days prior to delivery, and immediately upon diagnosis if her chicken pox started within 2 days after delivery. If untreated, about half of these neonates will develop serious varicella as early as 1 day of age. If a normal full-term newborn is exposed to chicken pox 2 or more days postnatally, VZIG and isolation are not necessary because these babies appear to be at no greater risk for complications than older children. Acyclovir may be used in patients at risk for severe varicella, such as those with chronic pulmonary conditions, skin infections, or patients older than 12 years of age.

106. The answer is e. (*Hay et al, p 1236. Kliegman et al, p 1666. Rudolph et al, p 95.*) There are few contraindications to breast-feeding. Active pulmonary tuberculosis and HIV are two examples of infectious contraindications in developed countries, as well as malaria, typhoid fever, and septicemia. In underdeveloped countries, the risk of infectious diarrhea due to use of contaminated water to mix formula or the unavailability of formula can preclude this recommendation; however, if infected mothers continue to breast-feed, the WHO recommends either mother or baby continue to take antiretroviral medication for the duration of breast-feeding. All medications taken by the mother will be secreted in breast milk, but usually not in amounts significant enough to affect the infant. Mothers taking antineoplastic agents should not breast-feed. Mothers with mastitis can continue to breast-feed; frequent feedings may help the condition by preventing engorgement. Mothers with mild upper respiratory or other mild viral illness may also continue to breast-feed. Cracked or bleeding nipples may make breast-feeding uncomfortable, but are not contraindications. Inverted nipples usually can be remedied, and only rarely prohibit breast-feeding.

107. The answer is a. (*Hay et al, p 35. Kliegman et al, pp 838, 860-862. Rudolph et al, pp 207-209.*) The low Apgar scores, meconium staining, and ensuing respiratory distress suggest perinatal asphyxia. During a period of asphyxia, the resulting hypoxemia, acidosis, and poor perfusion can damage a neonate's brain, heart, kidney, liver, and lungs. The resulting clinical abnormalities include cerebral edema, irritability, seizures, cardiomegaly, heart failure, renal failure, poor liver function, disseminated intravascular coagulopathy, and respiratory distress syndrome. Neonates that have experienced asphyxia develop excessively high pulmonary arterial pressure while simultaneously having a drop in their systemic blood pressure. The result is a persistent right-to-left shunt across a patent ductus arteriosus or foramen ovale. This condition is known as persistent pulmonary hypertension of the newborn (PPHN).

Although Apgar scores are not precise indicators of long-term outcome, 5-minute scores of 3 or lower are associated with an increased risk of cerebral palsy and death in the first year of life. Induced hypothermia has been shown to improve outcomes in infants with birth asphyxia.

108. The answer is a. (*Hay et al, pp 1209-1212. Kliegman et al, pp 1592-1593. Rudolph et al, pp 905-906.*) The child described has many features of congenital cytomegalovirus (CMV) infection. CMV infection is the most common cause of congenital infection, occurring in 0.2%-2.4% of all live births. Cytomegalic inclusion disease is a constellation of findings including hepatomegaly, splenomegaly, jaundice, petechiae, purpura, microcephaly, and periventricular calcifications on brain imaging. In the United States, 70%-90% of adult women have serologic evidence of a past infection with CMV. Symptomatic congenital disease usually occurs when a mother has a primary CMV infection in the first trimester of pregnancy. Many of these babies die, and those who survive are severely affected. In the event of reactivation of CMV infection during pregnancy, maternal IgG passed transplacentally, protects the infant from serious infection. Although most infants infected during this secondary maternal infection are asymptomatic, about 10% of them eventually manifest sensorineural hearing loss and neurologic problems. Some recommend keeping a child with congenital CMV infection away from susceptible pregnant (or about to become pregnant) women because CMV excretion can persist for months to years; at the very least, good hand-washing practices should be instituted. If infected shortly after birth, the younger sibling will probably be asymptomatic since he or she has maternal IgG in the circulation. CMV is primarily an occult infection. Of toddlers in day-care centers, 20%-80% acquire CMV and shed it in saliva and urine for years. Diagnosis is made with isolation of the virus from urine, saliva, or other secretions, although several rapid tests are also available. A CMV vaccine is in trials, and current studies are investigating different approaches to mitigate *in utero* infection.

109. The answer is b. (*Hay et al, p 51. Kliegman et al, p 867. Rudolph et al, pp 1389-1391.*) The neonate described was born vaginally with a pregnancy complicated by marginal placental separation. The physical examination and laboratory data are completely normal. The most likely source of the blood is ingested maternal blood. Hematemesis and melena are not uncommon in the neonatal period, especially if gross placental bleeding has occurred at the time of delivery. The diagnostic procedure that should be done first is the alkali denaturation, or Apt-Downey, test, which differentiates fetal from adult hemoglobin in a bloody specimen. Initially described in 1955, the test is based on the finding that fetal hemoglobin is alkali resistant, while adult hemoglobin will convert to hematin upon exposure to alkali. If the blood in an affected neonate's gastric contents or stool is maternal in origin, further workup of the newborn is obviated. If the blood proves to be of fetal origin, any of the other choices may prove to be appropriate.

A barium enema might identify bleeding from a lower gastrointestinal sources such as ulcers in older patients, but these conditions are extremely rare in the newborn. The placement of an orogastric tube and lavage of the stomach is a common practice in older patients with a suspected, ongoing gastric bleed. If the Apt-Downey test proves negative, this might be an appropriate next step. An upper gastrointestinal series may also be an appropriate choice should the Apt-Downey test be negative; it might help identify gastric ulcer disease or hemangioma. Isolated rectal bleeding from a coagulation disorder (hinted at by the option with measuring platelet count, prothrombin time, and partial thromboplastin time) is not an expected finding; bleeding from the nose, circumcision site, or from venipunctures would be more likely.

110. The answer is c. (*Hay et al, p 293. Kliegman et al, p 801. Rudolph et al, p 95.*) Most medications are secreted to some extent in breast milk, and some lipid-soluble medications may be concentrated in breast milk. Although the list of contraindicated medications is short, caution should always be exercised when giving a medication to a breast-feeding woman. Medications that are clearly contraindicated include lithium, cyclosporin, antineoplastic agents, illicit drugs (including cocaine and heroin), amphetamines, ergotamines, and bromocriptine (which suppresses lactation). Although some suggest that oral contraceptives may have a negative impact on milk production, the association has not been proven conclusively. In general, antibiotics are safe, with only a few exceptions (such as tetracycline). While sedatives and narcotic pain medications are probably safe, the infant must be observed carefully for sedation. All of the medications listed in the question are considered safe in breast-feeding, except for methamphetamine. Caution is advised when using methamphetamine in a seizure patient, in that stimulants tend to lower the seizure threshold and make seizures more likely.

111. The answer is b. (*Hay et al, p 65. Kliegman et al, pp 897-899. Rudolph et al, pp 195-198.*) The neonate in the question is a large-for-gestation age newborn to a diabetic mother; both are risk factors for hypoglycemia. The initial glucose was low, but subsequent levels have been normal. The physical examination is normal except for the tremors. Infants born to diabetic mothers are at risk for a variety of other problems including congenital heart disease, neural tube defects, small left colon, and metabolic derangements. Hypoglycemia in these infants is usually seen in the first 24 hours of life. *In utero* exposure to the mother's hyperglycemia leads to fetal islet cell hypertrophy and beta cell hyperplasia, resulting in increased insulin production. After the umbilical cord is cut, that glucose supply is abruptly terminated and the elevated insulin levels cause hypoglycemia. Between 48 and 96 hours of life, these neonates have usually achieved glycemic control as did the newborn in the case presented. However, many subsequently develop hypocalcemia and hypomagnesemia. Hypocalcemia is thought to result from delayed parathormone (PTH) synthesis and/or responsiveness in the infant of a diabetic mother. Symptoms of hypocalcemia may include irritability, sweating, tremors, twitches, seizures, and arrhythmias. In the vignette, the newborn was showing symptoms of hypocalcemia in the appropriate time frame after delivery. Treatment of symptomatic infants is intravenous calcium gluconate.

112. The answer is b. (*Hay et al, pp 19-20. Kliegman et al, pp 886-887. Rudolph et al, pp 230-232.*) The neonate in the case is normal except for jaundice. A major blood-group incompatibility is present (the mother is O positive and her baby is A positive). Hemolytic disease and jaundice caused by a major blood-group incompatibility are usually less severe than with Rh incompatibility. The hematocrit of affected neonates with a major blood-group incompatibility usually is normal as it is in this case, but an elevated reticulocyte count and the presence of nucleated RBCs and microspherocytes in the blood smear would provide evidence of hemolysis. The presence of a positive direct Coombs test adds further evidence for risk of hemolysis. Petechiae are usually associated with decreased number of platelets. Crescent-shaped (sickled) RBCs are found with sickle cell disease and would not be expected in a newborn due to fetal hemoglobin protection.

113. The answer is d. (*Hay et al, pp 41-42. Kliegman et al, pp 869-871. Rudolph et al, pp 246-249.*) The neonate presented in the question has the typical course of a child with necrotizing enterocolitis (NEC), a potentially life-threatening disease of the neonate. The radiograph demonstrates distended loops of bowel with air in the bowel wall (pneumatosis intestinalis). NEC is more common in premature newborns, but has been occasionally described in term neonates as well. Although several organisms have been isolated from NEC patients, no clear cause for this condition has been identified. Patients present with feeding intolerance and a distended abdomen; about a quarter have grossly bloody stool. Pneumatosis intestinalis is found on plain radiograph of the abdomen and is diagnostic for NEC in this age group. Management depends initially on the presence or absence of perforation; if no evidence of free peritoneal air is found, the newborn should be put on bowel rest with nasogastric decompression, and systemic antibiotics are initiated. Electrolytes and vital signs should be monitored closely, and serial abdominal films should be performed to evaluate for perforation. If free air is identified on plain radiographs or if the newborn clinically worsens with medical management, surgical consultation is required. An exploratory laparotomy is usually performed, and any necrotic intestinal tissue is removed. Occasionally, removal of necrotic gut will result in neonate without adequate intestinal surface area to absorb nutrition, a condition known as *short bowel syndrome.*

114. The answer is d. (*Hay et al, p 36. Kliegman et al, pp 798-799. Rudolph et al, pp 171-172.*) The radiograph is normal. However, the vignette describes an otherwise normal neonate who is cold (35°C [95°F]). A room temperature of 24°C (~75°F) provides a cold environment for newborn babies. Aside from the fact that these neonates emerge from a warm, 37.6°C (99.5°F) intrauterine environment, at birth newborns (and especially preterm neonates) are wet, have a relatively large surface area for their weight, and have little subcutaneous fat. Within minutes of delivery, the neonates are likely to become pale or blue and their body temperatures will drop. In order to bring body temperature back to normal, they must increase their metabolic rate; ventilation, in turn, must increase proportionally to ensure an adequate oxygen supply. Because a preterm neonate is likely to have respiratory problems and be unable to oxygenate adequately, lactate can accumulate and lead to a metabolic acidosis. Newborn babies rarely shiver in response to a need to increase heat production. If the tachypnea persists after warming the neonate, sepsis, pneumonia, and primary surfactant deficiency are all possible; several of the alternative answers then may be appropriate.

115. The answer is a. (*Hay et al, pp 38-39. Kliegman et al, pp 849-850. Rudolph et al, pp 1938-1939.*) Apneic episodes are characterized by an absence of respirations for more than 20 seconds and may be accompanied by bradycardia and cyanosis. A large number of conditions can cause central apnea. In an otherwise well premature neonate, apnea is thought to be secondary to an incompletely developed respiratory center. Although seizures, hypoglycemia, septicemia, and pulmonary disease accompanied by hypoxia can lead to apnea, these causes are less likely in the newborn described, given that no unusual movements occur during the apneic spells, the blood sugar level is more than 40 mg/dL, the electrolytes and calcium levels are normal, and the newborn appears well between episodes. Other less common explanations for central apnea include congenital central hypoventilation syndrome (formerly known as Ondine's curse), Arnold-Chiari malformations, and congenital infections. Periodic breathing, a common pattern of respiration in low-birth-weight babies, is characterized by recurrent breathing pauses of 3-10 seconds without heart rate changes or cyanosis.

116. The answer is d. (*Hay et al, p 1069. Kliegman et al, pp 726-727. Rudolph et al, pp 607-608.*) The description is of a neonate who is normal and has lost minimal weight. All 50 states in the United States, as well as most developed countries, screen in the neonatal period for a variety of conditions, among them galactosemia. The condition is autosomal recessive (about 1:40,000 live births); if not identified on newborn screening, affected neonates can present with jaundice, hepatomegaly, vomiting, hypoglycemia, convulsions, lethargy, irritability, feeding problems, poor weight gain, aminoaciduria, cataracts, liver cirrhosis/failure, and developmental delay. Early treatment is essential and consists of galactose avoidance by using soy or casein hydrolysate infant formula. Classic galactosemia is one of the few true contraindications to breast-feeding. With appropriate diet, many of the features listed can be avoided or reversed. However, affected children often have ovarian failure, reduced bone-mineral density, and developmental delay. A referral to a metabolic geneticist is appropriate.

117. The answer is b. (*Hay et al, pp 28-29, 841. Kliegman et al, p 848. Rudolph et al, p 178.*) The description is of a normal pregnancy and forceps-assisted delivery. The physical examination is normal other than commonly seen subconjunctival hemorrhage and the mid-clavicular callus formation after a fracture, both suggestive of a possibly difficult delivery. Osteosarcoma is not a condition seen in newborns; a biopsy, MRI, and orthopedic consultation are premature. The clavicle is the most commonly fractured bone in the delivery process. While some fractures are identified at birth by finding crepitus on physical examination of the shoulder, others may not be identified until callus formation is noted at about a week of age. Clavicular fracture may happen in any delivery, although there is higher risk with large-for-gestational-age neonates. Initial presentation of a fractured clavicle may include a pseudoparalysis, in which the neonate refuses to move the ipsilateral arm, mimicking an Erb-Duchenne paralysis. In the vast majority of cases no treatment is needed; the bone heals well without intervention. The presentation of osteogenesis imperfecta would be multiple fractures as opposed to an isolated clavicular fracture, thus negating the immediate need for an evaluation for this condition.

118. The answer is c. (*Hay et al, pp 885-886. Kliegman et al, pp 3406-3408. Rudolph et al, pp 2233-2234.*) The case describes a difficult delivery of a large baby. The examination demonstrates molding and bruising of the scalp and also abnormal positioning of the arm with reduced left arm reflexes. The pupils are normal as is the chest examination. In a difficult delivery in which traction is applied to the head and neck, several injuries, including all those listed in the question, may occur. Erb-Duchenne paralysis affects the fifth and sixth cervical nerves; the affected arm cannot be abducted or externally rotated at the shoulder, and the forearm cannot be supinated. Injury to the seventh and eighth cervical and first thoracic nerves (Klumpke paralysis) results in palsy of the hand and also can produce Horner syndrome. Fractures in the upper limb are not associated with a characteristic posture, and passive movement usually elicits pain. Spinal injury causes complete paralysis below the level of injury. When paralysis of an upper extremity from injury to the brachial plexus is found in a neonate, injury to the phrenic nerve should also be suspected because the nerve roots are close together and can be injured concurrently. The paralyzed diaphragm can be noted to remain elevated on a chest x-ray taken during deep inspiration when it will contrast with the opposite normal diaphragm in its lower normal position; on expiration, this asymmetry cannot be seen. On inspiration, not only is breathing impaired since the paralyzed diaphragm does not contract, but also the negative pressure generated by the intact diaphragm pulls the mediastinum toward the normal side, impairing ventilation further. The diagnosis can easily be made with fluoroscopy or ultrasound, where these characteristic movements on inspiration and expiration can be seen. Rarely, both diaphragms can be paralyzed, producing much more severe ventilatory impairment. Fortunately, these injuries frequently improve spontaneously.

119. The answer is a. (*Hay et al, p 29. Kliegman et al, p 834. Rudolph et al, p 177.*) Three types of birth trauma related scalp swelling are seen in a newborn: 1) caput succedaneum, edema that can be located anywhere on the scalp and typically resolving within 48 hours; 2) cephalohematoma, blood trapped under the periosteal layer of the skull and as such unable to cross suture lines, and; 3) subgaleal or subaponeurotic hemorrhage. The baby in the vignette developed tachycardia, a large, fluid-filled lesion over the scalp and a head circumference that has increased by 14 cm at 6 hours of life. The newborn has a subgaleal hemorrhage, which can be life-threatening; neonates may lose a third or more of their blood volume into this potential space, leading to hypovolemic shock. A subgaleal hemorrhage will feel like a cephalohematoma that crosses the midline, but rapidly expands and can have cardiovascular complications. Dependent pooling of blood in the occipital area of the scalp may be observed when the newborn is lying on his back. Careful monitoring is essential. Although some newborns require fluid resuscitation, observation alone in this case may be appropriate, but should be accomplished in an ICU setting. Like cephalohematomas, subgaleal hemorrhages will tamponade and do not require surgical drainage.

120. The answer is a. (*Hay et al, p 61. Kliegman et al, pp 887-888. Rudolph et al, p 227.*) A neonate of 2100 g (4 lb, 10 oz) at 38 weeks would be considered SGA, a not uncommon consequence of maternal preeclampsia. Pregnancy-induced hypertension can produce a decrease in uteroplacental blood flow and areas of placental infarction. This can result in fetal nutritional deprivation and intermittent fetal hypoxemia, with a decrease in glycogen storage and a relative erythrocytosis, respectively. Hence, neonatal hypoglycemia and polycythemia are common clinical findings in these neonates. However, a newborn is very unlikely to have a seizure as a result of a glucose level of 50 mg/dL, which is approximately what most clinicians consider normal on the first day of life. Serum calcium levels usually decline during the first 2-3 postnatal days, but will only be considered abnormally low in a term neonate when they fall below 7.5-8 mg/dL. Neonatal hypermagnesemia is common in a newborn whose mother has received $MgSO_4$ therapy, but is usually asymptomatic or produces decreased muscle tone or floppiness. A persistent venous hematocrit of greater than 65% in a neonate is regarded as polycythemia and will be accompanied by an increase in blood viscosity.

Manifestations of the "hyperviscosity syndrome" include tremulousness or jitteriness that can progress to seizure activity because of sludging of blood in the cerebral microcirculation or frank thrombus formation; renal vein thrombosis; NEC; and tachypnea. Simple phlebotomy, while decreasing blood volume, will also decrease systemic arterial pressure and thus increase viscosity (based on the Poiseuille law of flow) and is thus contraindicated. Therapy by partial exchange transfusion with saline or lactated Ringer solution is preferred, and may be more likely to be useful if performed prophylactically before significant symptoms have developed, but literature evaluating outcomes in these neonates is lacking.

121. The answer is b. (*Hay et al, p 35. Kliegman et al, p 846.*) In the description provided, the most likely cause of the neonatal respiratory depression is maternal analgesic narcotic drug administration. While controlling the pain of the delivery in the mother, use of narcotics can result in respiratory depression of the newborn by crossing the placenta. The appropriate first step in the management of this neonate (after managing the ABCs of airway, breathing, and circulation) is the administration of naloxone, 0.1 mg/kg, IM, IV, or endotracheal. The other possibilities are unlikely, given the clinical information provided.

122. The answer is a. (*Hay et al, pp 1291-1292. Kliegman et al, pp 1349-1352. Rudolph et al, pp 164-168.*) The mother has evidence of an infection and the delivery was notable for brown amniotic fluid. The preterm neonate's physical examination includes hypothermia, pallor, evidence of pneumonia, delayed capillary refill, hepatosplenomegaly, and pinkish-gray granulomas on the skin. These findings are suggestive of *Listeria* infection. *Listeria* infection is seen most commonly in immunocompromised patients and in pregnant women; a history of eating soft cheeses or processed meats such as hot dogs and deli meat is helpful. In adults the signs and symptoms the woman was having in the vignette are typical. Third trimester seeding of uterine contents results in fetal infection and preterm delivery. The rash is termed granulomatosis infantisepticum and is seen in severe cases. Treatment of the newborn is ampicillin, with an aminoglycoside for synergy in serious cases; mortality is high (around 25%) even with early treatment.

Passage of meconium occurs prior to delivery and results in green amniotic fluid; neonates born in such environments are at risk for meconium aspiration syndrome. This condition is seen after about 34 weeks' gestation when meconium is developed in the newborn. Affected neonates have hypoxia, evidence of respiratory distress (grunting, nasal flaring, subcostal and intercostal retractions) and a patchy infiltrate on chest radiograph. Excessively high pulmonary arterial pressure due to the hypoxic event at the same time systemic blood pressure typically begins to fall postnatally results in a persistent right-to-left shunt across a patent ductus arteriosus or foramen ovale. This condition is known as persistent pulmonary hypertension of the newborn (PPHN).

Respiratory distress due to surfactant deficiency presents in the premature neonate (especially those less than 28 weeks' gestation) soon after birth with tachypnea, evidence of respiratory distress, cyanosis, and chest radiographic findings of a "ground-glass" appearance and air bronchograms due to the collapsed alveoli. Exogenous surfactant is often provided to reduce the symptoms. Neonates may require supplemental oxygen, CPAP or mechanical ventilation.

Pneumothorax in a newborn classically presents with the sudden onset of respiratory distress and unilaterally decreased breath sounds. It may be seen in an otherwise normal delivery, but also can be seen as a complication of air trapping with meconium aspiration syndrome or as a complication of stiff lungs associated with surfactant deficiency.

Herpes simplex virus presents in the first week or so of life with overwhelming sepsis and pneumonia if the maternal infection is primary. A woman's primary infection classically presents with flu-like symptoms and with painful genital lesions.

123. The answer is d. (*Hay et al, pp 439-440. Kliegman et al, p 3038. Rudolph et al, p 1070.*) The time of onset of symptoms is somewhat helpful in the diagnosis of ophthalmia neonatorum. Chemical conjunctivitis is a self-limited condition that presents within 6-12 hours of birth and lasts for the first day or so of life as a consequence of ocular silver nitrate prophylaxis (no longer available in the United States). As most nurseries use erythromycin prophylaxis now, chemical conjunctivitis is less common. Both of these ocular medications prevent gonococcal (GC) conjunctivitis.

Gonococcal conjunctivitis has its onset within 2-5 days after birth and is the most serious of the bacterial infections. Prompt and aggressive topical treatment and systemic antibiotics are indicated to prevent serious complications such as corneal ulceration, perforation, and resulting blindness. Parents should be treated to avoid the risk to the newborn of reinfection. The primary goal of erythromycin prophylaxis, as recommended in the United States and other countries, is to prevent gonococcal conjunctivitis.

Chlamydial conjunctivitis occurs 5-14 days after birth; to avoid the risk of chlamydial pneumonia, treatment of the neonate with conjunctivitis is with systemic antibiotics (parents, too, require treatment). However, asymptomatic neonates born to chlamydia-positive mothers are not routinely treated with oral antibiotics at birth as prophylaxis, but rather watched closely for signs of infection, due to an increased incidence of hypertrophic pyloric stenosis among neonates having received macrolide antibiotics.

124. The answer is b. (*Hay et al, pp 39-40. Kliegman et al, pp 850-858. Rudolph et al, pp 233-238.*) For the neonate described in the question, prematurity and the clinical picture presented make the diagnosis of hyaline membrane disease (HMD, also known as infant respiratory distress syndrome or primary surfactant deficiency) likely. Surfactant decreases surface tension in the alveoli; production by type II pneumocytes is not fully mature until about 35 weeks' gestation. HMD is caused by surfactant deficiency, and the incidence is increased with decreasing gestational age and birth weight. Without sufficient surfactant, lung compliance is reduced. Lung volume is also reduced, and a significant right-to-left shunt of blood can occur. Some of the shunt can result from a patent ductus arteriosus or foramen ovale, and some can be due to shunting within the lung. Minute ventilation is higher than normal, and affected neonates must work harder to sustain adequate respiration. Radiographs demonstrate diffuse atelectasis resulting in a "ground-glass" appearance. Treatment with exogenous surfactant has significantly decreased the mortality in these premature infants.

125. The answer is c. (*Hay et al, pp 1235-1236. Kliegman et al, pp 1665-1666. Rudolph et al, pp 1164-1170.*) The transmission of HIV from mother to newborn has significantly decreased in recent years, due in large part to perinatal administration of antiretroviral medications to the mother and a course of zidovudine to the exposed neonate. Studies suggest that for a mother adherent to combination antiretroviral therapy the risk of perinatal transmission is less than 2%, and in mothers with a viral load less than 1000, the risk is less than 1%.

Intravenous immune globulin (IVIG) has not been shown to have a role in decreasing perinatal transmission. Healthy asymptomatic term neonates born to HIV-infected mothers do not need special monitoring, nor do they need routine radiographs.

An HIV ELISA is an antibody test and will be positive in the infant born to an HIV-infected mother due to maternal antibodies that are passed through the placenta; it is not a useful test in the newborn to determine neonatal infection because of this expected transfer of maternal immunoglobulin. The confirmatory Western blot also assays for antibodies to HIV and is similarly unhelpful in the newborn period.

A term neonate exposed to a primary HSV infection during a vaginal delivery (or one delivered by cesarean section after prolonged ROM) is at risk for acquiring a severe HSV infection since the neonate has no protective IgG antibody. A recurrent maternal infection, however, results in a reduced incidence of severe infection in a term baby as compared to a primary maternal infection due to passed maternal IgG antibody. The preterm neonate exposed to either primary (no antibody formation) or recurrent HSV infection (passage of protective maternal IgG occurs in the last trimester) may require intravenous acyclovir.

Neonatal group B streptococcal disease incidence is reduced to low levels with administration of penicillin at least 4 hours prior to delivery of the neonate. Prophylaxis in this case was indicated based on the maternal history of a group B strep UTI during the pregnancy.

126. The answer is c. (*Hay et al, p 1108. Kliegman et al, pp 621-622. Rudolph et al, pp 2068-2069.*) The description is of a girl with features of Turner syndrome. Turner syndrome is a genetic disorder; the 45,XO karyotype is the most common. Prenatally, neonates may have nuchal cystic hygroma and horseshoe kidneys. At birth, affected neonates have low weight, short stature, edema over the dorsum of the hands and feet, and loose skin folds at the nape of the neck. Some other findings of this syndrome include sexual infantilism, streak gonads, typical faces, shield chest, low hairline, coarctation of the aorta, hypertension, bicuspid aortic valve, and high palate. Coarse, tremulous movements accompanied by ankle clonus; vascular instability as evidenced, for example, by a harlequin color change (a transient, longitudinal division of a body into red and pale halves); softness of parietal bones at the vertex (craniotabes); and a liver that is palpable down to 2 cm below the costal margin are all findings often demonstrated by normal neonates and are of no diagnostic significance in the clinical situation presented.

127. The answer is b. (*Hay et al, pp 255-258. Kliegman et al, pp 1948-1949. Rudolph et al, p 186.*) The only vaccine routinely given in the newborn nursery is the hepatitis B vaccine. The other vaccines listed typically are administered beginning at 2 months of age. The other injection typically included on standardized order sheets and given to all hospitalized newborns is vitamin K, which is provided prophylactically to prevent a dangerous drop in vitamin K-dependent coagulation factors. Failure to provide vitamin K (especially to those fed human milk) can result in vitamin K levels low enough to produce classic hemorrhagic manifestations (melena, hematuria, bleeding from circumcision site, intracranial hemorrhage, hypovolemic shock) on the second to seventh day of life; this condition is classically referred to as hemorrhagic disease of the newborn. Hib, DTaP, rotavirus, and IPV cannot be given before 6 weeks of age.

128. The answer is b. (*Hay et al, p 402. Kliegman et al, pp 794-795. Rudolph et al, p 1275.*) The lesion in this completely normal baby is congenital dermal melanocytosis (Mongolian spot), a bluish-gray lesion located over the buttocks, lower back, and occasionally, the extensor surfaces of the extremities. These occur in more than 50% of African Americans, Asians, Native Americans and Latin Americans. They tend to disappear by 1-2 years of age, although those on the extremities may not fully resolve. Child abuse is unlikely to present with bruises alone; children frequently present with more extensive injuries. Subcutaneous fat necrosis, which may ultimately result in subcutaneous calcifications in the affected area, is usually found as a sharply demarcated, hard lesion on the cheeks, buttocks, and limbs but it usually is red. Hemophilia (the choice hinted by obtaining factor levels) and vitamin K (administering Vitamin K) deficiency rarely present with subcutaneous lesions as described and are more likely to present as a bleeding episode.

129. The answer is c. (*Hay et al, pp 635-636. Kliegman et al, pp 862-864. Rudolph et al, pp 209-211.*) Diaphragmatic hernia occurs with the movement of abdominal contents across a congenital or traumatic defect in the diaphragm. In the newborn, this condition results in profound respiratory distress with significant mortality. Prenatal diagnosis is common and, when found, necessitates that the birth take place at a tertiary-level center. In the neonate, respiratory failure in the first hours of life, a scaphoid abdomen, and presence of bowel sounds in the chest are common findings. Intensive respiratory support, including high-frequency oscillatory ventilation and extracorporeal membrane oxygenation (ECMO), has increased survival. Overall survival is around 70% with traditional post-delivery management; while surgery may correct the diaphragmatic defect, the lung on the affected side remains hypoplastic and continues to contribute to morbidity. Fetal surgery centers initially trialed open repair with limited success. The most promising prenatal intervention currently is the placement of a fetal tracheal occlusion device (fetoscopic endoluminal tracheal occlusion, or FETO). The balloon is left in place for several weeks, trapping the fluid the lung produces, causing expansion of the lung and gradually pushing the abdominal structures back into the abdomen. The balloon is removed prior to delivery.

Pneumonia and pneumothorax may cause respiratory distress with decreased breath sounds, but the radiograph in diaphragmatic hernia shows the nasogastric tube curving into the left thorax, clearly an abnormal placement. A congenital pulmonary airway malformation (CPAM) will frequently look like a diaphragmatic hernia on radiographs, but the nasogastric tube would be in the correct location. Choanal atresia is an upper airway abnormality and does not cause these radiographic changes; it would have been difficult to place the nasogastric tube in the first place with this condition, in which there is a bony or membranous septum between the nose and pharynx.

130. The answer is d. (*Hay et al, p 48. Kliegman et al, pp 1783-1784. Rudolph et al, pp 1401-1403.*) The newborn has abdominal distention, choking, tachypnea, retractions, drooling, and coughing associated with feedings. These are symptoms of esophageal anomalies. The anomaly illustrated by sketch D (proximal atresia with distal fistula) is the most common (~87%); that of sketch A (isolated H-type fistula) can be diagnosed after repeated episodes of pneumonia and represents about 4% of these malformations. The anomalies in sketches E (isolated esophageal atresia) and C (proximal fistula with distal atresia) are associated with all the same symptoms except abdominal distention, which cannot develop because air cannot enter the gastrointestinal tract. Sketches B (double fistula with intervening atresia) and C are the least common at 1% each; in these, the upper esophageal segment is connected directly to the trachea, and massive entry of fluid into the lungs occurs.

VACTERL (Vertebral, Anorectal, Cardiac, Tracheo-Esophageal fistula, Renal, and Limb) association has tracheoesophageal fistula as a common finding.

131. The answer is d. (*Hay et al, p 58. Kliegman et al, pp 1948-1949. Rudolph et al, p 186.*) The neonate of a mother who is a carrier of hepatitis B surface antigen has a significant risk of acquiring infection. This usually occurs at the time of delivery, but infection can also be acquired during pregnancy and postnatally. A small percentage of infected neonates develop acute icteric hepatitis, but the majority remains asymptomatic. Of these infected asymptomatic neonates, 80% or more will develop chronic infection, the long-term consequences of which are chronic liver disease and, possibly, hepatocellular carcinoma. Combined passive-active immunoprophylaxis in the form of hepatitis B immunoglobulin and hepatitis B vaccine affords protection not only from immediate perinatal infection but also from infection that may be acquired as a result of continued exposure in the household of a chronic carrier.

Immunization in this neonate is indicated regardless of the presence of hepatitis B "e" antigen (HBeAg) in the mother. Although the presence of HBeAg, especially in the absence of antibody to HBeAg, is associated with high rates of transmission to neonates, any woman positive for hepatitis B surface antigen (HBsAg) is potentially infectious. It is not necessary to isolate newborn to carriers of HBsAg, and screening of neonates for HBsAg is not indicated. Testing for HBsAg and anti-HBsAg at least 1 month after the third dose of hepatitis B vaccine will determine the efficacy of the combined passive-active immunoprophylaxis described.

Hepatitis B is currently a reportable disease in the United States. Local health departments frequently track babies born to hepatitis B positive mothers and ensure the child receives appropriate follow-up.

132. The answer is b. (*Hay et al, p 30. Kliegman et al, pp 893-894.*) Neonatal abstinence syndrome (NAS) is typically seen with mothers addicted to narcotics; infant withdrawal symptoms are similar with maternal use of both prescription medications (including methadone or buprenorphine/naloxone) and illegal substances. Symptoms typically present between 1 and 3 days of life. Most nurseries employ a structured scoring system to monitor these babies; a version of the Finnegan NAS score is currently used by most facilities. Initial therapy is focused on frequent small feedings, quiet dark rooms and swaddling. Pharmacological management, most commonly with morphine or methadone, may be required.

While narcotics are the most common cause of neonatal withdrawal, there are reports of symptoms with prenatal exposure to benzodiazepines and alcohol. Infants born to mothers using marijuana tend to have lower birth weight, but there are no consistent withdrawal findings. Cocaine can cause premature labor, abruption, fetal asphyxia, and long-term neurodevelopmental problems, but withdrawal is unusual.

133. The answer is b. (*Hay et al, pp 18-25. Kliegman et al, pp 871-875. Rudolph et al, pp 229-233.*) The case represents a normal neonate who is eating well, has appropriate weight loss, and mild jaundice. The laboratory data show a normal CBC and reticulocyte for age, a lack of ABO or Rh incompatibility, and a mild indirect hyperbilirubinemia. The development of jaundice in a healthy full-term baby may be considered the result of a normal physiologic process in certain circumstances. It may be normal if the time of onset and duration of the jaundice and the pattern of serially determined serum concentrations of bilirubin are in conformity with currently accepted safe criteria. Physiologic jaundice becomes apparent on the second or third day of life, peaks to levels no higher than about 12 mg/dL on the fourth or fifth day, and disappears by the end of the first week of life. The rate of rise is less than 5 mg/dL per 24 hours and levels of conjugated bilirubin do not exceed about 1 mg/dL.

Hyperbilirubinemia associated with breast-feeding can be separated into two categories. Breast-feeding jaundice typically occurs in the first week of life and is associated with suboptimal milk intake, leading to decreased passage of meconium and increased resorption of bilirubin in the intestines. Increased feedings will usually resolve breast-feeding jaundice. Breast milk jaundice, on the other hand, starts in the second week of life and is believed to be caused by a substance in the breast milk that interferes with bilirubin metabolism. Breast-feeding is typically continued, and phototherapy initiated for markedly elevated bilirubin levels.

Concern about neonatal jaundice relates to the risk of the neurotoxic effects of unconjugated bilirubin. The precise level and duration of exposure necessary to produce toxic effects are not known, but chronic bilirubin encephalopathy, or kernicterus, is rare in term infants whose bilirubin level is kept below 18-20 mg/dL. Certain risk factors affecting premature or sick newborns increase their susceptibility to kernicterus at much lower levels of bilirubin. The diagnosis of physiologic jaundice is made by excluding other causes of hyperbilirubinemia by means of history, physical examination, and laboratory determinations. The website *http://bilitool.org* can help provide guidance regarding risk factors, risk zones, and phototherapy.

Jaundice appearing in the first 24 hours is usually a feature of hemolytic states and is accompanied by an indirect hyperbilirubinemia, reticulocytosis, and evidence of red-cell destruction on smear. In the absence of blood group or Rh incompatibility, congenital hemolytic states (eg, spherocytic anemia) or G6PD deficiency should be considered. With infection, hemolytic and hepatotoxic factors are reflected in the increased levels of both direct and indirect bilirubin. Studies should include maternal and newborn Rh types and blood groups and Coombs tests to detect blood group or Rh incompatibility and sensitization.

Examination of the blood smear is useful in differentiating common hemolytic disorders. Except for determinations of total and direct bilirubin, tests of liver function are not particularly helpful in establishing the cause of early onset jaundice. Transient elevations of transaminases (AST and ALT) related to the trauma of delivery and to hypoxia have been noted.

Biliary atresia and neonatal hepatitis can be accompanied by elevated levels of transaminases, but characteristically present as chronic cholestatic jaundice with mixed hyperbilirubinemia after the first week of life. A conjugated hyperbilirubinemia should prompt further investigation.

134. The answer is d. (*Hay et al, pp 636-637. Kliegman et al, pp 1800-1803. Rudolph et al, pp 1421-1422.*) The finding of polyhydramnios suggests highintestinal obstruction, signs of which typically include abdominal distention and early and repeated regurgitation. Distention can be inconsistent, as vomiting keeps the intestine decompressed. The bile-stained vomitus of the neonate places the obstruction distal to the ampulla of Vater, eliminating esophageal atresia from consideration. Pyloric stenosis usually presents between 2 and 4 weeks of life with nonbilious emesis. The "double-bubble" sign on the x-ray is characteristic of duodenal atresia, which is compatible with the history. Midgut volvulus, which may obstruct the bowel in the area of the duodenojejunal junction, most often produces signs after the affected neonate is 3-4 days old with acute onset of bilious vomitus. Gastric duplication does not usually produce intestinal obstruction; a cystic mass may be palpated on abdominal examination. Patients with duodenal atresia should be examined closely for evidence of other conditions such as Down syndrome or heart disease.

135. The answer is b. (*Hay et al, p 292. Kliegman et al, p 2320.*) Goat's milk, by itself, is not an ideal source of infant nutrition as it contains inadequate folate and iron, potentially contributing to anemia. Caloric content is actually denser than cow's milk-based formulas (about 30 kcal/oz, compared to ~20 kcal/oz for formula and breast milk). Casein and whey are the protein sources in goat's milk, as they are for many formulas. Some manufacturers produce a goat milk-based formula that contains supplemental vitamins and iron. Unpasteurized goat's milk should never be used as an infant formula because of the risk of brucellosis.

136. The answer is d. (*Hay et al, pp 507-508. Kliegman et al, pp 1771-1772. Rudolph et al, pp 705-710.*) The infant pictured has bilateral cleft lip and palate. The incidence in the general population is about 1:1000 live births, but occurs in about 4% of the siblings of affected infants. Evaluation for other structural and chromosomal abnormalities is indicated. Although affected infants are likely to have feeding problems initially, these problems usually can be overcome by feeding in a propped-up position and using special nipples. Complications include recurrent otitis media and hearing loss as well as speech defects, which may be present despite good anatomic closure. Repair of a cleft lip usually is performed within the first 2-3 months of life; the palate is repaired later, usually between the ages of 6 and 18 months, before significant speech development occurs.

137. The answer is a. (*Hay et al, pp 1027-1028. Kliegman et al, pp 2668-2672. Rudolph et al, pp 2035-2036.*) The clinical findings of congenital hypothyroidism are subtle, and may not be present at all at birth; this is thought to be a result of passage of some maternal T_4 transplacentally. Neonates such as that in the vignette with examination findings will usually have an umbilical hernia and a distended abdomen. The head may be large, and the fontanelles will be large as well. The newborn may be hypothermic and have feeding difficulties; constipation and jaundice may be persistent. Skin may be cold and mottled, and edema may be found in the genitals and extremities. The heart rate may be slow, and anemia may develop. Essentially all of these findings are presented in the case. As these findings may be subtle or nonexistent, neonatal screening programs are extremely important for early diagnosis of these neonates.

Sepsis can cause hypothermia and poor feeding, but the 2-week course makes this choice unlikely. Hirschsprung disease may cause chronic constipation and abdominal distension, but not the other findings. Botulism can cause a flaccid paralysis and poor feeding, but the large fontanelles and umbilical hernia are not caused by this infection.

138. The answer is d. (*Hay et al, pp 118-119. Kliegman et al, pp 818, 2802-2803. Rudolph et al, pp 739, 2154-2155.*) Diseases that are due to defects in a single gene are designated as autosomal or X-linked, depending on whether the affected gene is located on an autosome or an X chromosome. Genetically determined diseases that are multifactorial in origin (ie, neural tube defects) do not conform to the Mendelian pattern of inheritance but exhibit a variable outcome that reflects the interaction between a particular genotype and an environment. The relatives of persons with diseases of multifactorial origin have an increased risk of having similar abnormalities.

The recurrence risk for most single primary defects of multifactorial inheritance (eg, neural tube defects) is increased with each child affected. This increased risk forms the basis for assuming that genetic factors play a role in the occurrence of these abnormalities. Other factors, such as race, sex, and racial background, influence the frequency with which an abnormality of multifactorial inheritance occurs in relatives.

The prenatal diagnosis of neural tube defects (anencephaly and meningomyelocele) can be made by the detection of elevated levels of alpha-fetoprotein in the amniotic fluid. To reduce the risk of neural tube defects, the U.S. Preventive Services Task Force recommended that all women capable of becoming pregnant take between 400 mcg and 800 mcg of folic acid daily.

139. The answer is e. (*Hay et al, p 26. Kliegman et al, pp 858-859. Rudolph et al, pp 201-203.*) Transient tachypnea of the newborn (TTN) is seen most commonly after a scheduled cesarean delivery, but can be seen in infants born via cesarean after a trial of labor, as well as in spontaneous vaginal deliveries. Infants born to diabetic mothers have a 2-3 times risk of developing TTN. The condition is a result of retained fetal lung fluid. These patients have tachypnea, retractions, grunting, and sometimes cyanosis. The chest examination is usually normal; the chest radiograph demonstrates prominent pulmonary vascular markings with fluid in the fissures and hyperexpansion (flat diaphragms). Therapy is supportive, with maintenance of normal oxygen saturation. Resolution usually occurs in the first 12-24 hours of life, but symptoms can last up to 3 days.

Diaphragmatic hernia would demonstrate intestinal contents located in the chest on plain radiograph. Meconium aspiration would present in a patient who is born with meconium at the delivery and the radiograph would have patchy infiltrates. Pneumonia in a patient of this age is more likely to have diffuse infiltrates on radiograph and clinical findings of temperature instability. Infant respiratory distress syndrome (RDS, also known as hyaline membrane disease, or primary surfactant deficiency) occurs in premature infants; radiographs demonstrate a "ground-glass appearance."

140. The answer is d. (*Hay et al, pp 1302-1305. Kliegman et al, pp 1475-1477. Rudolph et al, pp 1101-1103.*) The newborn in the question has pallor, jaundice, hepatosplenomegaly, a diffuse rash, and a constant nasal discharge, all features of congenital syphilis infection. While the clinical presentation is varied, many newborns appear normal at birth and continue to be asymptomatic for the first few weeks or months of life. Most untreated neonates will develop skin lesions, typically an infiltrative, maculopapular peeling rash that is most prominent on the face, palms, and soles. Involvement of the nasal mucous membranes causes rhinitis with a resultant serous, and occasionally purulent, blood-tinged discharge (snuffles). This, as well as scrapings from the skin lesions, contains abundant viable treponemes. Hepatosplenomegaly and lymphadenopathy are common, and early jaundice is a manifestation of syphilitic hepatitis. Liver function tests are elevated; hemolytic anemia and thrombocytopenia are common. Among the later manifestations, or stigmata, of congenital syphilis is "saddle nose" deformity, a result of destruction of bone from syphilitic rhinitis, occurring after the age of two in untreated patients; and interstitial keratitis, which is an acute inflammation of the cornea that begins in early childhood (most commonly between 6 and 14 years of age). Interstitial keratitis represents the response of the tissue to earlier sensitization. Findings include marked photophobia, lacrimation, corneal haziness, and eventual scarring. Hutchinson teeth (peg or barrel-shaped upper central incisors), abnormal enamel, and mulberry molars (first lower molars with an abnormal number of cusps) are dental manifestations of syphilis.

Toxoplasmosis causes the classic triad of hydrocephalus, chorioretinitis, and intracranial calcifications. These neonates may also display symptoms similar to other congenital infections, such as anemia, a petechial rash, organomegaly, jaundice, and seizures. The imaging finding of this condition is calcifications scattered throughout the cortex of the brain.

Glycogen storage disease type I (von Gierke disease) presents in the newborn period with hypoglycemia and lactic acidosis. Clinical findings of hypoglycemia such as irritability, apnea, hypotonia and especially seizures are common.

Congenital hypothyroidism may present with subtle or no findings, but classically is described as infants with examination findings of an umbilical hernia and a distended abdomen. The head may be large, and the fontanelles will be enlarged as well. The child may be hypothermic and have feeding difficulties; constipation and jaundice may be persistent. Skin may be cold and mottled, and edema may be found in the genitals and extremities. The heart rate may be slow, and anemia may develop. Neonatal screening programs are extremely important for early diagnosis of these neonates.

CMV infection can cause hepatomegaly, splenomegaly, jaundice, petechiae, purpura, and microcephaly. Many babies exposed early *in utero* to this virus die; of those who survive without prenatal findings, about 10% will have symptoms at birth. The classic CT finding of this condition shows periventricular calcifications.

141. The answer is b. (*Kliegman et al, pp 3307-3309. Rudolph et al, p 864.*) The newborn is completely normal other than fifth-finger, or post-axial, polydactyly which is 10 times more common in African American than in white children and is typically familial. This finding in otherwise healthy African American children should raise no special concern. In a white child, careful examination of the cardiac system is warranted. Similarly, preaxial (or thumb-side) polydactyly is unusual and should be further investigated in any ethnic background. Some syndromes that are associated with polydactyly are trisomy 13, Rubinstein-Taybi syndrome, Meckel-Gruber syndrome, and Ellis-van Creveld syndrome. Simple pedunculated postaxial polydactyly without bone involvement may be surgically removed shortly after birth; simply tying these appendages off with string will usually leave a nub.

142. The answer is a. (*Kliegman et al, pp 2586-2587. Rudolph et al, 1745-1746.*) Hypospadias is one of the more common birth defects, occurring in as many as 1 in 250 newborn males. In this condition there is incomplete formation of the prepuce, and the urethral meatus can be located anywhere from just below the end of the penis to the scrotum. The underlying problem is failure of fusion of the urethral folds. With this failure, the ventral side of the penis grows more slowly than the dorsal side, leading to ventral curvature, or chordee. Chordee and abnormal foreskin development are the most common findings associated with hypospadias, with inguinal hernia and undescended testes occurring less commonly. Hydrocele is not associated with hypospadias, and Peyronie disease is a penile curvature seen in adults, typically after trauma leads to the formation of scar tissue.

143. The answer is b. (*Hay et al, pp 38-39. Kliegman et al, pp 849-850. Rudolph et al, p 185.*) The newborn in the question has features concerning for congenital heart disease that is becoming evident as the ductus arteriosus is closing. Of the choices, immediate pulse oximetry and an echocardiogram are indicated. Neonatology consultation, transfer to the NICU, and the initiation of prostaglandin E are also likely indicated.

Blood type and Coombs testing is appropriate for the jaundiced newborn whose routine bilirubin levels are higher than expected for age. Idiopathic apnea is common in premature neonates but is not expected in the full-term newborn. When apnea occurs in the term infant, there is almost always an identifiable cause. Home monitoring without evaluation for the cause (sepsis, gastroesophageal reflux, congenital heart disease, seizures, RSV, hypoglycemia, central hypoventilation [Ondine's curse], and airway obstruction) is dangerous. Harlequin syndrome is an example of a condition where observation and reassurance may be appropriate. It is a transient change in the skin color of the otherwise asymptomatic newborn (usually preterm) in which the dependent side of the entire body turns red while the upper side remains pale. Clinical findings of hypoglycemia include irritability, apnea, hypotonia and especially seizures. Serum glucose and more extensive testing that might include insulin levels are indicated if the condition does not resolve with supplemental feeding.

144. The answer is d. The abstract suggests that obese women who become pregnant, and those who are obese and have excessive weight gain during the pregnancy have large infants. The infants who are products of these pregnancies gain weight rapidly through the first 3 months of life and remain large through the first year of life.

This is a retrospective study. Gestational weight gain alone was not associated with increased infant growth. Since these children were not followed beyond the first year, it is not known if they remain obese adolescents or adults.

145. The answer is b. (*Hay et al, p 32. Kliegman et al, pp 817-818. Rudolph et al, pp 190-191.*) The incidence of twin-to-twin transfusion syndrome

(TTTS) is around 1 in 50 for twin pregnancies; it is a common cause of fetal loss. This disorder should be suspected when the hematocrits of twins differ by more than 15%. The donor twin is likely to have oligohydramnios, anemia, and hypovolemia with evidence of shock if the hematocrit is significantly reduced; the recipient twin is likely to have polyhydramnios and plethora and to be larger than the donor twin. A 20% difference in body weight may result. As the central venous hematocrit rises above 65%, infants can develop hyperviscosity, respiratory distress, hyperbilirubinemia, hypocalcemia, renal vein thrombosis, congestive heart failure, and convulsions.

146. The answer is c. (*Hay et al, p 1119. Kliegman et al, pp 2554-2555. Rudolph et al, p 174.*) It is generally presumed that duodenal atresia and tracheoesophageal fistula lead to polyhydramnios by interference with reabsorption of swallowed amniotic fluid. Polyhydramnios is also associated with approximately 80% of infants who have trisomy 18. Approximately 50% of women with anencephalic fetuses have polyhydramnios. In addition to GI track obstruction, conditions associated with polyhydramnios include multiple congenital anomalies and fetal hypotonia. Oligohydramnios occurs in association with congenital abnormalities of the fetal kidneys or other parts of the genitourinary tract, such as renal agenesis or obstruction that impede normal formation or excretion of fetal urine.

147. The answer is b. (*Hay et al, pp 56, 1209-1212. Kliegman et al, pp 1590-1594. Rudolph et al, pp 902-907.*) Although hypothyroid neonates may develop hyperbilirubinemia, they typically do not develop a rash. The patient described has severe jaundice, hepatosplenomegaly, and a diffuse purpuric rash. He most likely has a congenital or acquired infection requiring immediate diagnosis and, if possible, treatment. Hospital personnel can acquire some of these conditions if appropriate isolation measures are not instituted. Exposure of pregnant healthcare workers to such conditions as CMV is to be avoided.

Among the important causes of neonatal sepsis are prenatal infections, including congenital syphilis, toxoplasmosis, CMV infection, and rubella. Useful diagnostic studies, in addition to cultures for bacteria, include specific serologic tests for pathogens, viral cultures, lumbar puncture, and x-rays of the chest and long bones. Longitudinal striations in the metaphyses are characteristic of congenital rubella, whereas osteochondritis or periostitis usually indicates congenital syphilis. Congenital syphilis, CMV, and rubella can be highly contagious. Urine can contain rubella virus for more than 6 months and is, therefore, a special hazard to nonimmune pregnant women.

148 to 151. The answers are 148-c, 149-e, 150-a, 151-d. (*Hay et al, pp 56-58, 1317-1318. Kliegman et al, pp 1550-1551, 1576-1577, 1592-1593, 1723-1733. Rudolph et al, pp 902-907, 1102, 1153, 1179, 1240.*) Congenital rubella infection affects all organ systems. Infants will be small, with intra-uterine growth retardation. They may also manifest cataracts, microphthal-mia, myocarditis, and a red or purple macular rash ("blueberry muffin" rash). Structural heart defects (such as a patent ductus arteriosus, pulmo-nary artery stenosis, and septal defects) are typical of congenital rubella, but not in the other TORCH infections. Laboratory anomalies may include a hemolytic anemia with thrombocytopenia, elevated liver functions, and pleocytosis in the spinal fluid. Affected children do not have a good prog-nosis. Congenital rubella is not commonly seen in developed countries with high immunization rates.

Transmission of HSV from mother to newborn can happen *in utero*, intrapartum, and postnatally. Intrapartum transmission is most common. Neonates born vaginally to a mother with a primary genital herpes infec-tion are at highest risk for disease, with up to a 50% possibility of perinatal transmission; the risk to a baby born to a mother with a recurrent HSV infection is much lower. About half the infants with congenital HSV are born to mothers who are unaware of their infection; thus, a negative mater-nal history does not preclude the diagnosis. Infants can display isolated CNS involvement, isolated cutaneous infection, or systemic generalized infection. Treatment usually is with acyclovir; even with therapy, morbidity is high in infants with CNS involvement.

Toxoplasmosis can cause symptoms similar to other congenital infections, but the combination of hydrocephalus, chorioretinitis, and intracranial calcifications is considered the "classic triad" of toxoplasma infection in a neonate. Infection usually occurs during primary infection of the mother or as a reactivation of infection in an immune-compromised host. These infants may also display symptoms similar to other congenital infections, such as anemia, a petechial rash, organomegaly, jaundice, and seizures.

CMV is a common congenital infection, with infection estimates rang-ing from 0.4% to 2.4% of all live births. Many cases are asymptomatic; oth-ers may develop cytomegalic inclusion disease, a multiorgan manifestation of disease including intrauterine growth restriction (IUGR), hepatospleno-megaly, jaundice, petechiae or purpura, microcephaly, chorioretinitis, and intracranial calcifications. More than half of infants with this congenital infection develop sensorineural hearing loss.

152 to 155. The answers are 152-i, 153-f, 154-e, 155-d. (*Hay et al, pp 538-539, 552-553, 885-886, 1119. Kliegman et al, pp 846-847, 2045-2048, 2554, 3406-3408. Rudolph et al, pp 178, 206-207, 256, 961-966.*) Neonates with upper brachial plexus injury (cervical nerves 3, 4, and 5) can also have ipsilateral phrenic nerve paralysis. These infants can present with labored, irregular breathings and cyanosis; the injury is usually unilateral. Confirmation of the diagnosis is made with ultrasound or fluoroscopy, which will demonstrate "seesaw" movements of the diaphragm during respiration.

Pneumothoraces occur with a frequency of about 1%-2% of births, but they are rarely symptomatic. Incidence is higher in infants born with meconium-stained fluid, and the chest radiograph is as described. Transillumination may assist in the diagnosis while awaiting radiograph; immediate treatment for infants with significant distress is with a 23-gauge butterfly needle attached to a stopcock inserted through the chest wall, and removal of the air. For those without significant distress and who are not requiring high levels of oxygen, 100% oxygen therapy can assist in "nitrogen washout" of the pneumothorax.

Pulmonary hypoplasia due to oligohydramnios (Potter sequence) includes a dysmorphic child (widely spaced eyes, low-set ears, broad nose, receding chin, limb abnormalities) and bilateral renal agenesis. These infants have immediate respiratory distress; the condition is not compatible with life.

Bronchiolitis is a very common viral infection most often caused by respiratory syncytial virus. It is most often seen in the winter months with symptoms of fever, wheezing, hypoxia, and respiratory distress seen in younger children; often an older sibling has milder, upper respiratory symptoms. Premature infants, infants with congenital heart disease, infants with a variety of lung disorders, and infants with immune system defects are at higher risk of severe complications. Diagnosis is made by clinical history and/or detection of the viral antigen in nasal secretions; treatment is supportive. Premature infants in their first year of life will typically receive monthly injections of palivizumab during RSV season. Palivizumab is a monoclonal antibody that provides passive immunity to high risk infants, decreasing the risk of severe RSV disease.

156 to 159. The answers are 156-a, 157-a, 158-c, 159-a. (*Hay et al, pp 1069, 1074-1077, 1081. Nelson et al, pp 637-638, 650-652, 726-727, 730. Rudolph et al, pp 561-563, 565-566, 591-592, 1504.*) In galactosemia, an enzyme deficiency (galactose-l-phosphate uridyl transferase) results in a block in the metabolic pathway of galactose and leads to the accumulation of galactose-l-phosphate in the tissues. Infants with this condition develop serious damage to liver, brain, and eyes after being fed milk containing lactose (a disaccharide compound of glucose and galactose). Clinical manifestations include lethargy, vomiting and diarrhea, hypotonia, hepatomegaly and jaundice, failure to thrive, and cataracts. The course of the disease in untreated patients is variable; death from liver failure and inanition can occur; most untreated patients develop physical and developmental delay. Treatment consists of prompt elimination of lactose-containing milk from the diet in infancy and, as a more varied diet is introduced, exclusion of foods that contain casein, dry milk solids, whey, or curds.

Phenylketonuria, a genetically determined disorder with an autosomal recessive pattern of inheritance, is caused by the absence of an enzyme that metabolizes phenylalanine to tyrosine. The resultant accumulation of phenylalanine and its metabolites in the blood leads to severe developmental delay in untreated patients. Treatment consists of a diet that maintains phenylalanine at levels low enough to prevent brain damage but adequate to support normal physical and mental development. Careful supervision of the low-phenylalanine diet and monitoring of blood levels are necessary. Special formulas are available for the infant; older children have difficulty following the diet. It is not clear when and if the diet can be discontinued.

Biotinidase is the enzyme responsible for breakdown of biocytin (the lysyl precursor of biotin) to free biotin. Deficiency of the enzyme, which is inherited as an autosomal recessive trait, results in malfunctioning of the biotin-dependent mitochondrial enzymes and in organic acidemia. Clinical problems related to the deficiency appear several months or years after birth and include dermatitis, alopecia, ataxia, hypotonia, seizures, developmental delay, deafness, immunodeficiency, and metabolic acidosis. The treatment is lifelong administration of free biotin.

Maple syrup urine disease presents early in life, frequently before the state metabolic screen results are back. Symptoms begin several days after birth and rapidly progress to convulsions and death in 2-4 weeks if not treated. The distinctive odor of caramel or maple syrup starts after 1-2 days of life, but is variable in intensity. The diet consists of careful regulation of the intake of leucine, isoleucine, and valine.

160 to 163. The answers are 160-c, 161-a, 162-b, 163-b. (*Hay et al,
pp 489-490, 789-790, 793, 972-973. Kliegman et al, pp 2464-2468, 2877-2879,
2881, 3138. Rudolph et al, pp 1266, 1644, 2269-2271.*) Aniridia is found in
1%-2% of children with Wilms tumor. Genitourinary anomalies are found
in 4%-5%, and hemihypertrophy is associated with this tumor in 2%-3%
of patients. Wilms tumor is the most common primary renal malignancy
in childhood. Presentation is usually an abdominal mass, sometimes with
hypertension, hematuria, abdominal pain, and fever. Prognosis is generally
good.

Waardenburg syndrome is inherited as an autosomal dominant trait
with variable penetrance. It includes, in decreasing order of frequency, the
following anomalies: lateral displacement of the medial canthi, broad nasal
bridge, medial hyperplasia of the eyebrows, partial albinism commonly
expressed by a white forelock or heterochromia (or both), and deafness in
20% of cases.

A flat capillary vascular malformation in the distribution of the tri-
geminal nerve is the primary cutaneous lesion in the Sturge-Weber syndrome. The malformation also involves the meninges and results in atrophy
to the underlying cerebral cortex. The damage is manifested clinically by
seizures, mental deficiency, and hemiparesis or hemianopsia on the contra-
lateral side. The cause is unknown.

Infants who have tuberous sclerosis are often born with hypopigmented oval or irregularly shaped skin macules (ash leaf spots). Cerebral
sclerotic tubers also present from birth and become visible radiographically
by the third to fourth year of life. Myoclonic seizures, present in infancy,
can convert to grand mal seizures later in childhood. Adenoma sebaceum
appears at 4-7 years of age. The disease, which also affects the eyes, kidneys,
heart, bones, and lungs, is inherited as an autosomal dominant trait with
variable expression; new mutations are very common.

The Cardiovascular System

Questions

164. A 14-year-old girl became angry at her mother for taking away her iPhone and ingested an unknown quantity of a friend's pills. She is an otherwise healthy adolescent without known medical problems. On physical examination she is sleepy but arousable. The temperature is 37°C (98.5°F), heart rate is 99 beats per minute, respiratory rate is 21 breaths per minute, and blood pressure is 75/50 mm Hg. The electrocardiogram (ECG) shows a widened QRS complex of 130 ms. Which of the following is the most appropriate next step?

a. *N*-acetylcysteine (Mucomyst)
b. Naloxone (Narcan) and *N*-acetylcysteine (Mucomyst)
c. Intensive care unit (ICU) admission and sodium bicarbonate
d. Intravenous ethanol
e. Intravenous deferoxamine

165. A 10-year-old boy had a sore throat about 2 weeks ago but did not tell anyone because he was afraid he would miss his school field trip. Since several children have been diagnosed with rheumatic fever in the area, his mother is worried that he may be at risk as well. You tell her that several criteria must be met to make the diagnosis, but which of the following is the most common finding?

a. Carditis
b. Polyarthritis
c. Erythema marginatum
d. Chorea
e. Subcutaneous nodules

166. A 2-year-old boy is seen by the pediatrician for routine care. The family has recently moved to the area, and the father denies any significant past medical or surgical history. He reports that the child's day care recently called asking about several episodes, usually after the child does not get what he wants, when he "breathes funny" and sits in a corner with his knees under his chin for a few minutes. On physical examination, the temperature is 37°C (98.5°F), heart rate is 100 beats per minute, respiratory rate is 22 beats per minute, and blood pressure is 100/70 mm Hg. Heart has a right ventricular impulse, a systolic thrill along the left sternal border, and a harsh systolic murmur (loudest at the left sternal border but radiating through the lung fields). His chest radiograph and ECG are shown (Photographs A and B). Which of the following is the most likely diagnosis?

a. Patent ductus arteriosus
b. Right ventricular outflow obstruction
c. Atrial septal defect (ASD)
d. Transposition of the great vessels with a patent foramen ovale
e. Hypoplastic left heart

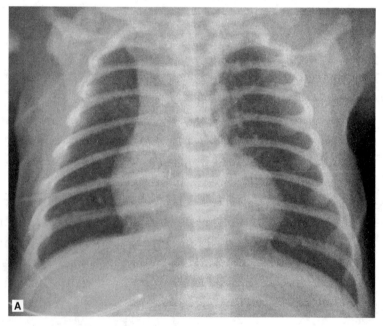

(Used with permission from Susan John, MD.)

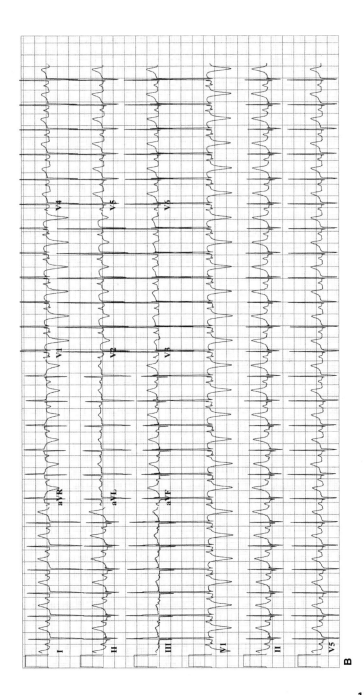

B

159

167. A 12-year-old boy is seen by the pediatrician for recurrent swelling of his face, hands, and feet over the last year, worsening recently. The family notes that these episodes occur following exercise and emotional stress, last for 2-3 days, and resolve spontaneously. The most recent episode was accompanied by abdominal pain, vomiting, and diarrhea. His past medical history is otherwise negative. Family history is positive for an older sister and a maternal uncle having similar episodes. On physical examination the vital signs are normal. Height and weight are at the 35th percentile for age. The mucous membranes are moist, pink, and without lesions. The chest is clear. Heart has normal S1 and S2 without murmur. Abdomen is soft, non-tender, and without hepatosplenomegaly. Swelling is noted in the hands, fingers, feet, and face. The skin is somewhat sensitive to touch over these areas. Laboratory data show:

Hemoglobin: 15 g/dL
Hematocrit: 45.2%
WBC: 5000/mm^3
    Segmented neutrophils: 60%
    Band forms: 1%
    Lymphocytes: 39%
Platelets: 185,000/mm^3
Urinalysis without protein, WBCs or RBCs

Which of the following is the most appropriate next step?

a. Obtain serum antinuclear antibody (ANA) titers, and anti-dsDNA and anti-Smith (Sm) antibodies
b. Measurement of ejection fraction on echocardiogram
c. Perform genetic testing for the NPHS1 and NPHS2 mutations
d. Obtain serum levels of C1, C4 esterase inhibitor, and C1q
e. Biopsy skin for electronic microscopy of vessels for vasculitis

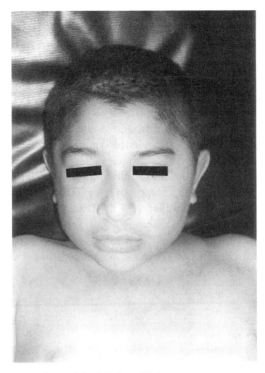

(Used with permission from Adelaide Hebert, MD.)

168. A 15-year-old girl is seen by the pediatrician for no menstrual cycles and short stature. She reports that she has always been a bit shorter, but that she has not had an adolescent growth spurt like her peers despite having pubic hair development at about 12 years of age. Her past medical history is significant for occasional upper respiratory illnesses with otitis media and the placement of orthodontia. She does well in school and is an accomplished member of the band. Family history is negative for delayed pubertal development. On physical examination the vital signs are normal. Height is less than 5th percentile (50th percentile for a 10-year old), and weight is 25th percentile for age. Head is normocephalic with redundant neck skin and low-set hairline. The mucous membranes are moist, pink, and without lesions with good dentition and braces in place. The chest is clear with good air movement. Nipples are widely set with Tanner 1 breast development. Heart has normal S1 and S2 without murmur. Perfusion is normal. Lower extremity pulses are diminished. Neurologic development is normal. Tanner 3 pubic hair is noted. A chromosomal analysis likely would demonstrate which of the following?

a. Mutation at chromosome 15q21.1
b. Trisomy 21
c. XO karyotype
d. Defect at chromosome 4p16
e. Normal chromosome analysis

169. An 8-year-old child is seen for a routine well-child visit. The mother reports the child has been in good health with seasonal allergies for which he takes over-the-counter loratadine. He is active in sports and does well in school. On physical examination the temperature is 37°C (98.5°F), heart rate is 85 beats per minute, respiratory rate is 22 breaths per minute, and blood pressure is 105/70 mm Hg. Height and weight are at the 75th percentile for age. The chest is clear. Heart has a loud S1 and a fixed, widely split S2. A grade II/VI midsystolic ejection murmur is present in the second intercostal space along the left sternal border. Abdomen is soft, nontender, and without hepatosplenomegaly. Extremities show no clubbing or cyanosis. Which of the following is the most likely diagnosis?

a. Atrial septal defect (ASD)
b. Ventricular septal defect (VSD)
c. Isolated tricuspid regurgitation
d. Tetralogy of Fallot (TOF)
e. Mitral valve prolapse

170. A 2-year-old boy is seen by the ED physician for fever, rash, and limp. The mother reports that the child has had a high, spiking fever up to 39.7°C (103.5°F), for 6 days, a limp over the previous 2 days, and a diffuse rash over the previous 3 hours. She also reports reduced oral intake, as well as decreased activity. Past medical history is unremarkable. On physical examination, the temperature is 39.2°C (102.5°F), heart rate is 115 beats per minute, respiratory rate is 26 breaths per minute, and blood pressure is 110/72 mm Hg. Height and weight are at the 50th percentile for age. He is awake, alert, but somewhat irritable. Skin shows diffuse, maculopapular rash (Photograph A). Head is normocephalic with prominent cervical adenopathy. Eyes are moist with bright red conjunctivae. Mouth is moist, pink, with red throat and tongue. The lips are dried and cracked. The chest is clear. Heart has a normal S1 and S2. A 2/6 vibratory midsystolic ejection murmur is noted at left lower sternal border. Abdomen is soft, nontender, and without hepatosplenomegaly. Extremities show edema and some peeling (Photograph B). Laboratory data show:

Hemoglobin: 13 g/dL
Hematocrit: 39.2%
WBC: 25,000/mm^3
    Segmented neutrophils: 80%
    Band forms: 5%
    Lymphocytes: 15%
Platelets: 425,000/mm^3
Erythrocyte sedimentation rate (ESR): 110 mm/h

Which of the following is the most likely diagnosis?

a. Scarlet fever
b. Rheumatic fever
c. Kawasaki disease
d. Juvenile rheumatoid arthritis
e. Infectious mononucleosis

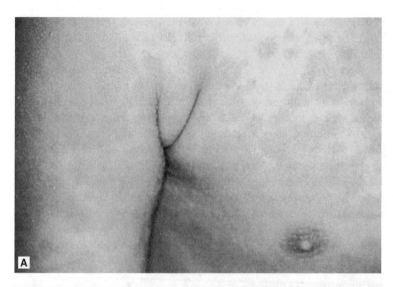

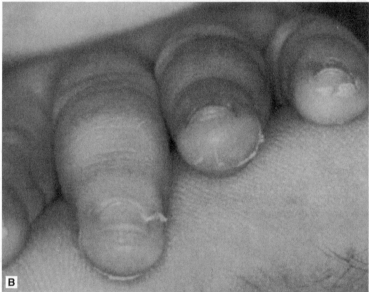

(Used with permission from Adelaide Hebert, MD.)

171. A 9-week-old girl is seen in the ED for 2 days of difficulty eating and fast breathing. The family notes that she has had an upper respiratory infection for the last 3 days, but is taking no medications other than daily vitamin D. She has one sick contact, a 2-year-old sibling, who had an upper respiratory infection that has since resolved. Birth was vaginal at term; the mother was group B *Streptococcus* (GBS) positive with incomplete treatment prior to delivery. On physical examination, the temperature is 36.7°C (98.0°F), heart rate is 195 beats per minute, respiratory rate is 80 breaths per minute, and blood pressure is 70/50 mm Hg. Height, weight, and head circumference are at the 50th percentile for age. She is irritable and somewhat difficult to arouse. Skin is pale and mottled. Head is normocephalic with tacky mucous membranes. Chest shows subcostal and intercostal retractions. Occasional crackles are noted over both lung fields. Heart sounds are distant. An S3 gallop is heard. Distal pulses are diminished; capillary refill time is 5 seconds. Extremities have no clubbing or edema. The ECG is shown (Photograph). The chest radiograph shows cardiomegaly. The echocardiogram demonstrates poor ventricular function, dilated ventricles, and dilation of the left atrium. Which of the following is the most likely diagnosis?

a. Myocarditis
b. Endocardial fibroelastosis
c. Pericarditis
d. Aberrant left coronary artery arising from pulmonary artery
e. Late-onset GBS infection

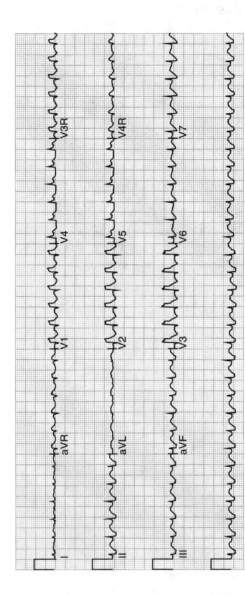

(Used with permission from John P. Breinholt III.)

172. A 5-month-old infant is seen by the pediatrician in follow-up from an emergency room visit. The family reports 2 weeks of intermittent low-grade fever, runny nose with cough, malaise, weight loss, and irritability with movement. His past history is positive for unrepaired TOF, and the family has been trained to watch for but have not noted any "tet spells." The emergency room evaluation from 48 hours prior shows:

Hemoglobin: 13.2g/dL
Hematocrit: 40.2%
WBC: 9600/mm^3
    Segmented neutrophils: 60%
    Band forms: 2%
    Lymphocytes: 38%
Platelets: 175,000/mm^3
Blood culture positive with *Kingella kingae*.

Which of the following is the most appropriate next step?

a. Repeat the blood culture and reassure the parents that the infant has a viral illness, and that the organism in the blood culture is a typical skin contaminant.
b. Increase the caloric density of his formula to help with weight gain and follow-up next week.
c. Arrange an evaluation by his cardiologist for next week.
d. Initiate oral clindamycin therapy and follow-up in 2 days.
e. Admit directly to the hospital, get two more blood cultures, and start vancomycin.

173. For the previous 24 hours an otherwise normal 3-month-old term infant has become less interested in feeding and seems to be more sleepy than normal. On physical examination, the temperature is 36.7°C (98.0°F), heart rate is unable to be counted, and respiratory rate is 60 breaths per minute. She is listless but arousable. Skin is pale and mottled. Chest has good air movement with minimal retractions and nasal flaring. A rare crackle is occasionally noted over both lung fields. Heart is tachycardic without variability with stimulation. S1 and S2 are difficult to distinguish; no murmur is noted. Distal pulses are diminished; capillary refill is 4-5 seconds. The ECG is shown (Photograph). Which of the following is the most appropriate initial management?

a. Begin a rapid verapamil infusion.
b. Initiate transthoracic pacing of the heart.
c. Initiate carotid massage.
d. Perform DC cardioversion.
e. Perform a precordial thump.

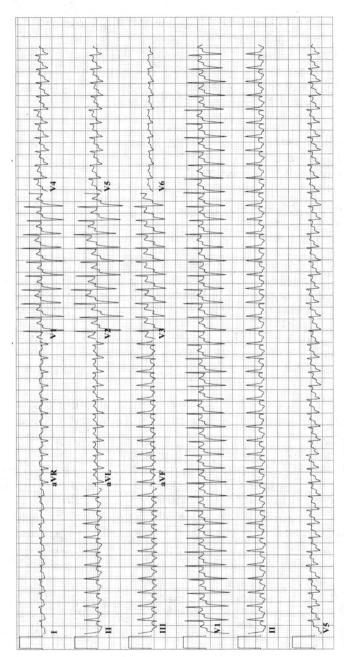

(Used with permission from Steven Lorch, MD.)

174. A 2-year-old child is seen by the pediatrician for "looking blue." The mother reports that over the previous week he appears to have less energy and to be a bit blue around the lips, especially when he gets upset. He was delivered vaginally at term to a 23-year-old woman whose pregnancy was complicated by type II herpes simplex virus. He has never been hospitalized and takes no medications. On physical examination vital signs are normal. Weight, length, and head circumference are 50th percentile for age. He is awake, alert, and in no distress but has slight cyanosis of the mouth and on the extremities. Head is normocephalic with moist mucous membranes. Chest has good air movement without distress. Heart has a normal S1, fixed split 2, and an S4 gallop. A 3 out of 6 systolic murmur in the pulmonic area is noted. Distal pulses are normal and capillary refill time is less than 3 seconds. Abdomen is soft, nontender, and without hepatosplenomegaly. Extremities have mild clubbing and no edema. The ECG is shown (Photographs A, B, and C). Which of the following is the most likely diagnosis?

a. Tricuspid regurgitation and pulmonic stenosis
b. Pulmonic stenosis and a VSD (TOF)
c. Atrioventricular canal
d. Ebstein anomaly
e. Wolff-Parkinson-White (WPW) syndrome

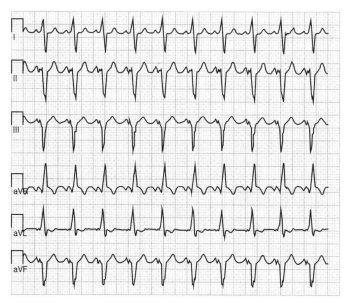

(Used with permission from John P. Breinholt III.)

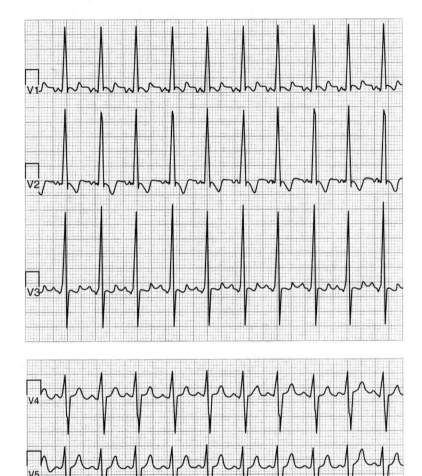

175. A 4-year-old girl is seen by the pediatrician in the office for pallor. Her father reports that she suddenly became pale and stopped running while he was playfully chasing her and her pet Chihuahua. He states that after 30 minutes, she was no longer pale and wanted to resume the game. Past medical history is negative for previous episode of pallor, cyanosis, serious illnesses, hospitalization, or medications. On physical examination vital signs are normal. Weight, length, and head circumference are 50th percentile for age. She is awake, alert, and in no distress, and her examination is completely normal. The chest x-ray and echocardiogram are also normal. An ECG tracing is shown in the photograph. Which of the following is the most likely diagnosis?

a. Paroxysmal ventricular tachycardia
b. Paroxysmal supraventricular tachycardia (SVT)
c. WPW syndrome
d. Stokes-Adams pattern
e. Excessive stress during play

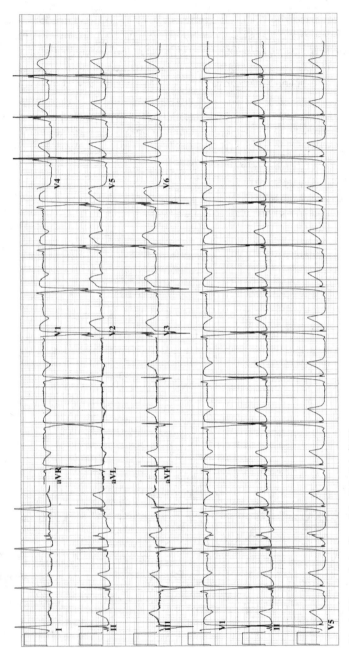

176. A 7-year-old girl is seen by the pediatrician for a 2-week history of spiking fevers as high as 40°C (104°F). Her mother reports that she has a slightly pink rash each time the fever subsides. The child complains of intermittent upper sternal pain and swollen fingers. She denies other symptoms. Past medical history is positive for a broken arm secondary to an auto-pedestrian accident. She takes no medications other than occasional over-the-counter antipyretics which have had variable effectiveness in reducing her fever. On physical examination vital signs and growth parameters are normal. Heart has muffled S1 and S2 with pulsus paradoxus but no murmur. Distal pulses are normal. Capillary refill time is less than 3 seconds. Extremities are without clubbing. The fingers are swollen and spindle shaped. A faint salmon-colored rash over the chest and back is noted. Which of the following is the most likely associated finding?

a. Positive streptococcal antibody testing
b. Hepatosplenomegaly
c. Elevated neutrophil count on fluid from a joint aspiration
d. Gram-positive cocci in fluid from joint aspiration
e. Elevation of serum anti-DNase B titer

177. A 48-hour-old neonate in the normal newborn nursery develops deep cyanosis with crying. He was born vaginally at term to a 19-year-old mother with scant prenatal care. She reports no problems during the pregnancy. On physical examination vital signs and growth parameters are normal. Chest has good air movement without distress. Heart has increased apical impulse that is displaced to the left. Left ventricular impulse is prominent. The first heart sound is increased in intensity; the second heart sound is single. A 4 out of 6 holosystolic murmur along the left sternal border is found. Distal pulses are normal. Capillary refill time is less than 3 seconds. Abdomen is soft, nontender, and the liver is felt 3 cm below the costal margin. Which of the following is the most likely diagnosis?

a. Transposition of the great arteries
b. Truncus arteriosus
c. Tricuspid atresia
d. TOF
e. Hypoplastic left heart syndrome

178. A 6-hour-old neonate has developed cyanosis which worsens with crying. The neonate was born at 37 weeks' gestation by cesarean section for nonreassuring heart tones to a 33-year-old woman whose pregnancy was complicated by preterm labor at 28 weeks' gestation. Apgar scores were 8 and 9 at 1 and 5 minutes, respectively. He was placed skin-to-skin and breast-fed well shortly after birth. On physical examination vital signs and growth parameters are normal. Head is normocephalic. Fontanelles are flat. Chest has good air movement without distress. Heart has normal S1 and S2. No murmur is heard. Distal pulses are normal. Capillary refill time is less than 3 seconds. Abdomen is soft and nontender. No hepatosplenomegaly is noted. An ECG shows an axis of 120° and right ventricular prominence. The chest radiograph is shown in the photograph. Which of the following is the most likely diagnosis?

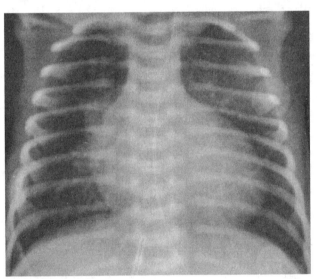

(Used with permission from Susan John, MD.)

a. TOF
b. Transposition of the great vessels
c. Tricuspid atresia
d. Pulmonary atresia with intact ventricular septum
e. Total anomalous pulmonary venous return below the diaphragm

179. A 16-year-old girl is seen by the pediatrician for a preparticipation sports evaluation. She reports no illness and takes no medications. Family history is positive for adult-onset diabetes in the paternal grandparents and "a heart murmur" in her mother. On physical examination, the temperature is 36.7°C (98.0°F), heart rate is 75 beats per minute, respiratory rate is 16 breaths per minute, and blood pressure is 110/70 mm Hg. Weight is at the 25th percentile and length is at the 50th percentile for age. Chest has good air movement without distress. Heart has normal S1 and S2 with a late apical systolic murmur preceded by a click noted. Pulses are normal. Capillary refill time is less than 3 seconds. Which of the following is the most likely diagnosis?

a. ASD
b. Aortic stenosis
c. Tricuspid regurgitation
d. Mitral valve prolapse
e. VSD

180. A 4-hour-old neonate in a rural normal newborn nursery develops cyanosis and an oxygen saturation of 65%; the neonatal transport team is en route to transfer the infant to the local children's hospital. The neonate was born vaginally at term to a 37-year-old woman whose pregnancy was complicated by hypertension and gestational diabetes. Apgar scores were 9 and 9 at 1 and 5 minutes, respectively. The newborn bottle-fed well initially but has since had decreased intake. On physical examination, the temperature is 36.7°C (98.0°F), heart rate is 145 beats per minute, respiratory rate is 60 breaths per minute, and blood pressure is 90/65 mm Hg. Oxygen saturation is 66% on 10 L/min oxygen face mask. Weight, length, and head circumference are at the 25th percentile for gestational age. Head is normocephalic. Fontanelles are flat. Chest has good air movement without distress. Heart has normal S1 and S2. No murmur is heard. Distal pulses are normal. Capillary refill time is less than 3 seconds. Abdomen is soft and nontender. No hepatosplenomegaly is noted. Arterial blood gas shows:

pH: 7.38
PaO_2: 33 mm Hg
$PaCO_2$: 43 mm Hg
HCO_3: 22 mEq/L
Base excess: −2 mmol/L

Which of the following is the most appropriate next step in management?

a. Indomethacin infusion
b. Saline infusion
c. Adenosine infusion
d. Prostaglandin E_1 infusion
e. Digoxin infusion

Questions 181 to 183

For each case presented, select the cardiovascular defect with which the examination findings are most likely to be associated. Each lettered option may be used once, more than once, or not at all.

a. Coarctation of the aorta
b. ASD
c. Mitral valve prolapse
d. Pulmonic stenosis
e. Patent ductus arteriosus

181. An infant has micrognathia and mild hypertelorism. The arms are bilaterally shortened, especially distally, with small hands that are deviated radially but with normal-appearing thumbs. The lower extremities are essentially normal; the hips are dislocated. Laboratory data show:

Hemoglobin: 16.2g/dL
Hematocrit: 48.2%
WBC: 25,000/mm^3
    Segmented neutrophils: 60%
    Band forms: 2%
    Lymphocytes: 28%
    Eosinophils: 10%
Platelets: 15,000/mm^3

182. A 15-year-old boy is seen in the pediatrician's office for a Special Olympics preparticipation sports physical. Past medical history is positive for frequent nosebleeds. On physical examination his height is 152 cm (50 in) and weight 63.5 kg (140 lb). Head has a high anterior hairline, low posterior hairline, prominent nasolabial folds, and low-set, posteriorly rotated ears. Chest has prominent superior sternum and depressed lower sternum and wide-set nipples. He has prominent split S2 and a II/VI crescendo-decrescendo murmur at the left upper sternal border that radiates to the back. Testes are undescended.

183. A 10-year-old girl is seen in the pediatrician's office for a well-child visit. Past history is positive for frequent joint dislocations and a recent visit to the ED for a bad ankle sprain. Her mother reports that she bruises easily. On physical examination the skin is lax and the joints are hypermobile. She can easily dislocate the joints of her fingers; relocation is painless.

The Cardiovascular System

Answers

164. **The answer is c.** (*Hay et al, pp 345-346. Kliegman et al, p 462. Rudolph et al, pp 461-462.*) The clinical presentation is that of a tricyclic antidepressant ingestion. In smaller children, the central nervous system (CNS) symptoms of drowsiness, lethargy, coma, and seizures are more commonly seen; the cardiac effects of tachycardia, initial hypertension followed by hypotension, widening of the QRS complex and ventricular dysrhythmias, are more often seen in adolescents. While therapy is mostly supportive, patients with a QRS complex wider than 100 ms, intractable hypotension, or ventricular dysrhythmias are candidates for alkalinization with an initial 1-2 mEq/kg of sodium bicarbonate followed by a continuous infusion, with the goal serum pH of 7.45-7.55.

Acetaminophen ingestion results initially in nausea, vomiting, and diaphoresis. These early symptoms often resolve in about 24-48 hours progressing to right upper quadrant abdominal pain and liver enzyme elevation. By 2-3 days after the ingestion, the peak liver function abnormalities are noted, and by 4 days to about 2 weeks, either recovery of liver function is noted or complete liver failure ensues. Therapy is with *N*-acetylcysteine. Narcotic ingestions result in respiratory depression as a major symptom during an acute ingestion as described; naloxone (repeated doses may be necessary) is the therapeutic choice. Ethanol is used to compete with methanol (which is not a pill); methanol ingestion causes mild inebriation, visual disturbances, nausea and vomiting, drowsiness, and profound acidosis. Iron overdose (treated with deferoxamine) leads to early nausea, vomiting, diarrhea, abdominal pain, bloody stools, hypotension, and ultimately gastric scarring.

165. **The answer is b.** (*Hay et al, pp 599-601. Kliegman et al, pp 1332-1335. Rudolph et al, pp 941-944.*) The diagnosis of rheumatic fever can be difficult because no single clinical manifestation or laboratory test is confirmatory. However, an accurate diagnosis must be made since treatment of the acute problems promptly and effectively is required, and long-term antibiotic prophylaxis to prevent recurrences must be instituted. To assist in diagnosis, the American Heart Association identified a set of major and minor standards relating to the manifestations of the disease, called the *Jones criteria* (revised), and recommends these criteria be applied in the diagnosis of every patient with possible rheumatic fever. The major criteria are carditis, polyarthritis, erythema marginatum, chorea, and subcutaneous nodules. The minor criteria are arthralgia (joint pain with no objective findings), fever, history of rheumatic fever, increased ESR or C-reactive protein (CRP), leukocytosis, and prolonged PR intervals on ECG. To make the diagnosis of rheumatic fever, the following criteria should be met: two major manifestations, or one major and two minor manifestations plus strong evidence of a preceding group A β-hemolytic streptococcal infection (positive culture or rapid antigen, or antibody elevation) or scarlet fever. The presence of Sydenham chorea is an exception in that, by itself, it is enough to make the diagnosis of rheumatic fever.

Of the major criteria, polyarthritis is the most common finding (75%), followed by carditis (50%-60%), chorea (10%-15%), erythema marginatum (<3%), and subcutaneous nodules (≤1%). Effective treatment of streptococcal pharyngitis can prevent rheumatic fever.

166. The answer is b. (*Hay et al, pp 588-590. Kliegman et al, pp 2211-2216. Rudolph et al, pp 1826-1828.*) This child has tetralogy of Fallot (TOF), which consists of right ventricular outflow obstruction (pulmonary stenosis), VSD, dextroposition of the aorta, and right ventricular hypertrophy. The radiograph shows the typical "boot-shaped" heart, while the ECG demonstrates the increased right ventricular forces. Children with TOF may have cyanotic episodes ("tet spells") associated with acute reduction in pulmonary blood flow. Typically, these spells are self-limited, lasting no more than 30 minutes. Assuming the knee-chest position is thought to increase peripheral resistance, decreasing the amount of right-to-left shunting and thus increasing pulmonary blood flow. Alternative therapies include morphine sulfate and propranolol. Prolonged hypoxia can lead to acidosis; correction may require infusion of sodium bicarbonate. Surgical correction is the definitive treatment in infancy when the defect is severe, and between 4 and 6 months when less so.

Patent ductus arteriosus is likely to present in this aged child with a constant, machine-like murmur, and if the flow is big enough, with evidence of progressive congestive heart failure. An ASD will have a fixed split second heart sound and a pulmonic stenosis murmur; it can also present with progressive evidence of heart failure if the flow across the ASD is large enough. Transposition of the great vessels with a patent foramen ovale and hypoplastic left heart syndrome invariably present with symptoms in the newborn period.

167. The answer is d. (*Hay et al, pp 1152-1154. Kliegman et al, pp 1126-1131. Rudolph et al, p 1196.*) Although hereditary angioedema is relatively rare as a cause of edema, the recurrent episodes in late childhood, the normal laboratory results, and the family history in the vignette make the other choices less likely. Hereditary angioedema, transmitted as an autosomal dominant trait, is a result of inadequate function (owing to either deficient quantity or quality) of C1 esterase inhibitor (C1-INH), involved in the first step in the complement cascade, which results in the excessive production of a vasoactive kinin. In addition to otherwise asymptomatic subcutaneous edema, edema can occur in the gastrointestinal tract and produce the symptoms mentioned in the question. Laryngeal edema with airway obstruction can also occur; a change in the tone of the voice and difficulty in swallowing secretions are symptoms of impending airway compromise and require emergent medical care.

ANA titers and anti-dsDNA and anti-Smith (Sm) antibodies are appropriate measures for a patient suspected to have systemic lupus erythematosus. In children this condition often presents with malar rash, mucocutaneous ulcers, renal abnormalities (urine with casts and protein), thrombocytopenia, anemia, fever, and lymphadenopathy.

Heart failure can cause swelling of dependent body parts, but typically not just of the hands and feet. Historical findings of fatigue, shortness of breath and poor growth, and physical examination findings of cardiac abnormalities might be seen.

Congenital nephrotic syndrome is caused by NPHS1 and NPHS2 gene mutations; the classic finding is edema, hypercholesterolemia, and proteinuria.

Electronic microscopy evidence of vasculitis would suggest Henoch-Schönlein purpura, a condition that presents with fever, headache, anorexia, and then rash of the legs and buttocks, abdominal and joint pain, and often bloody stools.

168. The answer is c. (*Hay et al, p 1108. Kliegman et al, pp 2744-2746. Rudolph et al, pp 2068-2069.*) Short stature, neck webbing, low hairline, sexual infantilism with absent menses but normal pubic hair development, and a shield-like chest with widely spaced nipples are signs of Turner syndrome, which is usually associated with an XO karyotype. Other features include high-arched palate (dental braces) and frequent otitis media. A bicuspid aortic valve is noted on echocardiography in 30%-50%, and aortic coarctation occurs in about 15%-20% of those with this disorder. Down syndrome is most commonly associated with endocardial cushion defects or VSD. Marfan syndrome (mutation 15q21.1) is associated with dilatation of the aorta root and mitral and aortic regurgitation. Ellis-van Creveld syndrome (defect 4p16) is associated with ASD.

169. The answer is a. (*Hay et al, pp 574-575. Kliegman et al, pp 2189-2191. Rudolph et al, pp 1811-1813.*) The child in the question has a normal history and physical examination with the exceptions of the fixed, split S2 and a murmur in the pulmonic area. Most children with an ASD are asymptomatic; the lesion is found during a routine examination. In older children, exercise intolerance can be noted if the lesion is of significant size. On examination, the pulses are normal, a right ventricular systolic lift at the left sternal border is sometimes palpable, and a fixed splitting of the second heart sound is audible. The murmur is caused by increased flow across the pulmonic valve from the left-to-right shunt through the ASD. For lesser degrees of ASD, surgical treatment is controversial.

VSD commonly presents as a harsh or blowing holosystolic murmur best heard along the left lower sternum, often with radiation throughout the precordium. The auscultatory finding of tricuspid regurgitation is typically a blowing holosystolic murmur, augmented during inspiration, and best heard at the left lower sternal border; a middiastolic rumble may also be heard. A history of birth asphyxia or findings of other cardiac lesions may be present. TOF is a common form of congenital heart disease. The four abnormalities include right ventricular outflow obstruction, VSD, dextroposition of the aorta, and right ventricular hypertrophy; cyanosis presents in infants and in young children. Mitral valve prolapse occurs with the billowing into the atria of one or both mitral valve leaflets at the end of systole. It is a congenital abnormality that frequently manifests only during adolescence or later. It is more common in girls than in boys and seems to be inherited in an autosomal dominant fashion. On clinical examination, an apical murmur is noted late in systole, which can be preceded by a midsystolic click. The diagnosis is confirmed with an echocardiogram that shows prolapse of the mitral leaflets during mid to late systole.

170. The answer is c. (*Hay et al, pp 601-602. Kliegman et al, pp 1209-1214. Rudolph et al, pp 1855-1858.*) The child in the question has high spiking fever for several days, limp, diffuse rash, conjunctivitis, oral changes (red tongue and fissured lips), cervical adenopathy, edema of the extremities with some peeling, and laboratory findings of an elevated WBC with left shift, thrombocytosis, and an elevated ESR.

Many conditions can be associated with prolonged fever, a limp caused by arthralgia, exanthem, adenopathy, and pharyngitis. Conjunctivitis, however, is suggestive of Kawasaki disease (KD). The fissured lips, although common in KD, could occur after a long period of fever from any cause if the child became dehydrated. For the laboratory results, the predominance of neutrophils and high ESR (and CRP) are common to all. An increase in platelets with this constellation of symptoms, however, is found typically in KD. KD typically presents with prolonged fever, a polymorphous rash, extremity changes (including swelling in the early period of the illness with peeling from the fingertips coming later), nonpurulent conjunctivitis, lymphadenopathy, and oral mucosal changes including fissured lips and oropharyngeal mucosal erythema. Although these are considered the diagnostic criteria, the diagnosis is still possible in the absence of one or two of these physical findings. Other clinical findings may include vomiting and diarrhea with abdominal pain, hydrops of the gallbladder, arthritis or arthralgias, sterile pyuria, irritability, and aseptic meningitis. Coronary artery aneurysms can develop, as can aneurysms in other areas. Baseline echocardiography is generally performed at the time of diagnosis, as coronary artery aneurysms are the most significant long-term complication of KD. Initial treatment is typically intravenous immunoglobulin (IVIG) and high-dose aspirin; IVIG significantly reduces the risk of aneurysms. The child will usually defervesce shortly after the infusion. Aspirin is typically kept at a higher dose until the platelet count begins to decrease, and then is continued at a lower dose for several weeks. While bacterial infection is in the differential diagnosis for this patient's presentation and blood cultures are usually part of the evaluation, IV vancomycin should be reserved for a culture-proven susceptible organism resistant to other antibiotics, or as empiric therapy in a critically ill patient.

171. The answer is a. (*Hay et al, pp 608-609. Kliegman et al, pp 2277-2279. Rudolph et al, pp 1858-1860.*) The history of poor feeding and respiratory distress along with physical examination findings of pallor, dyspnea, tachypnea, tachycardia, and cardiomegaly are common in congestive heart failure regardless of the cause. The ECG shows generalized low-voltage QRS, T-wave flattening, and ST elevation in the precordial leads, and the chest radiograph shows cardiomegaly. The constellation of findings in the question suggests myocarditis as the etiology of this infant's condition. The most common causes of myocarditis include adenovirus and coxsackievirus B, although many other viruses can cause this condition.

The echocardiogram in the question shows ventricular and left atrial dilatation as well as poor ventricular function. The echocardiogram findings in this case are not consistent with an aberrant origin of the left coronary artery, although the origin of the coronary arteries can be difficult to visualize. On ECG, the voltages of the ventricular complexes seen with aberrant origin of the left coronary artery are not diminished, and a pattern of myocardial infarction can be seen. Voltages from the left ventricle are usually high in endocardial fibroelastosis, and both right and left ventricular forces are high in glycogen storage disease of the heart. Late-onset GBS infection most commonly presents with signs and symptoms of meningitis or sepsis, including extreme irritability, lethargy, poor feeding, fever, and bulging fontanelle.

172. The answer is e. (*Hay et al, pp 602-603. Kliegman et al, pp 2263-2269. Rudolph et al, pp 1861-1863.*) The laboratory work is normal, but the blood culture is positive for a pathogen. Infective endocarditis may present as fulminant disease with shock and overwhelming sepsis, but the subacute form presents with more subtle findings, including low-grade fever, weight loss, lethargy, sleep disturbances, arthralgias, and myalgias. The much discussed Osler nodes (small tender nodules in the tips of fingers and toes), Janeway lesions (nontender hemorrhagic lesions on the hands and feet), and splinter hemorrhages (dark lines under nails) are uncommon findings. Children at the greatest risk of endocarditis are those with unrepaired cyanotic heart disease, those with prosthetic material from a repair, or those with a prior history of infectious endocarditis.

In children, endocarditis is typically caused by streptococcus organisms in the viridans group and *Staphylococcus aureus*. Other potential pathogens include coagulase-negative staphylococcus, *Streptococcus pneumoniae*, and the HACEK organisms including *Haemophilus* sp, *Actinobacillus actinomycetemcomitans*, *Cardiobacterium hominis*, *Eikenella corrodens*, and *Kingella* species.

Diagnosis may be confirmed with serial positive blood cultures and echocardiogram findings of vegetations and myocardial abscesses.

Treatment is an appropriate antibiotic for 4-8 weeks. Surgical intervention is reserved for patients with valvular obstruction, congestive heart failure (CHF), or abscess; persistent bacteremia may also result in surgery.

173. The answer is c. (*Hay et al, pp 616-620. Kliegman et al, pp 2254-2257. Rudolph et al, pp 1843-1845.*) The infant in the question has pallor and listlessness, poor feeding, mild respiratory distress, and slightly delayed capillary refill. The infant also has tachycardia that is too rapid to be counted, and the heart rate is not variable with crying. SVT, as shown on the ECG, is characterized by rapid heart rate (in this case about 250 beats per minute), little rate variability, and a consistent P wave for each QRS complex. Prolonged SVT can lead to heart failure with hepatomegaly and respiratory compromise. Fetal SVT can lead to hydrops fetalis. The first-line treatment is to stimulate the vagus nerve using techniques such as carotid massage, immersion of the face in cold water, or voluntary straining. Rapid infusion of IV adenosine can affect resolution if the maneuvers are not successful. Verapamil is contraindicated in this age group, as it may cause acute hypotension and cardiac arrest. Synchronized DC cardioversion may be performed in patients in shock or with heart failure; it must, however, be synchronized to the QRS complex. Transthoracic pacing is typically useful in bradyarrhythmias. A precordial thump might help individuals with an acute arrest from ventricular fibrillation but does not resolve SVT.

174. The answer is d. (*Hay et al, p 581. Kliegman et al, pp 2221-2222. Rudolph et al, p 1825.*) An S3 or S4 rhythm caused by volume overload or heart failure along with the murmur of tricuspid regurgitation and a mid-diastolic murmur at the lower left sternum suggests the diagnosis of Ebstein anomaly (downward displacement of the tricuspid valve). The presence of right atrial hypertrophy and right ventricular conduction (block) defects on the ECG shown confirms the diagnosis. Both tricuspid regurgitation with pulmonic stenosis and TOF give ECG evidence of right ventricular enlargement. WPW syndrome, which is frequently associated with Ebstein anomaly, is not associated with murmurs or cyanosis as an isolated entity, but is associated with SVT; the typical ECG finding is a curved upstroke of the QRS complex, termed a "delta wave."

175. The answer is c. (*Hay et al, pp 616-620. Kliegman et al, pp 2254-2255. Rudolph et al, pp 1843-1844.*) The child described in the question has no cyanosis or murmur, no cardiac or pulmonary vascular abnormalities by chest x-ray, and no evidence of structural anomalies by echocardiogram, and therefore is unlikely to have an underlying gross anatomic defect. The ECG pattern in the photograph shows the configuration of preexcitation, the pattern seen in the WPW syndrome. These patients have an aberrant atrioventricular conduction pathway, which causes the early ventricular depolarization appearing on the ECG as a shortened PR interval. The initial slow ventricular depolarization wave is referred to as the *delta wave.* Seventy percent of patients with WPW syndrome have single or repeated episodes of paroxysmal SVT, which can cause the symptoms described in the question. The preexcitation ECG pattern and WPW syndrome can occur in Ebstein malformation, but this is unlikely in the absence of cyanosis and murmur, and with a normal echocardiogram. If ventricular tachycardia were present, the symptoms would likely be more profound. Active play and exposure to over-the-counter medications containing sympathomimetics in a healthy 4-year-old child can cause symptoms such as those described in the question in children with WPW syndrome by precipitating paroxysmal SVT.

176. The answer is b. (*Hay et al, pp 889-892. Kliegman et al, pp 1160-1170. Rudolph et al, pp 800-806.*) Juvenile idiopathic arthritis (JIA) is the most common rheumatic disease in the pediatric population and includes systemic arthritis (5%-15%), oligoarthritis (40%-50%), polyarthritis (25%-30%), psoriatic arthritis, and enthesitis-related arthritis. The description of the case includes high, spiking fever, evanescent rash, swollen fingers, chest and finger pain, and muffled heart sounds with pulsus paradoxus, suggesting systemic-onset JIA. In addition to these findings, patients with systemic-onset JIA may have generalized myalgia, hepatosplenomegaly, lymphadenopathy, and evidence of heart failure if the pericardial effusion is severe. Systemic JIA can occur throughout childhood but peaks between 1 and 5 years of age. There is no diagnostic test specific for systemic JIA, so the diagnosis is only made after the exclusion of other possible diagnoses.

Rheumatic fever (which is associated with positive streptococcal antibody testing or elevation of serum anti-DNase B titers as minor criteria) typically presents in the febrile, toxic child 2-6 weeks after a streptococcal pharyngitis with major criteria of carditis, migratory polyarthritis (common), subcutaneous nodules (rare), erythema marginatum (rare), and Sydenham chorea (rare). Although septic arthritis can affect any joint, it would not be likely to affect finger joints by causing spindle-shaped swellings. The laboratory findings for septic arthritis include joint fluid findings of elevated neutrophils and positive Gram stain for bacteria.

177. The answer is c. (*Hay et al, pp 592-593. Kliegman et al, pp 2218-2220. Rudolph et al, pp 1824-1825.*) The patient in the question clearly has congenital heart disease. Patients with tricuspid atresia typically have a hypoplastic right ventricle, and therefore the ECG shows left-axis deviation and LVH; this translates to a left ventricular impulse on physical examination and likely notably diminished deflections of right ventricular forces. Additionally, right atrial overload may manifest as tall P waves in lead II. Almost all other forms of cyanotic congenital heart disease are associated with elevated pressures in the right ventricle and increased right ventricular impulse. In those conditions, the ECG will show right-axis deviation and right ventricular hypertrophy.

178. The answer is b. (*Hay et al, pp 594-596. Kliegman et al, pp 2223-2226. Rudolph et al, pp 1828-1829.*) Transposition of the great vessels with an intact ventricular septum presents with early cyanosis, a normal-sized heart (classic "egg on a string" radiographic pattern in one-third of cases as shown on the radiograph), normal or slightly increased pulmonary vascular markings, and an ECG showing right-axis deviation and right ventricular hypertrophy. In TOF, cyanosis is often not seen in the first few days of life. Tricuspid atresia, a cause of early cyanosis, causes diminished pulmonary arterial blood flow; the pulmonary fields on x-ray demonstrate a diminution of pulmonary vascularity, and left-axis deviation and LVH are shown by ECG. Total anomalous pulmonary venous return below the diaphragm is associated with obstruction to pulmonary venous return and a classic radiographic finding of marked, fluffy-appearing venous congestion with a "snowman" or "figure of eight" appearance to the mediastinum; the body of the snowman is formed by the enlarged right atrium, and the head of the snowman is formed by the dilated vertical vein, brachiocephalic vein, and the superior vena cava. In pulmonary atresia with an intact ventricular septum, cyanosis appears early, the lung markings are normal to diminished, and the heart is large.

179. The answer is d. (*Hay et al, pp 585-586. Kliegman et al, p 2210. Rudolph et al, p 1815.*) Mitral valve prolapse occurs with the billowing into the atria of one or both mitral valve leaflets at the end of systole. It is a congenital abnormality that frequently manifests only during adolescence or later. It is more common in girls than in boys and seems to be inherited in an autosomal dominant fashion as outlined in the case. On clinical examination, an apical murmur is noted late in systole, which can be preceded by a click. The diagnosis is confirmed with an echocardiogram that shows prolapse of the mitral leaflets during mid to late systole. The ECG and chest x-ray are usually normal. β-Blockers and digitalis are unlikely to be required, and penicillin prophylaxis for dental procedures for patients with mitral valve prolapse is no longer recommended by the American Heart Association.

Classic findings of ASD are fixed and split second heart sound with systolic murmur over the pulmonary area due to increased blood flow across a normal valve. Aortic stenosis typically presents with a harsh, systolic murmur over the aortic area. Tricuspid regurgitation presents with a high-pitched, pansystolic murmur located over the fourth intercostal space in the parasternal region. The murmur worsens with inspiration and diminishes with expiration and Valsalva. A VSD typically presents with a harsh murmur over the left lower sternal border with preservation of the normal splitting of the heart sounds when the lesions are small and heart failure is not present.

180. The answer is d. (*Hay et al, pp 590-592. Kliegman et al, pp 2217-2218. Rudolph et al, pp 1825-1826.*) The vignette describes a neonate with a ductal-dependent cyanotic congenital heart lesion. The blood gas has hypoxia but normal pH and CO_2 levels. In this example, the newborn had pulmonary atresia without a corresponding VSD; a patent ductus arteriosus is the only source of pulmonary blood flow with this defect. Another example of a ductal-dependent lesion is transposition of the great vessels with an intact ventricular septum. In this condition, blood flows in two parallel circuits: desaturated blood comes into the right atrium and ventricle and re-enters the systemic circulation through the aorta, while oxygenated blood enters the left atrium and ventricle and returns to the lungs through the pulmonary artery. Without a septal defect, a patent ductus arteriosus is the only route to mix oxygenated and deoxygenated blood.

Cyanotic infants who do not improve their saturations with supplemental oxygen should be evaluated carefully for structural heart disease. The ductus arteriosus typically closes in the first few hours of life; thus, these neonates will develop their cyanosis in the same time frame. Prostaglandin E_1 (PGE_1) will help keep the ductus patent until a surgical procedure can be performed. PGE_1 does have the tendency to cause hypoventilation, so arrangements must be made for a potential artificial airway, if necessary. Indomethacin closes a patent ductus arteriosus. Adenosine is used for SVT.

181 to 183. **The answers are 181-b, 182-d, 183-c.** (*Hay et al, p 562. Kliegman et al, pp 2405, 2747-2748, 3179-3181. Rudolph et al, pp 1568-1569, 1585, 1778-1779.*) The patient in the first case has dysmorphic features and a low platelet count on the complete blood count (CBC). Thrombocytopenia-absent radius (TAR) syndrome is diagnosed in the newborn who demonstrates profound thrombocytopenia and bilateral absence of radius; thumbs are present (this distinguishes TAR from other syndromes that affect the radii). Other features of the condition include micrognathia, hypertelorism, small and posteriorly rotated ears, renal anomalies, short stature, and a variety of lower extremity changes. Cardiac lesions include TOF and ASD. Many of these infants have an allergy to cow's milk protein. About 40% of patients die in the newborn period as a result of low-platelet–induced bleeding.

Noonan syndrome, the "male Turner syndrome," occurs in both sexes. The most common features include short stature, downslanting palpebral fissures, ptosis, low-set and malformed ears, webbed neck, shield-like chest, pulmonic stenosis, and cryptorchidism. About 50% of patients with this condition have a history of abnormal bleeding tendencies. Mental retardation is seen in one-fourth of affected individuals. It is associated with advanced paternal age.

Mitral valve prolapse is seen in patients with Ehlers-Danlos syndrome (EDS), a group of genetically different connective tissue disorders. Patients with EDS have hyperextensibility and easy bruising, joint hypermobility (leading to joint dislocations and sprains), skin that is velvety to touch, and tissue fragility. Six recognized forms are described, along with several "unclassified" types; "classic" (EDS I and II) and "hypermobility" (EDS III) types predominate.

The Respiratory System

Questions

184. A 3-hour-old neonate is seen by the pediatrician for initial evaluation. The neonate was born vaginally, at term to a 33-year-old mother whose pregnancy was complicated by poorly controlled insulin-dependent gestational diabetes and gestational hypertension. On physical examination the temperature is 37°C (98.6°F), heart rate is 155 beats per minute, respiratory rate is 55 breaths per minute, O_2 saturation is 85% on room air, and 99% on 5 L/min nasal cannula. Weight, length, and head circumference are at the 95th percentile. The head has molding and a left-sided cephalohematoma. The chest has irregular, labored breathing, and decreased breath sounds on the right side. Heart has normal S1 and S2 without murmur. Abdomen is soft, nontender, and without hepatosplenomegaly. Extremities show decreased tone and no spontaneous movement of the right arm. A stat portable chest radiograph is normal. Which of the following is the most appropriate next step?

a. Obtain nasal wash for viral culture.
b. Perform fiberoptic bronchoscopy of the airways.
c. Order chest CT.
d. Obtain ultrasound of chest and diaphragm.
e. Start antibiotics for presumed group B *Streptococcus* infection.

185. A 10-month-old infant is seen by the pediatrician for poor weight gain, a persistent cough, and a history of several bouts of pneumonitis. The mother also reports the infant as having a several months' history of very large, foul-smelling stools. The infant was born vaginally at term to a 29-year-old woman whose pregnancy was complicated by gestational diabetes. The infant was breast-fed, voided in the first day, and stooled just before discharge on the third day of life. On physical examination temperature is 37°C (98.6°F), heart rate is 90 beats per minute, and respiratory rate is 24 breaths per minute. Weight is at the 10th percentile; length, and head circumference are at the 50th percentile. Head is normocephalic. The chest has equal good air movement, equal breath sounds, and occasional crackles scattered over both lung fields. Heart has normal S1 and S2 without murmur. Abdomen is soft, nontender, and without hepatosplenomegaly. Which of the following is the most likely mechanism of disease?

a. Tumor of the airway
b. Deficiency of serum immunoglobulins
c. Infection with atypical bacteria
d. Aspiration of a foreign body
e. Mutation of a protein transmembrane conductance regulator gene

186. A 9-month-old infant has 2 days of runny nose, sneezing, and cough, worsening over the last 4 hours. Sick contacts include two other members of the family with similar cough and congestion and several children with similar symptoms in the day care. His past medical history is positive for occasional upper respiratory infections, but no hospitalizations. He takes no medications. Family history is positive only for coronary artery disease in the maternal grandparents. On physical examination temperature is 38.4°C (101.1°F), heart rate is 110 beats per minute, and respiratory rate is 45 breaths per minute. Nose has clear nasal discharge. Chest has moderate respiratory distress with slightly reduced air movement. Mild nasal flaring, subcostal, and intercostal retractions are seen. Diffuse wheezing and scattered crackles are noted bilaterally. Arterial blood gas on room air shows:

pH: 7.46
PaO_2: 75 mm Hg
$PaCO_2$: 34 mm Hg
HCO_3: 18 mEq/L
Base excess: −4 mmol/L

His chest radiographs are shown in the photographs. Which of the following is the most appropriate next step?

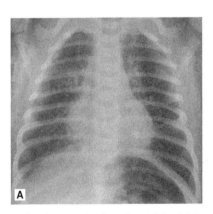
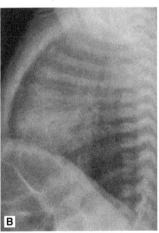

(Used with permission from Susan John, MD.)

a. Monitoring oxygenation and fluid status
b. Inhaled epinephrine and a single dose of steroids
c. Acute-acting bronchodilators and a short course of oral steroids
d. Emergent intubation, mechanical ventilation, and antibiotics
e. Chest tube placement

187. A 6-year-old girl is seen by the pediatrician for a 2-day history of cough and fever. The mother reports that the child was in her normal state of good health until she suddenly developed cough and fever to 39.3°C (102.7°F) 2 days prior. Subsequently she has also developed decreased intake and is more lethargic. Her past medical history is positive for occasional otitis media and upper respiratory tract infections. She takes no routine medications. On physical examination she is asleep but arousable, and is oriented. The temperature is 39.4°C (103°F), heart rate is 120 beats per minute, and respiratory rate is 45 breaths per minute. Nose has clear nasal discharge and flaring. Chest has reduced air movement and some crackles are heard on the left side. Mild subcostal and intercostal retractions are seen. Her chest x-ray is shown in the photograph. Which of the following is the most appropriate initial treatment?

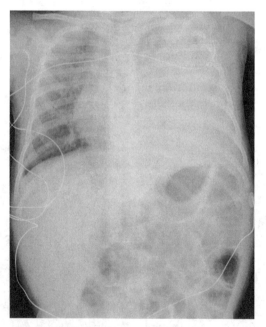

(Used with permission from Susan John, MD.)

a. *N*-acetylcysteine and chest physiotherapy
b. Vancomycin
c. Partial lobectomy
d. Postural drainage
e. Placement of tuberculosis skin test

188. A 2-year-old girl is seen in the emergency center for cough and respiratory distress. Her father reports that she was playing in the garage with her Chihuahua while he was weed-whacking around the garden gnomes in the front yard. He returned about 5 minutes later to find her gagging, vomiting, and smelling of gasoline. She vomited once, and then seemed fine. Over the subsequent 4 or 5 hours she developed cough and trouble breathing. On physical examination she is sleepy with frequent coughing. The temperature is 38.4°C (101.1°F), heart rate is 110 beats per minute, and respiratory rate is 55 breaths per minute. Chest has subcostal retractions. Scattered wheezes are heard throughout both lung fields. Heart has normal S1 and S2 without murmur. Which of the following is the most appropriate first step in management?

a. Administer charcoal.
b. Begin nasogastric lavage.
c. Administer ipecac.
d. Perform pulse oximetry and arterial blood gas.
e. Administer gasoline-binding agent intravenously.

189. A 3-year-old girl is seen in the hospital by the pediatrician for 10 days of cough and fever. The family reports she has been healthy until this illness began, noting that she has occasional upper respiratory tract infections only. They have not travelled. Family history reveals essential hypertension in both parents and adult onset diabetes in a paternal aunt. The child lives with her parents and her 6-week-old brother who is healthy. Her grandfather stayed with the family for 2 months before his return to the West Indies 1 month prior. He had had a 3-month history of weight loss, fever, and hemoptysis. The child's chest radiograph is shown in the photograph. Which of the following is the most appropriate next step?

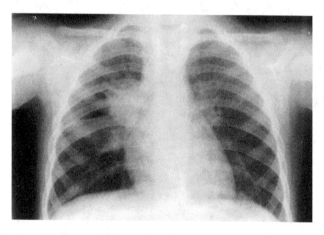

a. Order bronchoscopy and culture of washings for all family members.
b. Place a Mantoux test on the 6-week-old sibling and initiate pyrazinamide.
c. Isolate the 3-year-old patient for 1 month.
d. Treat the 3-year-old patient with isoniazid (INH), rifampin, and pyrazinamide.
e. Obtain HIV testing for all family members.

190. A pediatrician sees a 4-year-old boy who has been admitted to the children's hospital with pneumonia. The child has had multiple episodes of fever and respiratory difficulty over the previous 2 years. These episodes include cyanosis, wheezing, and dyspnea, and each episode lasts for about 3 days. During each event he has a small amount of hemoptysis, is diagnosed with left lower lobe pneumonia, and improves upon treatment. They state that with each episode, radiographs normalize several days after the events. A rheumatologic and immunologic evaluation has been normal. On physical examination he is awake, alert, and in no distress. The temperature is 38.4°C (101.1°F), heart rate is 90 beats per minute, and respiratory rate is 38 breaths per minute. Chest has minimal subcostal retractions. Scattered wheezes and a few crackles are heard over the left lower lobe. Heart has normal S1 and S2 without murmur. Fingers show digital clubbing. Which of the following is the most appropriate next step?

a. Begin intravenous cephalosporin and oral macrolide therapy.
b. Order a modified barium swallow study to evaluate for aspiration.
c. Send nasal swab for viral culture.
d. Initiate incentive spirometry.
e. Perform bronchoscopy with bronchoalveolar lavage.

191. An 18-month-old girl is seen by the pediatrician for foul-smelling nasal discharge. The mother reports the child to be healthy until about 4 days prior when she developed a slight upper respiratory tract infection and nasal discharge. She has had no fever, cough, sneezing, or sick contacts. Past medical history is benign; growth and development have been normal. On physical examination she is awake, alert, and in no distress. Vital signs are normal. Nose has left-sided, foul-smelling purulent drainage without air movement; the right side is normal. The ear canals are clear and the tympanic membranes are translucent. Chest is clear. Which of the following is the most likely diagnosis?

a. Foreign body
b. Nasal polyps
c. Frontal sinusitis
d. Deviated septum
e. Choanal atresia

192. A 7-year-old child is seen by the pediatrician for a school physical. His mother reports he often complains of headaches. His development has been normal, and although his grades are average, his teachers report he is sleepy in school and that he has become disruptive in class. Past medical history is negative except for loud snoring. On physical examination his height is 50th percentile for age, and his weight is more than 95th percentile for age. He has enlarged (3+) tonsils. Which of the following is the most appropriate next step in evaluating and managing this condition?

a. Refer to the in-school psychologist for diagnostic evaluation and counseling.
b. Refer to an otolaryngologist.
c. Check serum TSH, T4, and T_3U.
d. Start methylphenidate 5 mg PO in the morning before school and at lunchtime.
e. Arrange for polysomnography.

193. A 1-year-old boy presenting with cough, fever, and mild hypoxia was admitted to the hospital the previous evening. At that time, he had evidence of a right upper lobe consolidation on his chest radiograph. A blood culture has since become positive for *Staphylococcus aureus*. Approximately 20 hours into his hospitalization, he acutely worsens over a few minutes with markedly increased work in breathing, increasing oxygen requirement, and hypotension. Diminished breath sounds are noted on the right. Which of the following is the most appropriate next step?

a. Order a repeat chest radiograph to evaluate for pneumatocele formation.
b. Obtain a large-bore needle and chest tube kit for aspiration of a tension pneumothorax.
c. Change in antibiotics to include gentamicin.
d. Add a sedative to treat the child's attack of severe anxiety.
e. Order a thoracentesis kit to drain a pleural effusion.

194. A 2-year-old child is seen by the ED physician for cough and stridor. The family reports that the child has had several days of low-grade fever, a barking cough, and noisy breathing but had been drinking well. They state that over the previous few hours he has developed a fever of 40°C (104°F) and has become lethargic. Past medical history is positive for occasional upper respiratory infection; his immunizations are current. On physical examination he is sleepy and toxic in appearance. Temperature is 40°C (104°F), heart rate is 120 beats per minute, and respiratory rate is 35 breaths per minute. Mucous membranes are moist, and no drooling is noted. Oral examination shows normal epiglottis. Nose has clear discharge bilaterally. On chest examination he has biphasic stridor, along with subcostal and intercostal retractions. A few rales are heard throughout the lung fields. Which of the following is the most appropriate next step?

a. Intubate and initiate intravenous antibiotics.
b. Begin inhaled epinephrine and oral steroids.
c. Start intravenous methylprednisolone.
d. Place in a cool mist tent for observation.
e. Prescribe oral antibiotics and arrange outpatient follow-up.

195. A 6-year-old boy is seen by the emergency room physician for respiratory distress. His family reports that he has a 3-hour history of fever to 39.5°C (103.1°F) and sore throat. Past medical history is negative. His immunizations are current. On physical examination he is alert, but anxious and toxic. He is sitting on the examination table leaning forward with his neck extended. Temperature is 40°C (104°F), heart rate is 110 beats per minute, and respiratory rate is 38 breaths per minute. Drooling is noted. Nose has clear discharge bilaterally. Chest has mild inspiratory stridor and mild subcostal retractions. An occasional rale is heard throughout the lung fields. Laboratory data show:

Hemoglobin: 17 g/dL
Hematocrit: 51%
WBC: 17,000/mm^3
    Segmented neutrophils: 67%
    Band forms: 18%
    Lymphocytes: 15%
Platelet count: 278,000/mm^3

A lateral radiograph of his neck is shown in the photograph. Which of the following is the most appropriate immediate management?

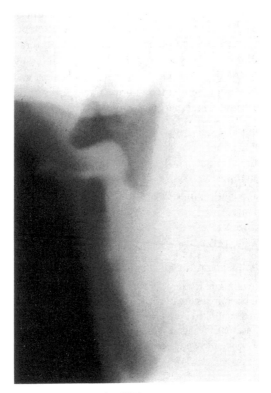

(Used with permission from Susan John, MD.)

a. Examine the throat and obtain a culture.
b. Obtain an arterial blood gas and start an IV line.
c. Administer a dose of nebulized epinephrine.
d. Prepare to establish an airway in the operating room.
e. Admit the child and place him in a mist tent.

196. A 4-year-old boy is seen by the pediatrician for coughing. His mother reports that he has been in good health without recent illnesses. She reports he has a regular diet although notes he tends to eat dirt when left alone. He has had no hospitalizations, recent travel nor day care exposure. On physical examination he is alert, active, and in no distress. Temperature is 37°C (98.6°F), heart rate is 90 beats per minute, and respiratory rate is 24 breaths per minute. Mild wheezing scattered throughout both lung fields is noted. No stridor or retractions are noted. Heart has normal S1 and S2. No murmurs are heard. Abdomen is soft and nontender. The liver edge is palpable 4 cm below the right costal margin. Laboratory data show:

Hemoglobin: 11.2 g/dL
Hematocrit: 33.1%
Platelet count: 215,000/mm^3
WBC: 18,500/mm^3
    Segmented neutrophils: 31%
    Band forms: 1%
    Lymphocytes: 15%
    Eosinophils: 43%

Which of the following is the most appropriate next step?

a. Place a tuberculin skin test.
b. Order a histoplasmin test for *Histoplasma capsulatum*.
c. Obtain an enzyme-linked immunosorbent assay (ELISA) for *Toxocara*.
d. Send gastric aspirate for methenamine silver stain for fungi.
e. Evaluate the stool for ova and parasites.

197. A 10-year-old girl is seen by the pediatrician for a 2-day history of fever and facial pain. The mother reports that she has had a "cold" for 14 days, but in the two previous days she has developed a fever of 39°C (102.2°F), purulent bilateral nasal discharge, facial pain, and a daytime cough. Past medical history is positive for seasonal allergies for which she takes over-the-counter antihistamines. Immunizations are current. On physical examination she is alert, active, and in no distress. Temperature is 37°C (98.6°F), heart rate is 90 beats per minute, and respiratory rate is 24 breaths per minute. Mucous membranes are moist and without lesions. Throat is clear. After instillation of a topical decongestant, the nasal examination shows pus in the middle meatus. Ear canals are patent with translucent tympanic membranes. Which of the following is the most likely diagnosis?

a. Brain abscess
b. Maxillary rhinosinusitis
c. Streptococcal throat infection
d. Sphenoid rhinosinusitis
e. Middle-ear infection

198. A 2-year-old child is seen in the ED for cough and respiratory distress. The father reports that he was awakened in the middle of the night by his son who had developed noisy breathing on inspiration, respiratory distress, and a new barking cough. He has had an upper respiratory infection for the previous 2 days with nasal discharge, sneezing, and a mild, dry cough. Past medical history is negative. His vaccines are current. On physical examination temperature is 38.4°C (101.1°F), heart rate is 90 beats per minute, and respiratory rate is 24 breaths per minute. Nose has clear nasal discharge. Ears canals are patent with translucent tympanic membranes. Chest has good, equal air movement, marked retractions of the chest wall and flaring of the nostrils. A prominent barking cough is heard. Which of the following is the most appropriate next step?

a. Short-acting bronchodilators and a 5-day course of steroids
b. Intubation and antibiotics
c. Observation for hypoxia and dehydration alone
d. Inhaled epinephrine and a dose of steroids
e. Rigid bronchoscopy

199. An 8-year-old girl with well-controlled moderate, persistent asthma visits the clinic for a routine well child check. Medications include about once a month use of short-acting β-agonists, daily inhaled steroids, and a leukotriene inhibitor. On physical examination she is alert, active, and in no distress. Vital signs and growth parameters are normal for age. Mucous membranes are moist with white patches on her buccal mucosa. Nose has slightly clear nasal discharge. Heart has normal S1 and S2 without murmur. Chest has good, equal air movement, without rales or wheezes. Extremities are without clubbing or edema. Which of the following is the most appropriate next step?

a. Order HIV testing.
b. Place a tuberculosis skin test.
c. Measure serum immunoglobulin levels.
d. Discontinue all asthma medications.
e. Suggest she rinse her mouth after use of her inhaled medications.

200. A 13-year-old boy is seen by the pediatrician for fever, malaise, sore throat, and a dry, hacking cough for the previous several days. His mother reports that he has been drinking well, and was more tired than normal, but has been able to manage his homework. On physical examination he does not appear sick. Temperature is 37.2°C (99.9°F), heart rate is 80 beats per minute, and respiratory rate is 24 breaths per minute. Mucous membranes are moist without lesions. Nose has slight clear nasal discharge. Chest has good air movement. Diffuse rales and rhonchi are heard. No retractions or nasal flaring is noted. The chest radiograph is shown in the photograph. Which of the following is the most appropriate therapy?

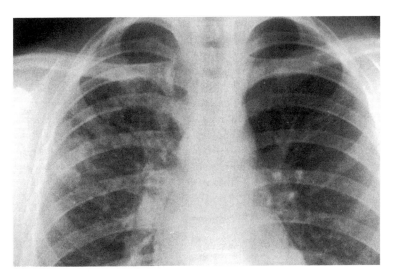

(Used with permission from Susan John, MD.)

a. Intravenous vancomycin
b. Oral isoniazid
c. Intravenous ceftriaxone
d. Intravenous penicillin G
e. Oral azithromycin

201. A 10-year-old boy is seen in the pediatrician's office for his weekly injection of pollen extract as prescribed by his allergist. Minutes after the injection he starts to complain about nausea and a funny feeling in his chest. On physical examination the face is flushed and the voice sounds muffled and strained. Which of the following is the first priority in managing this condition?

a. Preparation for endotracheal intubation
b. Intramuscular injection of diphenhydramine
c. Administration of oxygen
d. Intramuscular injection of 1:1000 epinephrine
e. Intravenous injection of methylprednisolone

202. An 18-month-old child is seen in the ED for drooling and refusal to eat. The family reports that he had been healthy when they heard him in the next room suddenly develop a cough which resolved after a few minutes. Subsequently, they noted him to be normal except for increased amounts of drooling and refusal to take foods. On physical examination he is happy, alert, and in no distress. Temperature is 37°C (98.6°F), heart rate is 100 beats per minute, and respiratory rate is 20 breaths per minute. Mucous membranes are moist and without lesions. Some drooling of saliva is noted. Nose is patent without discharge. Chest has good air movement bilaterally; no rales, wheezes, rhonchi, or retractions are noted. Which of the following tests is most likely to identify the cause of the problem?

a. Barium swallow
b. AP and lateral films of the upper airway
c. Sweat chloride test
d. Plain abdominal (KUB) radiograph
e. AP and lateral chest radiograph

203. A mother calls the clinic triage line, concerned that over the last few hours her 4-year-old child has started breathing fast, coughing, and running a temperature of 40°C (104°F). The past medical history is positive for sickle cell anemia for which the child takes daily penicillin and folate. Which of the following is the most appropriate advice?

a. Prescribe aspirin and ask her to call back if the fever does not respond.
b. Make an office appointment for the next available opening.
c. Make an office appointment for the next day.
d. Refer the child to the laboratory for an immediate hematocrit, WBC count, and differential.
e. Refer the child to the hospital ED.

204. A 5-year-old boy has a history of chronic and recurrent upper respiratory tract infections, several admissions to the hospital for pneumonia, and three surgeries for PE tubes for chronic otitis media. His most recent radiograph is normal other than a right-sided heart. Which of the following is the most likely mechanism of his disease?

a. Eosinophilic infiltrate of the nasal mucosa
b. Infection by *Bordetella pertussis*
c. Absence of nasal mucous glands
d. Random orientation of nasal cilia
e. Obstruction of the nares with nasal polyps

205. A 13-year-old girl is seen in the ED for respiratory distress. Past medical history is significant for sickle cell disease. In the ED, laboratory data show:

CBC
    Hemoglobin: 5 g/dL
    Hematocrit: 16%
  Platelet count: 100,000/mm^3
  WBC: 30,000/mm^3
    Segmented neutrophils: 60%
    Band forms: 1%
    Lymphocytes: 40%
  Arterial blood gas
    pH: 7.10
    PaO_2: 35 mm Hg
    $PaCO_2$: 28 mm Hg
    HCO_3: 16 mEq/L
    Base excess: 8 mmol/L

These values indicate which of the following?

a. Acidemia, metabolic acidosis, respiratory alkalosis, and hypoxia
b. Alkalemia, respiratory acidosis, metabolic alkalosis, and hypoxia
c. Acidosis with compensatory hypoventilation
d. Long-term metabolic compensation for respiratory alkalosis
e. Primary respiratory alkalosis

206. A 3-hour-old neonate is seen by the pediatrician in the low-risk nursery for respiratory distress. The neonate was delivered in the ED after the 24-year-old mother arrived in active labor and delivered the newborn vaginally in the triage area. The mother reported the pregnancy to be term, but that she received no prenatal care after 16 weeks of gestation when she lost her medical insurance. She reports taking daily vitamins containing folate; she denies alcohol, smoking, or other drugs. On physical examination temperature is 37°C (98.6°F), heart rate is 155 beats per minute, and respiratory rate is 60 beats per minute. Nose is patent with bilateral flaring. Heart has normal S1 and S2 with the PMI displaced toward the left. Chest has diminished breath sounds on the right. Subcostal retractions are noted. No rales, wheezes, or rhonchi are noted. The initial chest radiograph is shown in the photograph. A subsequent film shows an NG tube in the stomach to be below the diaphragm. Which of the following is the most likely diagnosis?

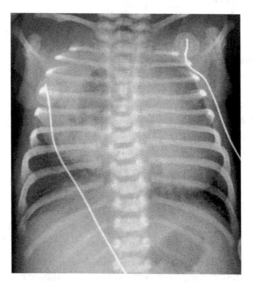

(Used with permission from Susan John, MD.)

a. Congenital pulmonary airway malformation
b. Congenital diaphragmatic hernia
c. Bronchogenic cysts
d. Congenital lobar emphysema
e. Congenital pneumonia

207. A 13-year-old boy is seen in the ED for the sudden onset of high fever, difficulty swallowing, and drooling. His mother reports that he has had a 3-day history of low-grade fever, runny nose, slight cough, and a sore throat. He indicates his throat is exquisitely sore. Temperature is 38.4°C (101.1°F), heart rate is 90 beats per minute, and respiratory rate is 22 breaths per minute. Oral evaluation demonstrates poor handling of oral sections. Teeth are without caries. Pharynx has a fluctuant bulge in the posterior wall. Nose has clear nasal discharge. Chest has good, equal air movement, without wheezes, rhonchi or retractions. A soft tissue radiograph of his neck is shown in the photograph. Which of the following is the most appropriate initial therapy?

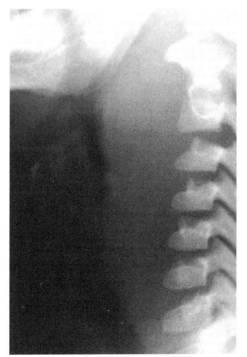

(Used with permission from Susan John, MD.)

a. Intravenous narcotic analgesics
b. Trial of oral penicillin V
c. Surgical consultation
d. Rapid streptococcal screen
e. Monospot test

208. A 6-week-old infant is seen by the pediatrician with the maternal complaint of "breathing fast" and a cough. The infant was born vaginally at term to a 19-year-old woman whose pregnancy was complicated by scant prenatal care. Past medical history includes a bilateral eye discharge at about 3 weeks of age for which antibiotics were prescribed. On physical examination temperature is 37°C (98.6°F), heart rate is 120 beats per minute, respiratory rate is 65 breaths per minute, and oxygen saturation is 94%. Nose is patent with minimal bilateral flaring. Heart has normal S1 and S2 with normal pulses. Chest has good air movement with some subcostal and minimal intercostal retractions. Diffuse rales and rhonchi are noted. Which of the following organisms is the most likely cause of this infant's condition?

a. *Neisseria gonorrhoeae*
b. *S aureus*
c. Group B *Streptococcus*
d. *Chlamydia trachomatis*
e. Herpes virus

209. A 5-year-old girl is seen by the pediatrician for well-child care. The mother reports daily coughing, especially with exercise, necessitating daily use of albuterol. She has coughing fits that awaken her from sleep about twice a week with additional use of her albuterol. Social history is positive for her grandmother recently entering the home. The grandmother had recommended a chihuahua as a "cure" for her asthma, but the child's mother has seen no difference since the arrival of the pet. On physical examination vital signs and growth parameters are normal for age. Nose is patent with slight clear discharge. Heart has normal S1 and S2 with normal pulses. Chest has good air movement without wheezes, rhonchi, or rales. Extremities are without clubbing. Which of the following is the most appropriate next step?

a. Begin as needed long-acting, inhaled β-agonists.
b. Initiate daily leukotriene modifier with as needed short-acting β-agonist.
c. Start inhaled nedocromil with scheduled short-acting β-agonists.
d. Begin medium-dose, inhaled corticosteroids with as needed short-acting β-agonists.
e. Start high-dose, inhaled corticosteroids with theophylline and scheduled short-acting β-agonists.

210. A previously healthy 2-year-old child is seen by the pediatrician for a 6 weeks' history of chronic cough. The family reports that he has been seen in different emergency rooms on two occasions during this period and has been placed on antibiotics for pneumonia. He was a term infant, he takes no medications, and growth and development have been normal. On physical examination vital signs and growth parameters are normal for age. Nose is patent without discharge. Heart has normal S1 and S2 with normal pulses. Chest has good air movement on the left. On the right decreased air movement during inspiration and no air movement upon expiration is found. No wheezes, rhonchi, or rales are heard. Extremities are without clubbing. Inspiratory (Photograph A) and expiratory (Photograph B) radiographs of the chest are shown. Which of the following is the most likely mechanism of disease?

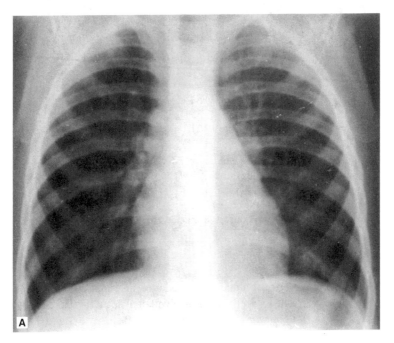

(Used with permission from Susan John, MD.)

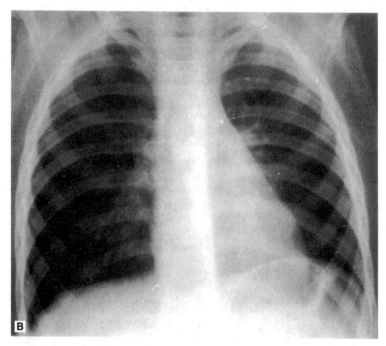

(Used with permission from Susan John, MD.)

a. Mutation of a protein transmembrane conductance regulator gene
b. Aspiration of a foreign body into the airway
c. Infection of the alveoli with bacteria
d. Hyperresponsiveness of the bronchial tree
e. Remodeling of the airways due to chronic obstruction

Questions 211 to 213

The following are arterial blood gases obtained on room air. Match each set of blood gas results with the most likely patient scenario. Each lettered option may be used once, more than once, or not at all.

Base	PCO$_2$ (mm Hg)	PO$_2$ (mm Hg)	Excess pH (mEq/L)
a. 7.20	28	95	16
b. 7.20	70	41	2
c. 7.64	18	94	1
d. 7.34	32	39	8

211. A 14-year-old girl is upset after receiving a text message that her boyfriend was seen with another girl. She begins to cry hysterically, complains of tingling in her hands and feet, and then faints.

212. A 12-year-old boy is admitted for pneumonia. He is awake, alert, and in no respiratory distress. Chest examination has decreased breath sounds in both lung bases. His oxygen saturation is 85%.

213. A 3-day-old newborn at 28 weeks' gestation being mechanically ventilated for infant respiratory distress syndrome suddenly develops worsening respiratory distress and unilaterally diminished breath sounds.

The Respiratory System

Answers

184. The answer is d. (*Hay et al, pp 885-886. Kliegman et al, pp 3406-3408. Rudolph et al, p 1998.*) Neonates born to mothers with gestational diabetes are at risk for being large for gestational age and thus at increased risk for difficult deliveries such as shoulder dystocia, leading to peripheral nerve injuries such as Erb palsy (C5-C6, upper trunk of the brachial plexus), Klumpke palsy (C8-T1, lower trunk) and phrenic nerve (C3, C4, and C5) paralysis. An ultrasound or fluoroscopy of the chest would reveal asymmetric diaphragmatic motion in a seesaw manner. While a chest film can be normal as in this case, an elevated hemidiaphragm may be observed. With a negative chest radiograph, a chest CT would not be helpful at this point. Bronchoscopy would help delineate airway abnormalities and foreign bodies, but would not identify phrenic nerve paralysis.

185. The answer is e. (*Hay et al, pp 526-527. Kliegman et al, pp 2098-2113. Rudolph et al, pp 1977-1986.*) The patient in the question had delayed stooling at birth, a history of large stools and frequent pneumonia, and current evidence of failure to thrive (low weight) and pneumonitis. This constellation of findings suggests cystic fibrosis (CF), a multisystem disease caused by an abnormally functioning CF transmembrane regulator (CFTR) protein. Over 1900 mutations that affect CFTR function have been associated with CF. The most common of these is a phenylalanine deletion at amino acid 508 (ΔF508). Abnormal secretions are produced as a result of decreased permeability of ionized chloride in the secretory epithelium of a number of organs. Progressive lung failure is caused by accumulation of viscid secretions that obstruct the airway and lead to infection, bronchiectasis, and inflammatory changes. Protein and fat malabsorption is related to diminished exocrine pancreatic function. Survival has improved markedly during the past few decades as a result of prompt recognition of CF and aggressive treatment; the median age at death has increased from less than 10 years to almost 40 years. Therapeutic approaches include inhalation therapy, airway clearance therapy (such as chest physiotherapy, flutter valves, or a vibrating vest), aggressive antibiotic administration, bronchodilators, oxygen, and nutritional support. Heart–lung transplants provide prolong life and improve quality of life for some terminal patients. Newer therapies for CF include the use of purified human plasma α_1-antitrypsin, recombinant DNAse, and gene therapy. The rationale for these therapeutic modalities is that they focus directly on ameliorating or correcting the basic deficit: α_1-antitrypsin by counteracting the effects on the lungs of neutrophil elastase, a proteolytic enzyme released by neutrophils; DNAse by reacting with DNA released by dead leukocytes to reduce sputum viscosity; and gene therapy by altering genetic material. Lung cancer does not appear to be associated with CF.

Unlike many other tests, there is almost no overlap in chloride values in sweat between patients with CF and normal control participants. A chloride concentration of more than 60 mEq/L is diagnostic, values less than 40 are normal, and values between 40 and 60 are intermediate. There are about 1700 known mutations in the CFTR gene that can cause CF; genetic studies are commercially available that assay for about 100 of the most common. All 50 states in the United States now test for CF as part of their newborn screen program, and when combined with confirmatory testing, the sensitivity has been reported to be as high as 95%.

Tumors of the airway and aspiration of foreign bodies cause evidence of obstruction with stridor or wheezes. Pneumonia may be seen, but failure to thrive and large stools would be unlikely. Immunoglobulin deficiencies result in frequent infections that are caused by unusual organisms. Failure to thrive may also be seen. Delayed stooling at birth and ongoing, large and malodorous stools are not common features. Atypical bacteria (tuberculosis) can cause acute pneumonitis but would not be expected to result in large stools or delayed stooling at birth.

186. The answer is a. (*Hay et al, pp 538-539. Kliegman et al, pp 2044-2048. Rudolph et al, pp 962, 963, 966.*) The infant in the question has exposure to a virus as well as fever, tachypnea, and mild respiratory distress on examination. The blood gas demonstrates respiratory alkalosis due to the increased respiratory rate. Based on the symptoms, examination findings, and the radiograph (patchy infiltrates with flat diaphragms), bronchiolitis is the most likely diagnosis, and monitoring oxygenation and hydration status (supportive care) is the most appropriate course of action. Bronchodilators and a short course of steroids are treatments for asthma, a less likely diagnosis in this patient without previous wheezing episodes and without a family history of atopy. A single dose of short-acting β-agonist might be trialed in this patient but would likely be of limited benefit. A single dose of steroids would be an appropriate treatment for viral croup; intubation and antibiotics would be the approach to a patient with epiglottitis, and her gas does not reflect impending respiratory failure. Chest tube placement for a pneumothorax may be required if unilateral breath sounds were absent or if the radiograph demonstrated collapse; neither is noted in this case.

The most likely cause of the illness is infection by respiratory syncytial virus, which causes outbreaks of bronchiolitis of varying severity, usually in the winter and spring. Other viruses, such as parainfluenza, influenza, and the adenoviruses have also been implicated in producing bronchiolitis. Treatment is generally supportive in this usually self-limited condition.

187. The answer is b. (*Hay et al, pp 536-537. Kliegman et al, pp 2134-2135. Rudolph et al, pp 997, 1092.*) The physical examination shows evidence of pneumonia with fever, tachypnea, retractions, and reduced air movement with crackles on the left. The x-ray reveals a lung empyema on the left side, characterized by nearly complete whiteout of that side by the pleural or extrapleural fluid collection. An empyema is usually caused by *S aureus*, *S pneumoniae*, or *S pyogenes* (group A strep). These organisms, previously sensitive to penicillin, now have a variety of resistance patterns requiring extended spectrum antibiotics or vancomycin. Patients who do not improve quickly with antibiotic therapy alone are also surgical candidates.

188. The answer is d. (*Hay et al, p 349. Kliegman et al, pp 2063-2064. Rudolph et al, pp 466-467.*) Hydrocarbons with low viscosity and high volatility are the most likely agents to cause respiratory symptoms. Gasoline, kerosene, and furniture polish are common causes of hydrocarbon aspiration. Initially these children often are asymptomatic. Symptoms usually develop within 6 hours of aspiration, and include fever, dyspnea, cyanosis, and respiratory failure. Treatment is symptomatic, sometimes requiring intubation and mechanical ventilation. Induction of emesis is contraindicated; the risk of aspiration with emesis is generally higher than systemic toxicity. Placement of a nasogastric tube is used only in high-volume ingestions or when the hydrocarbon is mixed with another toxin. Charcoal is not useful, and no intravenous binding agent is available.

189. The answer is d. (*Hay et al, pp 1293-1296. Kliegman et al, pp 1455-1461. Rudolph et al, pp 1049-1057.*) The key to controlling tuberculosis in children and eradicating the disease is early detection and appropriate treatment of adult cases; the child, once infected, is at lifelong risk for the development of the disease and for infecting others, unless given appropriate prophylaxis. The usual source of the disease is an infected adult, as is noted in this case. Household contacts of a person with newly diagnosed active disease have a considerable risk of developing active tuberculosis, and the risk is greatest for infants and children. Therefore, when tuberculosis is diagnosed in a child, the immediate family and close contacts should be tested with tuberculin tests and chest radiographs and treated appropriately when indicated. Bronchoscopy would be indicated only in unusual circumstances. Three to eight weeks is required after exposure before hypersensitivity to tuberculin develops. This means that the traditional tuberculin skin test must be repeated in exposed persons if there is a negative reaction at the time when contact with the source of infection is noted. TB skin tests (TSTs) are usually negative in children of this age, even when active disease is ongoing. A logical preventive measure for the 6-week-old baby is the administration of isoniazid for 3 months when a Mantoux (purified protein derivative, PPD) can then be placed. Transmission of tuberculosis occurs when bacilli-laden, small-sized droplets are dispersed into the air by the cough or sneeze of an infected adult. Small children with primary pulmonary tuberculosis are not considered infectious to others, and they are not capable of coughing up and aerosolizing sputum. Sputum, when produced in child of this age, is promptly swallowed, and for this reason specimens for microbial confirmation can be obtained by means of gastric lavage from smaller children.

Standard therapy for pulmonary disease is 6 months of isoniazid and rifampin, along with pyrazinamide and ethambutol for the first 2 months. However, drug resistance is increasing throughout the world. In the United States, approximately 10% of *Mycobacterium tuberculosis* isolates demonstrate resistance to at least one medication, and the rate of resistance is at least twice that in areas of Latin America and Asia. Therefore, isolation of the specific pathogenic organism is very helpful.

A newer TB testing modality, the interferon gamma release assay (IGRA), was FDA approved in stages between 2005 and 2008. These include the QuantiFERON-TB Gold In-Tube (GFT-GIT) test and the T-SPOT.*TB* test. Both screen whole blood for *M tuberculosis* proteins not found in BCG (thus avoiding false-positive skin tests in BCG [Bacillus Calmette–Guérin] vaccine recipients), but may cross react with proteins in nontuberculous mycobacteria (*M kansasii*, *M bovis*) and cause false-positives. White blood cells infected with *M tuberculosis* release interferon gamma (IFN-g) when infected blood is incubated with the synthetic peptides in QFT-GIT (quantifies amount of IFN-g released). In contrast, T-SPOT.*TB* measures the number of "spots" or cells with IFN-g release. Sensitivity and specificity for both are around 90% in children. Results are usually known within 2-3 days.

An IGRA can be used in place of the skin test, and preferentially should be considered in pregnant patients, patients having received BCG, and serial assessment of those infected and treated. In children older than 5 years and patients who may not return for traditional skin testing interpretation, GFT-GIT is the recommended modality. Skin testing or IGRA can be used in children older than 5 years of age and in patient contact evaluation. Performing both a TST and IGRA is not recommended in routine screening, except in select situations (initial negative or indeterminate independent testing but high clinical suspicion, independent testing delivers indeterminate results). IGRA results are reported as positive, negative, or indeterminate (QFT-GIT) or borderline (T-SPOT.*TB*), with indeterminate or borderline results warranting retesting; if results continue to be elusive, another modality such as skin testing should be considered. After noting a positive skin test or IGRA, a thorough physical examination and CXR should be performed.

190. The answer is e. (*Hay et al, pp 546-548. Kliegman et al, pp 2120-2123. Rudolph et al, pp 1992-1993.*) This child likely has idiopathic pulmonary hemosiderosis (IPH). While fever, respiratory distress, and localized chest radiograph findings as described should point initially toward an acute pneumonia, the history of recurrence, the rapid clearing of radiographic findings, and the hemoptysis suggest pulmonary hemorrhage. Digital clubbing suggests a chronic process. Other typical findings would include microcytic and hypochromic anemia, low serum iron levels, and occult blood in the stool (from swallowed pulmonary secretions). Bronchoalveolar lavage will reveal hemosiderin-laden macrophages and would be most likely to make the diagnosis. A distinct subset of patients with pulmonary hemosiderosis has hypersensitivity to cow's milk (the association is called Heiner syndrome) and may improve with a diet free of cow's milk products.

191. The answer is a. (*Hay et al, p 497. Kliegman et al, pp 2008-2009. Rudolph et al, p 1320.*) Young children frequently introduce any number of small objects into their noses, ranging from food to small toys. Initially, only local irritation occurs. Later, as prolonged obstruction is seen, symptoms increase to include worsening of pain, and a purulent, malodorous, bloody discharge can be seen. Unilateral nasal discharge in the presence of obstruction suggests the need to examine the patient for a nasal foreign body.

Polyps are a possible cause of unilateral nasal obstruction, but at 18 months of age they are unusual and would suggest a diagnosis of CF. Frontal sinusitis usually does not cause unilateral symptoms, and sinusitis in an 18-month-old child is unusual owing to poor sinus development. Similarly, a deviated septum is not found in small children. Choanal atresia would present in the newborn period with periods of respiratory distress at rest with improvement with crying.

192. The answer is b. (*Hay et al, pp 503-505. Kliegman et al, pp 114-118. Rudolph et al, pp 1940-1942.*) Obstructive sleep apnea (OSA) is fairly common, occurring in about 2% of normal children. Factors such as obesity and craniofacial abnormalities increase the risk. Symptoms suggestive of sleep apnea include snoring, frequent nighttime awakenings, changes in behavior, bedwetting, and of course witnessed apnea. While obesity contributes to OSA, poor growth may be a symptom. Chronic OSA can lead to cor pulmonale. Significant overlap is seen with the symptoms of OSA and attention-deficit/hyperactivity disorder (ADHD), and thyroid problems can cause behavioral disturbances. In this case, however, the reported snoring and daytime sleepiness suggests OSA. Snoring children with quality-of-life issues as in the patient described in the case should be evaluated by ENT (otolaryngology); tonsillectomy and adenoidectomy may be indicated. Children who just snore, do not have quality-of-life issues, do not have enlarged tonsils, and do not have gasping, apnea, or long pauses in breathing while sleeping may be observed. A polysomnogram would be most helpful in a snoring child with markedly enlarged (4+) tonsils but who did not have a history of gasping while sleeping nor quality-of-life issues during the day, as the results of the study in that situation would help guide further management.

193. The answer is b. (*Hay et al, p 1258. Kliegman et al, p 1317. Rudolph et al, pp 440, 959-961.*) Necrotizing pneumonitis, a recognized complication of staphylococcal (and other) pneumonia, is caused by toxin production by the bacteria leading to rupture of the alveoli into the pleural space. Tension pneumothorax may result, and can be quickly lethal if not recognized and treated; this makes a high index of suspicion and prompt diagnosis mandatory. The other complications (effusion, pneumatocele) can also occur but do not require so prompt a response. Immediate action to relieve the pressure of a tension pneumothorax is essential, usually accomplished by inserting a needle or catheter into the second or third intercostal spaces in the midclavicular line while the patient is supine. Administering a sedative to a patient with respiratory distress is not wise unless you are planning on immediate intubation.

194. The answer is a. (*Hay et al, p 521. Kliegman et al, pp 2035-2036. Rudolph et al, p 1952.*) Bacterial tracheitis is an uncommon but severe and life-threatening sequela of viral laryngotracheobronchitis. The typical story is that presented in the case, with several days of viral upper respiratory symptoms, followed by an acute elevation of temperature and an increase in respiratory distress. Inspiratory stridor is typical in croup; the biphasic stridor and high fever in this patient should be clues to consider alternative diagnoses. Children may also present acutely and without the initial viral symptoms. The differential must include epiglottitis; the lack of drooling and dysphagia (and the rarity of epiglottitis since the introduction of the *Haemophilus influenzae* type B vaccine) help make this less likely. Management for tracheitis includes establishing an airway with endotracheal intubation and IV antibiotics. Special attention is focused on preservation of the airway, as even intubated children with tracheitis can have secretions thick and copious enough to occlude the airway.

Oral antibiotics and outpatient follow-up for a patient with respiratory distress and toxic appearance are never appropriate. Inhaled epinephrine and oral steroids as well as observation in a cool mist tent suggest a diagnosis of croup, a disease that presents without high fever but with inspiratory stridor a few days into an upper respiratory infection. Note that cool mist tents, while for years a mainstay of hospital treatment for croup, do not seem to affect outcome, and may serve as a barrier to caregivers to properly assess the child. In the case presentation, the fever and toxic appearance differentiate this condition from viral croup. Intravenous methylprednisolone is a component of treatment for asthma, a diagnosis unlikely in a patient with high fever as outlined.

195. The answer is d. (*Hay et al, p 521. Kliegman et al, pp 2032-2033. Rudolph et al, p 1040.*) In the past, epiglottitis was most commonly caused by invasive *H influenzae* type B. Due to the widespread use of the Hib vaccine, this condition is now more commonly caused by group A β-hemolytic

Streptococcus, Moraxella catarrhalis, or *S pneumoniae.* The radiography shows the typical "thumb" sign of a swollen epiglottis. The CBC shows an elevated white blood count with left shift. Epiglottitis is a life-threatening form of infection-produced upper airway obstruction. The course of the illness is brief and prodromal symptoms are lacking. The patient experiences a sudden onset of sore throat, high fever, and prostration that is out of proportion to the duration of the illness. Drooling and difficulty in swallowing, a muffled voice, and preference for a characteristic sitting posture with the neck hyperextended may be noted. Radiography of the neck, which may delay definitive treatment, is often avoided. Rather, preparations are made for immediate intubation by skilled personnel, and any attempt to visualize mechanically the epiglottis should be avoided until these preparations are complete and the child is in a controlled environment. Morbidity and mortality are usually related to a delay in establishing an airway early in the disease. Croup was historically treated with a mist tent and inhaled epinephrine. Obtaining an arterial blood sample would cause significant pain and crying and could hasten airway compromise.

196. The answer is c. (*Hay et al, pp 1328-1329. Kliegman et al, pp 1743-1744. Rudolph et al, p 1197.*) The presentation described is characteristic of visceral larva migrans from infestation with a common parasite of dogs, *Toxocara canis.* Dirt-eating children ingest the infectious ova. The larvae penetrate the intestine and migrate to visceral sites, such as the liver, lung, and brain, but do not return to the intestine, so the stools do not contain the ova or parasites. The physical examination in this case shows complications of wheezes and hepatomegaly. The CBC shows mild anemia with significant eosinophilia. The diagnosis can be confirmed by a specific ELISA for *Toxocara.* Patients with minimal symptoms may be managed expectantly, while patients with more significant symptoms may be treated with albendazole. Some experts recommend concomitant therapy with steroids to decrease the inflammatory response from dying parasites. Ocular larval migrans, also caused by *T canis,* can present with unilateral vision loss, eye pain, and strabismus.

197. The answer is b. (*Hay et al, pp 493-495. Kliegman et al, pp 2014-2017. Rudolph et al, pp 1321-1324.*) Maxillary and ethmoid sinuses are large enough to harbor infections from infancy. Frontal sinuses are rarely large enough to harbor infections until the sixth to tenth year of life. Sphenoid sinuses do not become large until about the third to fifth year of life. In general, a "cold" lasting longer than 10-14 days with fever and facial pain is suggestive of rhinosinusitis. Examination of the nose can reveal pus draining from the middle meatus in maxillary, frontal, or anterior ethmoid sinusitis. Pus in the superior meatus indicates sphenoid or posterior ethmoid sinuses. Diagnosis is on clinical grounds and can be difficult. Positive findings on plain sinus films in a symptomatic child are supportive of sinusitis. CT scans are more sensitive but are usually reserved for the more complicated cases. The treatment is usually oral antibiotics for 10-14 days. Decongestants and antihistamines have not been shown to be helpful or necessary. Saline washes may help with symptoms; intranasal steroids have shown moderate benefit.

Brain abscess is unlikely in this patient who demonstrates no neurologic symptoms. A streptococcal throat infection classically presents with acute onset of sore throat without other signs and symptoms of upper respiratory infection. Sphenoid sinusitis usually does not cause facial pain or drainage from the middle meatus. The child might have a middle-ear infection coincident with a sinusitis, but her lack of ear pain and normal ear examination suggests otherwise.

198. The answer is d. (*Hay et al, pp 520-521. Kliegman et al, pp 2031-2034. Rudolph et al, pp 1951-1952.*) Subglottic edema that develops as part of an upper respiratory tract infection results in the inspiratory stridor commonly heard with laryngotracheobronchitis (croup). The extrathoracic airway tends to collapse on inspiration, producing the characteristic findings this patient demonstrates; therapy usually is with a single dose of steroids. Agents causing croup include parainfluenza types 1 and 3, influenza A and B, RSV, and occasionally other viruses. Affected children are typically between the ages of 6 months and 5 years. Treatment is usually supportive, but racemic epinephrine and corticosteroids reduce the length of time in the emergency room and hospitalizations. Inspiratory stridor at rest and/or hypoxia are indications for admission and close observation.

Intrathoracic airway diseases, such as asthma (bronchodilators and short course of steroids) or bronchiolitis (supportive therapy including observation for hypoxia or dehydration alone), produce breathing difficulty on expiration, with expiratory wheezing, prolonged expiration, and evidence of air trapping on radiographs.

Acute airway foreign body (rigid bronchoscopy) should result in differential air movement between the two lungs; a foreign object may create a ball-valve effect, leading to air trapping and hyperinflation on the affected side. The typical case of epiglottis (intubation and antibiotics) presents acutely and the child is toxic in appearance; it is now a rare disease with the widespread use of vaccines.

199. The answer is e. (*Hay et al, pp 1124-1141. Kliegman et al, pp 1095-1115. Rudolph et al, pp 1969-1970.*) The patient in the question is a normally appearing child who has well-controlled, moderate, persistent asthma for which the National Heart, Lung and Blood Institute of the US National Institutes of Health recommends daily inhaled corticosteroids as a controller medication. Failure to rinse her mouth after administration of this medication can result in localized candida infection (thrush). Discontinuation of her asthma medications is contraindicated. While it is possible she has an immune dysfunction, simply rinsing her mouth is more likely to be both diagnostic and therapeutic. A child over the age of one with thrush and no history of inhaled steroids should be evaluated for immunodeficiency.

200. The answer is e. (*Hay et al, pp 539-540. Kliegman et al, pp 1487-1490. Rudolph et al, pp 1066-1068.*) The clinical description is of a child with fever and diffuse pneumonic process. The radiograph shown has reticulonodular opacities in the right upper lobe and prominence of the right hilum (lymphadenopathy) consistent with *M pneumoniae*. Infections with *M pneumoniae* are common in older children and young adults, less so in infants and toddlers. Although the infection typically produces an interstitial infiltrate, its effects are characteristically nonspecific, and it can produce lobar pneumonia as well. It can produce upper respiratory infection, pharyngitis, otitis media and externa, bronchiolitis, hemolytic anemia, and Guillain-Barré syndrome. Treatment of choice is a macrolide antibiotic.

Intravenous vancomycin is used for severe pneumonia, usually when *S aureus* is suspected. Staphylococcal pneumonia is uncommon in the normal adolescent, but rather is traditionally seen in infants less than 6 months of age. Other organisms for which ceftriaxone or penicillin G might be used (*H influenzae* and *S pneumoniae*) present with more sudden onset of high fever and lobar pneumonia, often with pleural effusion. *H influenzae* was seen in younger children in the past but is rarely seen now because of the widespread use of *H influenzae* type B vaccine; it typically is resistant to penicillin G. A switch from a broad-spectrum antibiotic such as ceftriaxone to penicillin G would be appropriate for patients with *S pneumoniae* but only after the organism was proven in laboratory testing to be sensitive.

At this age, a child with *M tuberculosis* presents most typically with hilar adenopathy and localized lobar pneumonia in the upper lobe, and *S pneumoniae* causes the sudden onset of high fever and a lobar pneumonia, often with pleural effusion. A TB skin test for this patient would be reasonable.

201. The answer is a. (*Hay et al, pp 1154-1156. Kliegman et al, pp 1131-1136. Rudolph et al, pp 777-778.*) Anaphylaxis is a medical emergency that must be recognized and managed promptly. The onset of symptoms is usually dramatic. In the case presented, the change in voice suggests impending airway compromise, making airway stabilization your top priority. The other choices are all important in managing anaphylaxis and, in reality, may be occurring concurrently; of those listed, intramuscular epinephrine would be the first medication used, and should be repeated every 5-15 minutes as necessary to maintain blood pressures and manage symptoms. Additional treatment can include plasma expanders, diphenhydramine (an H1 antihistamine), and ranitidine (an H2 antihistamine), as indicated by the clinical course of the patient. Additional treatment such as administration of corticosteroids should be started early, but the effect will be delayed. Mortality from anaphylaxis occurs as a result of upper airway edema and asphyxiation, severe bronchial obstruction causing respiratory failure, or cardiovascular collapse. Children with anaphylaxis should always have an epinephrine auto-injector available. Many schools now maintain auto-injectors as part of the school nurse's supplies.

202. The answer is e. (*Hay et al, pp 631-632. Kliegman et al, pp 1793-1794. Rudolph et al, pp 449-450, 1412-1413.*) Many types of objects produce esophageal obstruction in young children, including small toys, coins, and food. Most are lodged below the cricopharyngeal muscle at the level of the aortic arch. Initially, the foreign body may cause cough, drooling, and choking. Later, pain, avoidance of food (liquids are tolerated better), and shortness of breath can develop. Diagnosis is by history (as outlined in the question) and by radiographs (especially if the object is radiopaque). The usual treatment is removal of the object via esophagoscopy; this is particularly urgent if the object is a button battery.

Severe gastroesophageal reflux, diagnosed with a barium swallow, would likely not present with acute findings as those outlined in the question, but rather with ongoing respiratory symptoms (asthma or pneumonia) or failure to thrive. Symptoms of foreign body in the airway, for which an AP and lateral film of the upper airway might be helpful, may present acutely as described with resolution as the offending object settles in the lung, but the patient's refusal to eat and drooling would not be expected. Sweat chloride testing is appropriate for the child with signs and symptoms of CF such as delayed passage of meconium at birth, ongoing large and bulky stools, failure to thrive and frequent pneumonia. A KUB would show a foreign body in or beyond the stomach and might show evidence of previous ingestion, but it would not be helpful as an initial test in identifying the reason for the acute symptoms described associated with refusal to eat.

203. The answer is e. (*Hay et al, pp 913-916. Kliegman et al, pp 2336-2345. Rudolph et al, pp 1531-1534.*) Fever, cough, and tachypnea in a patient with sickle cell anemia can be manifestations of pneumonia, pulmonary vaso-occlusive crisis, or sepsis. Aside from being relatively common in patients with sickle cell anemia, these diseases can be rapidly progressive and quickly fatal. It is therefore important for the patient to be evaluated and treated on an emergency basis. Children with sickle cell and fever are typically managed in the hospital with empiric antibiotics; without a functional spleen, they are at increased risk for serious bacterial infection.

204. The answer is d. (*Hay et al, pp 527-528. Kliegman et al, pp 2114-2115. Rudolph et al, pp 1955-1957.*) Patients with primary ciliary dyskinesia (PCD, also known as immotile cilia syndrome) have dysfunctional cilia and, as such, have abnormal airway clearance. Described structural aberrations include abnormal cytoskeletal proteins and defects in the dynein arms. Kartagener syndrome (the triad of situs inversus, chronic sinusitis and otitis media, and airway disease) is associated with PCD; approximately 50% of patients with the latter also have the former. Although it is a chronic disease, patients with PCD can have a normal life span.

Allergic rhinitis can cause polyps and eosinophilia on a nasal smear (seen with Hansel stain), but the history in the vignette is not an allergic one. *Bordetella pertussis* infection is not commonly found in immunized children, but it can be found in adults. Pertussis does not cause the chronic and recurrent findings in the vignette.

205. The answer is a. (*Hay et al, pp 724-725. Kliegman et al, pp 374-384. Rudolph et al, pp 1684-1686.*) While some texts use the terms acidosis and acidemia interchangeably, there are subtle differences. The low pH in the arterial blood can be called *acidemia* (the state of a low pH in the blood);

it is caused by a metabolic *acidosis* (the process leading to the low pH) that is a direct result of poor perfusion and lactic acid produced by anaerobic metabolism in tissues with inadequate oxygen delivery. Inadequate oxygenation is caused by the low PO_2, the low oxygen-carrying capacity of the blood (Hgb 5 g/dL), and circulatory inadequacy due to the sickling itself and to the vascular disease it produces. The low PCO_2 reflects the hyperventilation, which is secondary to the respiratory difficulty, and to the anemia, and is also respiratory compensation for the metabolic acidosis. Note that some texts distinguish the two terms by using acidemia to refer specifically to inborn errors of metabolism that lead to low serum pH.

206. The answer is a. (*Hay et al, p 532. Kliegman et al, pp 2057-2059. Rudolph et al, p 1931.*) The vignette is of a newborn with early onset respiratory distress. Large lesions in the lung (as that noted on the radiograph on the patient's right side) may compress the affected lung and cause pulmonary hypoplasia, and cause midline shift away from the lesion (note the heart is shifted toward the patient's left on the radiograph). Of the choices, congenital pulmonary airway malformation (CPAM, formerly referred to as congenital cystic adenomatoid malformation, or CCAM) is the most likely etiology. CPAM is thought to arise from an embryonic disruption before the 35th day that causes improper development of bronchioles. The cystic mass is usually identified on prenatal ultrasound around the 20th week, but this woman's lack of prenatal care precluded that early diagnosis. Treatment is typically surgical excision of the affected lobe. Although some CPAMs spontaneously resolve, there have been reports of malignant potential, so observation alone should be a very cautious choice. Intrauterine intervention options include placing a thoracoamniotic shunt to drain fluid and decrease the size of the mass, as well as open fetal surgical resection. The latter procedure is reserved for the fetus with a very large mass compressing the heart that would likely die in utero without intervention; even with this procedure, only about half of the affected infants survive.

Congenital diaphragmatic hernia results in the stomach's displacement into the thoracic cavity; the NG tube would be expected to be located above the diaphragm. A congenital bronchogenic cyst presents with signs of vital structure compression such as respiratory distress or esophageal obstruction; the radiograph might show a spherical mass off of the bronchus often located in the mediastinum around the carina. In older patients this lesion may result in chest pain and dysphagia or with recurrent chest infections. Congenital lobar emphysema is usually detected during prenatal care as an overinflated, fluid-filled mass on ultrasound. Postnatally it may present in the early period with respiratory distress, hyperresonance on examination, absent breath sounds over the lesion, and an area of hyperlucency on plain radiography, often with shift of the mediastinal structures. Congenital pneumonia would be expected to present with temperature instability, respiratory distress, crackles on examination, and radiographic evidence of bilateral infiltrates.

207. The answer is c. (*Hay et al, p 501. Kliegman et al, pp 2021-2022. Rudolph et al, pp 1327, 1952.*) Suppurative infection of the chain of lymph nodes between the posterior pharyngeal wall and the prevertebral fascia leads to retropharyngeal abscesses. The most common causative organisms are *S aureus*, group A β-hemolytic streptococci, and oral anaerobes. Presenting signs and symptoms include a history of pharyngitis, abrupt onset of fever with severe sore throat, refusal of food, drooling, and muffled or noisy breathing. Pain with flexion and extension of the neck may be confused with meningismus. A bulge in the posterior pharyngeal wall is diagnostic, as are radiographs of the lateral neck that reveal the retropharyngeal mass (the radiograph in the question demonstrates thickening of the prevertebral space). Palpation (with adequate provision for emergency control of the airway in case of rupture) reveals a fluctuant mass. Treatment should include incision and drainage if fluctuance is present. The other answers listed would delay definitive treatment and/or might be life-threatening.

208. The answer is d. (*Hay et al, pp 1299-1301. Kliegman et al, pp 1493-1496. Rudolph et al, pp 1033-1034.*) Chlamydiae organisms, sexually transmitted among adults, are spread to infants during birth from genitally infected mothers. The sites of infection in infants are the conjunctivae and the lungs, where chlamydiae cause inclusion conjunctivitis and afebrile pneumonia, respectively, in neonates between 2 and 12 weeks of age. Diagnosis is confirmed by culture of secretions and by antibody titers. In adolescents, chlamydial infections may be a cause of cervicitis, salpingitis, endometritis, and epididymitis and appear to be an important cause of tubal infertility. The most common treatment for this condition includes macrolide antibiotics orally, which clears both the nasopharyngeal secretions when conjunctivitis is present and prevents the pneumonia that can occur later. Topical treatment for chlamydia conjunctivitis is not effective in clearing the nasopharynx. Early treatment with oral macrolides is, however, associated with an increased incidence in the development of idiopathic hypertrophic pyloric stenosis; they must be used with caution in the neonatal period, and empiric prophylaxis is not recommended.

Neisseria gonorrhoeae can cause a sepsis syndrome in children (and not just respiratory symptoms), but its presentation would be in the first days of life and not at 6 weeks, and the infant would be toxic. *Staphylococcus aureus*, and more unusually group B *Streptococcus* (which more likely would occur in the first days of life), can cause pneumonia in a child of this age, but the presentation would more likely be of a toxic, febrile child. Herpes virus, when it causes pneumonia, does so more likely in a child in the first days of life; the infant is toxic.

209. The answer is d. (*Hay et al, pp 1124-1143. Kliegman et al, pp 1095-1115. Rudolph et al, pp 1962-1973.*) Asthma may be classified by severity based on the frequency of symptoms, and is stratified by age. Children 5-11 years old with *mild intermittent* asthma have symptoms less than two times a week and have less than two nighttime episodes a month. These patients do not require daily medication and only short-acting β-agonists are needed. The second classification is *mild persistent* asthma; these children have symptoms more than two times a week, and have three to four nights a month with symptoms. These patients are typically managed with daily low-dose inhaled corticosteroids for control and short-acting β-agonists as needed for rescue; daily mast cell stabilizers such as cromolyn, or leukotriene inhibitors such as montelukast, are listed as alternatives for controller therapy. This patient has *moderate persistent* asthma; she has daily symptoms and difficulty at night more than once a week. Her treatment should consist of medium-dose corticosteroids, or a combination of low-dose corticosteroids and a long-acting β-agonist; alternatives include a leukotriene modifier or sustained-release theophylline, although the latter is rarely used today due to its narrow therapeutic window and interactions with other medications. Patients with *severe persistent* asthma have continual symptoms and frequent nighttime symptoms. This group requires daily high-dose inhaled steroids as well as long-acting β-agonists; they may require oral steroids as well. Note that the latest guidelines make a distinction between 0-4 years and 5-11 years; the younger children require less frequent symptoms to be classified in a particular zone. Many unproven cultural "cures" exist for a variety of diseases. Among them is the false belief that chihuahua dogs will "take on" the child's asthma, thus transferring the disease from the child to the animal.

210. The answer is b. (*Hay et al, p 525. Kliegman et al, pp 2039-2040. Rudolph et al, pp 449-451.*) Recurrent unilateral pneumonias in an otherwise healthy child should suggest the potential for anatomic blockage of an airway. In the patient in this question, the findings on clinical examination suggest a foreign body in the airway. Inspiratory and expiratory films can be helpful. Routine inspiratory films are likely to appear normal or near normal (as outlined in the question and noted in the first radiograph). Expiratory films can identify air trapping distal to the foreign body (as noted on the second radiograph). It is uncommon for the foreign body to be visible on the plain radiograph; a negative radiograph does not eliminate the possibility of a foreign body, and a high index of suspicion is necessary to make the diagnosis. Suspected foreign bodies in the airway are potentially diagnosed with fluoroscopy, but rigid bronchoscopy is not only diagnostic but also the treatment of choice for removal of the foreign body. Recurrent unilateral pneumonia is unlikely to be CF (caused by a mutation of a protein transmembrane conductance regulator gene) which rather presents classically with delayed stooling at birth, recurrent pneumonias, nasal polyps, failure to thrive, and large, bulky, malodorous stools. Infection of the alveoli with bacteria (pneumonia) typically results in fever, cough, rales, and radiographic findings of infiltrates. Asthma is caused in part by hyperresponsiveness of the bronchial tree that ultimately causes remodeling of the airways due to chronic obstruction; signs and symptoms are of episodes of bilateral wheezing that are responsive to bronchodilator or steroid therapy.

211-213. The answers are 211-c, 212-d, 213-b. (*Hay et al, pp 724-725. Kliegman et al, pp 373-384. Rudolph et al, pp 1684-1686.*) The laboratory results of row C indicate a striking respiratory alkalosis. This could be secondary to voluntary hyperventilation or inappropriate respirator settings for a patient on a ventilator. The findings are also typical of acute hyperventilation syndrome secondary to anxiety; such a patient can complain of dyspnea, chest pain, tingling, and dizziness, and can even have generalized convulsions secondary to low ionized calcium levels (alkalosis increases binding of calcium to protein, resulting in decreased ionized calcium). Rebreathing into a paper bag can be both therapeutic and diagnostic.

The blood gases of row D are the only ones shown that are relatively normal, except for a low-oxygen partial pressure. The mild respiratory alkalosis and metabolic acidosis can be a consequence of the hypoxia. These results could be obtained in a patient with moderately severe pneumonia, bronchiolitis or asthma, or secondary to ventilation-perfusion inequality with some areas of the lung underventilated with respect to perfusion. This cause of hypoxia can be easily corrected by giving the patient relatively small increases in oxygen concentration to breathe. These results would also be typical of findings in patients with right-to-left shunting of blood, as in tetralogy of Fallot, in which case giving oxygen would not help.

The blood gases of row B demonstrate an uncompensated respiratory acidosis with hypoxia but with no metabolic acidosis. This is compatible with acute hypoventilation, which could be produced by a tension pneumothorax, for example, in a premature baby who is being ventilated for respiratory distress syndrome. This can be treated easily by placing a needle or catheter in the pleural space and evacuating the air.

The results in row A show fairly severe metabolic acidosis with respiratory compensation and without hypoxia. These would be typical for someone in early shock and would most commonly be seen in children with diarrhea. Treatment of this type of acidosis is hydration.

The Gastrointestinal Tract

Questions

214. A 4-year-old boy is seen by the pediatrician with the parental complaint of constipation since the child was about 6 months old. The family reports that he produces "large and hard" stools every 3-4 days. They deny nausea, vomiting, fever, change in behavior, or blood in his stools. He was born at term, voided and stooled in the first day of life, and was discharged to home on the third day of life. Subsequently he has been a healthy child and his immunizations are current. Today his temperature is 37°C (98.6°F), and his heart rate is 90. His weight is at the 75th percentile, length at the 65th percentile, and the head circumference at the 75th percentile. The abdomen is somewhat full but soft and nontender. Rectal examination reveals a large ampulla, poor sphincter tone but an intact anal wink, and stool in the rectal vault. The plain film of his abdomen is shown in the photograph. Which of the following is the most appropriate next step in management?

a. Obtain a lower gastrointestinal (GI) barium study.
b. Provide parental reassurance and dietary counseling.
c. Measure serum electrolytes.
d. Order an upper GI contrast study.
e. Initiate thyroid-replacement hormone.

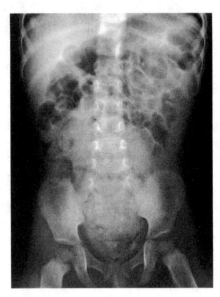

(Used with permission from Susan John, MD.)

215. A 10-year-old boy is seen by the pediatric nurse practitioner for "bellyaches" of 2 years' duration. He reports the pain to be dull and achy, especially in the epigastric area, predominantly at night. The family states that he occasionally vomits after the onset of pain, but has had no fever or weight loss. They report his stools are dark. He has tried over-the-counter antacid tablets with variable relief. He does well in school. Family history is positive for his father also having frequent, nonspecific stomachaches. Growth parameters are at the 50th percentile. The mucous membranes are pink, moist, and without lesions. His abdomen is soft and nontender. No hepatosplenomegaly or adenopathy is noted. Which of the following is most appropriate next step?

a. Endoscopic evaluation for *Helicobacter pylori.*
b. Obtain a CT scan of the abdomen.
c. Order a Meckel scan.
d. Provide reassurance to the patient and family.
e. Obtain early morning peri-rectal adhesive tape sample for microscopy.

216. An 8-year-old presents in clinic for follow up after an upper endoscopy; he was referred to GI for a 2-year history of intermittent vomiting, dysphagia, epigastric pain, and occasionally "getting food stuck in his throat." His father reports that the child has been taking oral calcium carbonate (Tums) for 18 months without symptom relief. He denies fever, headache, bloody stools, or weight loss. Past medical history is significant for eczema and a peanut allergy. His development and growth have been normal. On physical examination his oral pharynx is normal. Chest is clear. Abdomen is soft, nontender, and without hepatosplenomegaly. Endoscopy results show:

Normal anatomy without erosive lesions noted. Biopsy reveals many eosinophils.

Which of the following is the most appropriate next step?

a. Prescribe a fluticasone inhaler.
b. Initiate prolonged course of proton pump inhibitors.
c. Prescribe "swish and swallow" nystatin oral solution to use four times daily.
d. Surgical consultation for fundoplication.
e. Observation.

217. A 1-week-old neonate is seen in the emergency room for the acute onset of bilious vomiting. The neonate has been doing well at home, exclusively breast-feeding every 2½-3 hours, voiding and stooling, and without irritability or lethargy until the emesis and extreme irritability began about 2 hours previously. The family denies fever and diarrhea. The infant was born via vaginal delivery after a benign pregnancy. Discharge was at 48 hours of age and the 3-day early follow-up visit was unremarkable. On physical examination the newborn has a heart rate of 140 beats per minute, a respiratory rate of 40 breaths per minute, and is very irritable. The abdomen is distended and tender throughout without hepatosplenomegaly. A bloody stool is found in the diaper. The abdominal plain film in the emergency department (Photograph A) and a stat barium enema (Photograph B) are shown. Which of the following is the most likely diagnosis?

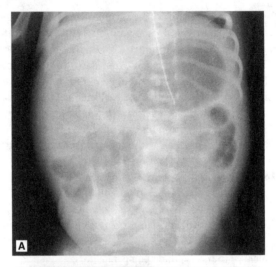

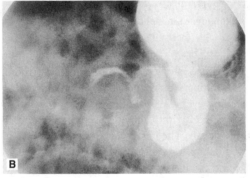

(Used with permission from Susan John, MD.)

a. Jejunal atresia
b. Hypertrophic pyloric stenosis
c. Malrotation with volvulus
d. Acute appendicitis
e. Intussusception

218. The newborn nursery nurse reports that a 1-day-old male newborn has developed abdominal distension and has had one bilious emesis. His mother reports that he initially fed infant formula by bottle well, but has since reduced intake. Delivery was a scheduled repeat cesarean section to a 31-year-old woman whose pregnancy was complicated by hypertension and fetal ultrasound findings of echogenic areas of bowel. Physical examination shows a normal appearing infant without dysmorphic features. The vital signs are normal. Chest is clear without rales, rhonchi, or retractions. Heart has normal S1 and S2 with normal pulses. Abdomen is nontender but distended. Bowel sounds are active. No hepatosplenomegaly is noted. Anus is patent, but the infant has not stooled yet. Genitourinary examination is normal. The plain abdominal radiograph and contrast enema are shown in photographs A and B. Which of the following is the most likely diagnosis?

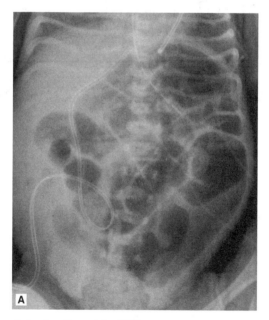

(Used with permission from Susan John, MD.)

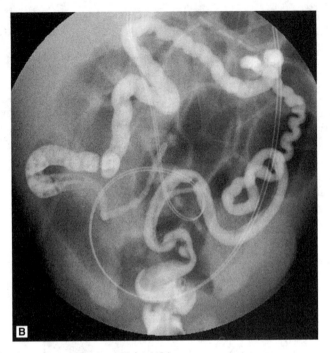

(Used with permission from Susan John, MD.)

a. Duodenal atresia
b. Cystic fibrosis (CF)
c. Gastroenteritis
d. Malrotation with volvulus
e. Hirschsprung disease

219. A 15-year-old girl is seen by the pediatrician for a 5-month history of weight loss of about 6 kg, intermittent bloody diarrhea, and intermittent fever. She reports cramping abdominal pain with bowel movements but no vomiting. Past medical history is positive for attention deficit disorder which is well controlled with daily oral stimulant medication. She denies smoking, alcohol, or other drug use except for occasional acetaminophen for the fever. She is sexually active with one partner and reports consistent barrier prophylaxis use. She began her menses at 13; her last cycle was about 12 days prior. On physical examination her heart rate is 75 beats per minute and her blood pressure is 101/68 mm Hg. Oral mucosa is pink and without lesions. Chest is clear. Heart has normal S1 and S2. Distal pulses are normal; no murmur is found. Abdomen is soft, minimally tender, and without hepatosplenomegaly. Bowel sounds are slightly hyperactive. Anus is patent without lesions. Genitourinary examination has normal external female genitalia; bimanual examination is without pain; no vaginal discharge is noted. Laboratory data show:

CBC
  Hemoglobin: 9.9 g/dL
  Hematocrit: 30.1%
  Mean corpuscular volume (MCV): 50 fL
  Many microcytes noted on smear
  WBC: 8000/mm^3
    Segmented neutrophils: 60%
    Band forms: 1%
    Lymphocytes: 39%
  Platelet count: 199,000/mm^3
Erythrocyte sedimentation rate (ESR): 70 mm/h

Serum:
  Anti-*Saccharomyces cerevisiae* antibodies (ASCA) negative
  Antineutrophil cytoplasm antibodies (p-ANCA) positive

Stool:
  Guaiac positive
  Routine cultures negative

Urine pregnancy test negative

Which of the following is the most appropriate next step in management?

a. Order serum lead levels.
b. Obtain stools culture on sorbitol MacConkey (SMAC) agar plates.
c. Assay stool for *Clostridium difficile* toxins A and B.
d. Perform CT scan of the abdomen.
e. Arrange for a colonoscopy.

220. A 4-year-old child is seen by the pediatric nurse practitioner for constipation. The mother reports the child has about one stool per week despite frequent use of stool softeners. She denies diarrhea and reports that he is becoming "potty trained" with only rare fecal soiling. He has had no emesis, fever, or weight loss. Growth and development are normal compared to her other children. He was born by repeat cesarean delivery at term, voided in the delivery room, passed stool at 48 hours of age, and was discharged at 72 hours of age with his mother. Past medical history is significant for occasional upper respiratory infections. On physical examination he is alert, awake, and in no distress. Mucous membranes are moist without lesions. Distal pulses are normal. Abdomen is distended with palpable dilated loops of bowel. Rectal examination results in forceful expulsion of feces. Which of the following is the most appropriate next step?

a. Counsel family about stool retention patterns and provide parental reassurance.
b. Arrange for a barium enema and rectal manometry.
c. Obtain plain films of the abdomen.
d. Increase fiber intake and maintain dietary log.
e. Begin an oral antispasmodic medication.

221. A 6-week-old boy is seen by the pediatrician for emesis. The mother reports that he had been doing well until the previous 10 days when he developed emesis that has increased in frequency and in forcefulness. Because of the emesis she has switched from breast milk to infant formula, and describes him as eating vigorously but within a few minutes of the feeding he has emesis consisting only of formula. He was born vaginally at term after an uncomplicated pregnancy. Birth weight was 3200 g (7 lb, 1 oz). He voided in the delivery room, passed stool at 12 hours of age, and was discharged at 48 hours of age with his mother. He takes vitamin D daily. Family history is unremarkable. On physical examination weight is 3300 g (7 lb, 3 oz). Mucous membranes are moist without lesions. Abdomen is soft, nontender, and with normal bowel sounds. No hepatosplenomegaly is noted. An ultrasound of the abdomen is shown (Photographs A and B). Which of the following is the most appropriate next step?

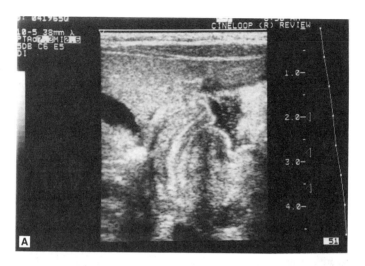

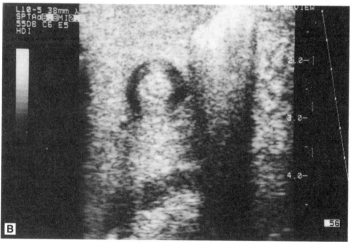

a. Surgical consultation
b. Upper GI with small-bowel follow-through
c. Intravenous (IV) fluids and switch to elemental formula
d. Air contrast enema
e. Computed tomography (CT) of the brain

222. A 17-year-old girl is seen in the emergency department (ED) for a 1 weeks' history of abdominal pain, nausea, low-grade fever, and occasional nonbilious vomiting. She states the pain is crampy in nature and is 6 out of 10 on a pain scale. She denies weight loss, diarrhea, or headache. Past history is positive for vaginal delivery of a term infant 6 weeks prior. She denies use of alcohol, tobacco, or other drugs. On physical examination vital signs are normal. Eyes are moist with icterus. Oral mucosa is moist without lesions. Chest is clear. Heart has normal S1 and S2. No murmur is heard. Distal pulses are normal. Abdomen has right upper quadrant pain with guarding. Which of the following tests is most likely to reveal the etiology of this pain?

a. Serum chemistries
b. Complete blood count (CBC) with platelets and differential
c. Ultrasound of the right upper quadrant
d. Upper GI series
e. Hepatitis panel

223. An 8-year-old boy is seen in the ED for abdominal pain. His mother reports that he was in good health until about 24 hours prior when he was accidentally hit in the abdomen by a baseball bat during a little league game. Over the ensuing 24 hours she reports that he has developed a fever, a return of the abdominal pain which is now radiating to the back, and the development of persistent vomiting. Vital signs include a temperature of 38.3°C (101.9°F), a heart rate of 120 beats per minute, a respiratory rate of 25 breaths per minute, and a blood pressure of 100/65 mm Hg. He appears quite uncomfortable. His abdomen is diffusely tender, especially in the midepigastric region where guarding is noted. Bowel sounds are decreased. Which of the following is the most appropriate next step in management?

a. Measure serum amylase levels.
b. Obtain a CBC with differential and platelets.
c. Measure serum total and direct bilirubin levels.
d. Order an abdominal radiograph.
e. Order an electrolyte panel.

224. A 7-month-old infant presents to the emergency center with vomiting and intermittent abdominal pain, crying and drawing his knees up to his chest during the pain. Between the episodes he is lethargic. Oral intake is significantly decreased. Past history is unknown, as he was recently adopted from Ecuador. The family reports that he had a loose stool while en route to the ED. On physical examination the temperature is 37°C (98.6°F), heart rate is 120 beats per minute, respiratory rate is 24 breaths per minute, and blood pressure is 100/70 mm Hg. He is very irritable with constant crying and is hard to console. Oral mucosa is moist and without lesions. Chest is clear. Heart is regular with no murmur. Abdomen is diffusely tender with a right upper quadrant mass. Bowel sounds are reduced. Which of the following is the most appropriate next step?

a. Send stool for routine culture.
b. Examine the stool for ova and parasites.
c. Obtain an air contrast enema.
d. Examine the blood smear for sickled cells.
e. Order ondansetron.

225. A 9-month-old girl is seen by the pediatric nurse practitioner for spitting up. The mother reports that since about 1 month of age the child has had frequent spitting of her meals. She denies the emesis to be bilious but rather a partial amount of her recent food intake. She has had no fever, change in behavior, nor diarrhea. The child was a vaginally born term infant. Past medical history is negative except for occasional upper respiratory infection. She sits independently, pulls to a stand, crawls, and is distrustful of anyone in the room other than her mother. Weight is 8.5 kg (95th percentile), height is 65 cm (50th percentile), and head circumference 42.3 cm (50th percentile). The child's physical examination is normal. Which of the following is the most appropriate next step?

a. Measure pyloric muscle thickness with ultrasound.
b. Obtain an upper GI with small-bowel follow-through.
c. Measure thyroid functions studies.
d. Provide family reassurance and dietary guidance.
e. Order a modified barium swallow with speech therapy present.

226. A 14-year-old girl is seen by the pediatrician with a 9-month history of diarrhea, periumbilical and postprandial abdominal pain, intermittent low-grade fever, and weight loss. She reports that the pain is crampy in nature, often partially relieved with defecation. She reports frequent episodes of blood in her stool. Past medical history is significant only for occasional upper respiratory infection and a single urinary tract infection 1 year prior. Menses began at 12 years, but have now become irregular. She denies sex as well as alcohol, smoking, or other drug use. On physical examination vital signs are normal. Oral mucosa is moist with a few ulcers noted. Abdomen is soft and minimally tender throughout. Bowel sounds are hypoactive. No hepatosplenomegaly is found. The right lower quadrant feels full. Genitourinary examination is normal. Which of the following is the most likely mechanism of disease?

a. Chronic inflammation of her appendix
b. Intermittent inflammation of the pancreas
c. Inflammatory infiltration and granuloma formation of the intestinal wall
d. Eating disorder with self-induced emesis
e. Functional constipation

227. A 4-year-old boy is seen in clinic for 2 weeks of diarrhea and abdominal pain. His parents report frequent non-bloody watery stools, nausea but no vomiting, frequent belching and passing of foul-smelling flatus, and generalized abdominal pain. Past history is unknown; he is a recent international adoption. On physical examination the vital signs are normal. Weight is 14 kg (29 lb; 5th percentile) and height is 102 cm (40 in; 50th percentile). He is awake, alert, and mildly cachectic. Head is normocephalic and without lesions. Oral mucosa is moist and without lesions. Chest is clear. Heart has normal S1 and S2. No murmur is heard. Distal pulses are normal. Abdomen is soft, minimally tender and without focality; bowel sounds are a bit hyperactive. No hepatosplenomegaly or masses are noted. Which of the following studies is most likely to identify the etiology of his condition?

a. CBC and differential
b. ESR
c. Abdominal ultrasound
d. Liver function studies
e. Stool microscopy for ova and parasites

228. A 6-month-old infant is seen by the pediatrician for a well-child evaluation. The family reports that he has had no recent problems, but is concerned about the "outie" belly button. They report he breast-feeds well, and has daily stools and voids. He was the product of a vaginal delivery at term to a 22-year-old woman whose pregnancy was uncomplicated. Vaccines are current; he has had no previous illnesses or hospitalizations. Development is normal. Height, weight, and head circumference are at the 75th percentile for age. He is awake, alert, and happy. Abdomen is soft and nontender. Bowel sounds are normal. A protuberant umbilical sac is noted. The contents of the umbilical sac are easily relocated into the abdominal cavity revealing a 0.75 cm underling abdominal wall defect. No hepatosplenomegaly or masses are noted. Which of the following is the most appropriate next step?

a. Tape a coin or use "belly band" over the defect to keep abdominal contents out of the sac.
b. Obtain pediatric surgical consultation for closure of the defect.
c. Provide parental counseling and reassurance.
d. Order abdominal ultrasound and measure thyroid function studies.
e. Order chromosomes for analysis.

229. A previously healthy 2-year-old boy is seen in the emergency center with several days of rectal bleeding. The mother reports that 2 days prior he had reddish-colored stools; these have transitioned to contain what appears to be only blood. She reports no fever, vomiting, or change in appetite or activity. He eats a regular toddler diet and takes no medications. Family history is negative. On physical examination temperature is 37°C (98.6°F), heart rate is 130 beats per minute, respiratory rate is 18 breaths per minute, and blood pressure is 105/70 mm Hg. Height, weight, and head circumference are at the 75th percentile for age. He is awake, alert, and in no distress. Head is normocephalic. Oral mucosa are pale, moist, and without lesions. Abdomen is soft and nontender. Bowel sounds are normal. No hepatosplenomegaly or masses are noted. Which of the following is the most appropriate next step to confirm the diagnosis?

a. Surgical consultation
b. Barium enema
c. Ultrasound of the abdomen
d. Radionuclide scan of abdomen
e. Stool for culture and parasite evaluation

230. A 15-year-old boy is seen by the pediatrician for routine care. He reports that he has been in good health other than having recently developed intermittent abdominal distention, crampy abdominal pain, and excessive flatulence. He reports the symptoms began about 2 weeks prior when his football coach suggested he "bulk up" by drinking milk shakes twice daily. Past medical history is positive for mild intermittent asthma for which he rarely requires an inhaled β-agonist. Vital signs are normal. Height, weight, and head circumference are at the 75th percentile for age. He is awake, alert, and in no distress. Head is normocephalic. Oral mucosa are pink, moist, and without lesions. Abdomen is soft and nontender. Bowel sounds are normal. No hepatosplenomegaly or masses are noted. Which of the following is the most appropriate study to diagnose his condition?

a. Barium swallow and upper GI
b. Hydrogen breath test
c. Esophageal manometry
d. Stool pH after 1-2 weeks of a lactose-free diet
e. Fasting serum lactose levels

231. A 4-week-old infant is seen by the pediatrician for well-child care. The mother reports the infant to be doing well and without complaints. He eats every 3-4 hours, stools and voids several times per day, and is developing normally compared to her other children. The infant was a product of a benign pregnancy, born at term vaginally, and was discharged at 2 days of age. Feeding has been by breast only; vitamin D supplements were started at hospital discharge. Past medical history shows the infant to have lost about 7% of birth weight by 5 days of age and to be back to birth weight by the 2-week visit. On physical examination temperature is 37°C (98.6°F), heart rate is 130 beats per minute, and respiratory rate is 35 breaths per minute. Height, weight, and head circumference are at the 50th percentile for age. He is awake, alert, and in no distress. Skin is mildly icteric. His examination is otherwise unremarkable.

Birth hospital laboratory data show:
Blood type:
    Mother: B+/antibody screen negative
    Baby: O–/Coombs negative
Serum bilirubin:
    Total 7.8 mg/dL; direct 0.2 mg/dL (24 hours old)
    Total 9.2 mg/dL; direct 0.3 mg/dL (48 hours old)

Office laboratory data show:
    Transcutaneous bilirubin: 10.1 mg/dL (96 hours old)
    Current (4-week old) total serum bilirubin: 12.2 mg/dL; direct 3.5 mg/dL

Which of the following disorders is most likely to be responsible?

a. ABO incompatibility
b. Biliary atresia
c. Rh incompatibility
d. Gilbert disease
e. Crigler-Najjar syndrome

232. A 2-year-old girl is seen in the emergency center after swallowing the battery from a piece of her grandmother's hearing aid. The mother reports that she had no coughing, vomiting, or other distress, and has been acting normally. Past medical history and family history are negative. Physical examination is unremarkable. Radiographs of the chest are shown (Photograph A and B). Which of the following is the correct next step?

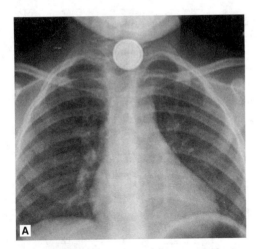

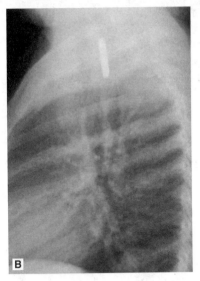

a. Induce emesis with syrup of ipecac.
b. Admit for observation, and obtain serial radiographs to document movement of the foreign body.
c. Discharge home with instructions to monitor the stool for the foreign material.
d. Immediate removal of the ingested object.
e. Encourage oral intake and a high fiber diet to assist in passage of the foreign body.

233. A 14-year-old girl has had 6 months of weight loss, intermittent bloody diarrhea, and intermittent fever. She had had cramping abdominal pain with bowel movements and occasional vomiting. She has undergone an extensive workup including a colonoscopy. The colonoscopy and pathology report show:

(a) *Inflammation of the rectum with erythematous, friable, and granular mucosa.*

(b) *Biopsy of lesion with many polymorphonuclear leukocytes at the base of the crypts. No granulomas noted.*

Which of the following statements about her condition is correct?

a. Inheritance is autosomal dominant.
b. Her risk of colon cancer is minimally elevated over the general population.
c. Intestinal strictures are common.
d. The most serious complication of her disease is toxic megacolon.
e. The intestinal involvement is separated by areas of normal bowel.

234. A 9-month old is brought to the emergency center by ambulance. The infant had been having emesis and diarrhea with decreased urine output for several days, and the parents noted that she was hard to wake up this morning. Her weight is 9 kg, down from 11 kg the week prior at her 9-month checkup. You note her heart rate and blood pressure to be normal. She is lethargic, and her skin is noted to be "doughy." After confirming that her respiratory status is stable, you send electrolytes, which you expect to be abnormal. You start an IV. Which of the following is the best solution for an initial IV bolus?

a. 0.25% sodium chloride (one-fourth normal saline, 38.5 mEq sodium/L)
b. 0.9% sodium chloride (normal saline, 154 mEq sodium/L)
c. 3% sodium chloride (hypertonic saline, 513 mEq sodium/L)
d. D10 water (100 g glucose/L)
e. Fresh-frozen plasma

235. A 4-month-old infant is seen by emergency room physician for a 3-day history of poor feeding, emesis, and diarrhea. She is given a fluid bolus via interosseous line, has subsequent urine output, and an intravenous line is obtained. Her care is transferred to the inpatient pediatric hospitalist team. Results from laboratories drawn in the ED are now available and show:

Sodium: 157 mEq/L
Potassium: 3.9 mEq/L
Chloride: 120 mEq/L
Bicarbonate: 14 mEq/L
Glucose: 195 mg/dL
Creatinine: 1.8 mEq/L
Blood urea nitrogen (BUN): 68 mEq/L

Which of the following is the most appropriate next step in her management?

a. Slow rehydration over 48 hours
b. Continued rapid volume expansion with one-fourth normal saline
c. Infuse packed red blood cells (RBCs)
d. Rehydration with free water
e. Obtain urinary electrolytes

236. A 6-month-old infant is seen by the pediatric nurse practitioner for well-child care. The mother reports the infant to be doing well and has no concerns other than the infant may be teething. Which of the following bits of anticipatory guidance regarding the typical first tooth eruption is correct?

a. Mandibular central incisors
b. Maxillary lateral incisors
c. Maxillary first molars
d. Mandibular cuspids (canines)
e. First premolars (bicuspids)

237. An 8-year-old boy is seen by the pediatrician for abdominal pain. He reports the pain to be 5 out of 10 on a pain scale and the pain to be diffuse across his abdomen. He denies nausea, vomiting, headache, fever, or weight loss. His mother reports the pain is worse during the week and seems to be less prominent during the weekends. She states that he has one soft stool daily and does not complain of painful defecation. Past medical history is unremarkable. He attends the second grade where he performs "average" per his mother. On physical examination vital signs are normal. Height and weight are in the 50th percentile for age. Oral mucosa is moist and without lesions. Chest is clear. Heart has normal S1 and S2. No murmur is heard. Abdomen is soft and nontender. Bowel sounds are normal. No hepatosplenomegaly or masses are noted. Laboratory data show:

Complete blood count:
   Hemoglobin: 14.2 g/dL
   Hematocrit: 41.5%
   WBC: 7500/mm^3
      Segmented neutrophils: 49%
      Band forms: 0%
      Lymphocytes: 51%
      Platelet count: 138,000/mm^3
Erythrocyte sedimentation rate: 9 mm/h

Electrolytes:
   Sodium: 140 mEq/L
   Potassium: 4.5 mEq/L
   Chloride: 100 mEq/L
   Bicarbonate: 24 mEq/L
   Glucose: 95 mg/dL
   Creatinine: 0.5 mEq/L
   Blood urea nitrogen (BUN): 12 mEq/L
Stool guaiac negative
Urinalysis negative for WBCs, RBCs, and protein

Which of the following is the best next step in the care of this patient?
a. Perform an upper GI series with small-bowel follow-through.
b. Perform CT of the abdomen with contrast.
c. Administer a trial of a proton pump inhibitor.
d. Observe the patient and reassure the patient and family.
e. Recommend a lactose-free diet.

238. A 4-year-old child is seen by the pediatric nurse practitioner for an initial child protective services placement evaluation. The foster mother knows of no concerns about his health. Court documents show his past medical history to be positive for occasional otitis media treated with unknown antibiotics and occasional upper respiratory infections. On physical examination the vital signs are normal. Height and weight are at the 90th percentile for age. Head is normocephalic. Oral mucosa is moist and without lesions; his teeth are shown (Photograph). Which of the following is the most likely explanation for the findings noted?

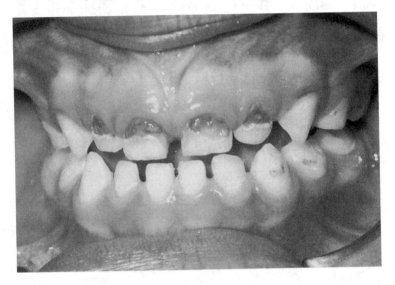

a. Excessive use of fluoride
b. Tetracycline exposure
c. Use of bottled water that lacks fluoride
d. Prolonged use of a baby bottle in the crib at night
e. Consumption of too much candy

239. A 2-month-old infant is seen by the pediatrician for a well-child visit. The infant was born prematurely at 27 weeks of gestation and was discharged the previous week. The hospital course was relatively uncomplicated with a short period of oxygen need, initial feeding intolerance, and a grade I interventricular hemorrhage. Eye examination prior to discharge noted no retinopathy of prematurity. The infant has been doing well at home taking regular feedings of fortified breast milk. On physical examination vital signs are normal. Height and weight are at the 50th percentile corrected for gestational age. A prominent bulge in the inguinal canal is noted (Photograph). The mass is not tender, firm, hot, or red, and it does not transilluminate. The mass resolves with pressure, but returns when the infant cries or strains. The rest of the examination is normal. Which of the following is the most appropriate next step?

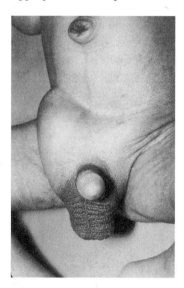

a. Obtain a surgical consultation.
b. Perform a needle aspiration.
c. Order a barium enema.
d. Order a KUB (plain radiographs of kidney, ureter, and bladder).
e. Observe the patient and reassure the patient and family.

240. An 18-month-old child is seen by the emergency room physician after having been found at home with the contents of a bottle of drain cleaner in his mouth. The family reports that they found him in the kitchen with the product opened and some of the contents dripping from his mouth. They deny coughing, vomiting, or change in color. On physical examination vital signs are normal. Oral mucosa is moist and without lesions. Chest is clear. Heart has normal S1 and S2. No murmur is heard. Distal pulses are normal. Abdomen is soft and nontender. Bowel sounds normal. Which of the following is the most appropriate next step?

a. Induce emesis immediately.
b. Admit and arrange for endoscopic examination in 12-24 hours.
c. Decontaminate stomach using activated charcoal.
d. Neutralization of the drain cleaner pH by drinking a solution of the opposite pH.
e. Have the patient drink copious amounts of milk or water.

241. A 16-year-old boy is seen by the ED physician about 30 minutes after he tries to commit suicide by taking an unknown quantity of an unknown material found at home. For which of the following household materials and medications should he be given activated charcoal as part of his emergency center treatment?

a. Drain cleaner
b. Ethylene glycol
c. Bleach
d. Phenobarbital
e. Lithium

Questions 242 to 246

For each of the patient descriptions mentioned later, choose the best initial diagnostic step in the evaluation of the patient's apparent GI hemorrhage. Each lettered option may be used once, more than once, or not at all.

a. Abdominal radiographs
b. Fiberoptic endoscopy
c. Apt test
d. Routine stool culture
e. Barium enema
f. No immediate intervention
g. Meckel scan
h. Stool culture on sorbitol-MacConkey medium

242. A 24-hour-old neonate is seen by the pediatric nurse practitioner in the normal newborn nursery. The staff reports that the newborn just had a grossly bloody stool. The neonate was the product of a term pregnancy with delivery by emergency cesarean section for partial placental previa. Apgar scores were 8 and 9 at 1 and 5 minutes, respectively. The newborn has been breast-feeding well. On physical examination the vital signs are normal. Oral mucosa is moist and without lesions. Chest is clear. Heart has normal S1 and S2. No murmur is heard. Distal pulses are normal. Abdomen is soft and nontender. Bowel sounds are normal.

243. A 7-day-old neonate in the NICU has a grossly bloody stool, abdominal distention, and increasing oxygen requirements. The neonate was born by cesarean section at 26 weeks' gestation for severe maternal pre-eclampsia. On physical examination temperature is 37°C (98.6°F), heart rate is 180 beats per minute, and respiratory rate is 55 breaths per minute. Oral mucosa is moist and without lesions. Chest is clear. Heart has normal S1 and S2. No murmur is heard. Distal pulses are normal. Abdomen is distended, tender, and no bowel sounds are noted. No hepatosplenomegaly is found.

244. A 2-year-old boy is seen by the pediatrician for 6 days of crampy abdominal pain and a 2-day history of grossly bloody diarrheal stool. Several other family members developed diarrhea 24 hours after eating at their favorite local restaurant on the way home from a trip to the petting zoo on an outing with their nursing-home-bound grandmother; the other family members' symptoms have resolved. On physical examination temperature is 38.8°C (101.8°F), heart rate is 120 beats per minute, respiratory rate is 24 breaths per minute, and blood pressure is 100/70 mm Hg. Oral mucosa is moist, pale, and without lesions. Chest is clear. Heart has normal S1 and S2. No murmur is heard. Distal pulses are normal. Abdomen is slightly distended and diffusely tender; bowel sounds are reduced. No hepatosplenomegaly or masses are found.

245. A 7-year-old boy is seen by the pediatrician for 2 days of vomiting and 1 day of diarrhea. His mother is concerned that she has noted small streaks of blood in his emesis. The rest of his family has had similar symptoms, but no blood in their emesis. On physical examination vital signs are normal. He is awake, alert, and in no distress. His abdominal examination is benign, and the rest of his examination is normal.

246. A 10-year-old boy is seen by the pediatrician for a 1-month history of intermittent epigastric pain that awakens him from sleep. The child notes that eating food sometimes helps reduce the pain. He reports black stools during the prior week, and also admits that he has occasionally vomited frank blood. On physical examination vital signs are normal. He is awake, alert, and in no distress. Oral mucosa is slightly pale but moist and without lesions. Chest is clear. Heart has normal S1 and S2. No murmur is heard. Distal pulses are normal. Abdomen is soft and nontender. Bowel sounds are normal. No hepatosplenomegaly or masses are found.

Questions 247 to 251

For each presented child, choose the one most appropriate vitamin or trace element replacement therapy to treat the described condition. Each lettered option may be used once, more than once, or not at all.

a. Vitamin A
b. Niacin (Vitamin B_3)
c. Pyridoxine (Vitamin B_6)
d. Folate (Vitamin B_9)
e. Vitamin C
f. Vitamin D
g. Vitamin E
h. Vitamin K
i. Iodine
j. Iron
k. Selenium

247. A 15-year-old girl has complaints of tingling and numbness of her feet, especially at night. She denies fever, nausea, vomiting, headache, or change in behavior. She has had no recent weight loss on her strictly vegetarian diet. She is in her sixth month of a planned 9-month course of antituberculosis medications for a positive tuberculosis screening test, and reports good compliance with taking her medications.

248. A 9-month-old infant is seen by the pediatric nurse practitioner for well-child checkup. The mother reports the infant has been healthy, has had no recent illnesses, and takes no medications. She states the infant has been taking about 32 oz of cow's milk for the previous 4 months and is developing normally as compared to her other children. On physical examination temperature is 37°C (98.6°F), heart rate is 130 beats per minute, and respiratory rate is 24 breaths per minute. Oral mucosa is moist, pale, and without lesions. Chest is clear. Heart has normal S1 and S2. No murmur is heard. Distal pulses are normal. Abdomen is soft, nontender, and with normal bowel sounds. No hepatosplenomegaly or masses are found.

249. A 3-day-old neonate is seen in the ED for a 1-day history of bloody stools, hematemesis, and purpura. He was a term infant born vaginally at home as had been planned; prenatal care provided by the nurse midwife was normal. His mother reports that he had been doing well at home, tolerating breast-feeding well until earlier that day. He has had no other medical care since birth.

250. A 17-month-old child is seen by the pediatrician on a missionary trip to a rural community. The mother reports that the child has been irritable over the previous month, to have developed a low-grade fever, and now refuses to walk. On physical examination vital signs are normal. The child seems to have tenderness in both of her legs. She has had a low-grade fever, petechiae on her skin and mucous membranes, and poorly healing cuts and abrasions. Radiographs of the legs done at the local safety-net hospital reveal generalized bony atrophy with epiphyseal separation.

251. A 2-year-old boy is seen by the ED physician for pain in his right leg after a fall. The mother reports the child to have been previously healthy without significant illnesses and requiring no medications. The delivery was vaginal after an uncomplicated pregnancy. He was exclusively breast-fed through 8 months of age with solids added at that time. He was recently weaned from breast milk to 2% cow's milk in addition to his other toddler foods. On physical examination his weight, height, and head circumference are at the 10th percentile. Head has a 3-cm anterior fontanelle, a flattened occiput, and a prominent forehead. The bilateral lower extremities are bowed. Radiographs reveal a greenstick fracture at the site of pain, along with fraying at the distal ends of the femur.

The Gastrointestinal Tract

Answers

214. The answer is b. (*Hay et al, pp 644-646. Kliegman et al, pp 1763-1764, 1765. Rudolph et al, pp 1386-1389, 1436-1437.*) This child has a normal past history and normal growth. The radiograph demonstrates a stool-filled megacolon. Finding a dilated, stool-filled anal canal with poor tone on the physical examination of a well-grown child supports the diagnosis of functional constipation. Hirschsprung disease is usually suspected in the chronically constipated child, but the vast majority of such children with the signs and symptoms described have functional constipation. The treatment of functional constipation emphasizes dietary changes and counseling of parents regarding proper toileting behavior. Effective stool softeners are available as a second-line option. An extensive workup of this patient with lab work or radiographic studies would likely be negative and expensive, and is not indicated. Hirschsprung usually presents in infancy with increasingly difficult defecation in the first few weeks of life. Typically no stool is found in the rectum, and anal sphincter tone is abnormal. Diagnosis of Hirschsprung disease may be made with rectal manometry and rectal biopsy.

215. The answer is a. (*Hay et al, pp 634-635. Kliegman et al, pp 1817-1819. Rudolph et al, pp 1454-1457.*) Although the majority of children with periumbilical or epigastric pain have a functional gastrointestinal disorder, the presence of nocturnal abdominal pain and GI bleeding in a patient with a positive family history supports a diagnosis of peptic ulcer disease (PUD). A dull or aching pain is the most common symptom; the classic complaint of epigastric pain relieved by eating is not typical in the pediatric population. Symptoms often persist for several years before diagnosis. The increased incidence of PUD in families (25%-50%) and concordance in monozygotic twins suggest a genetic basis for the disease. About half of the patients with PUD will have hematemesis or melena. Diagnosis may be made conclusively with endoscopy; stains and cultures obtained during endoscopy can diagnose the subset of PUD caused by *H pylori*. The serum test for *H pylori* has poor sensitivity and specificity, and typically does not distinguish between acute and past infection. The urea breath test is another noninvasive option for identifying the presence of *H pylori* infection. The mainstay of treatment of PUD is acid blockade. Antibiotic treatment for *H pylori* can cure this disease in infected patients, although the optimal combination of medications is still unclear.

Appendicitis is an acute event, and in suspected cases abdominal ultrasound (or CT if ultrasound not available) may be indicated. Pinworms produce perianal pruritus but do not commonly cause abdominal pain or other serious problems. Adult worms lay their eggs on the hosts' perirectal region at night; the eggs of this worm can be identified by microscopic examination of a piece of adhesive tape that has been applied to the rectum of an awakening child. Meckel diverticulum causes painless rectal bleeding, usually during early childhood. Functional, or recurrent, abdominal pain is a benign, self-limited diagnosis of exclusion; GI bleeding is not a typical finding.

216. The answer is a. (*Hay et al, pp 628-629. Kliegman et al, pp 1791-1792. Rudolph et al, pp 1411-1412.*) Information about eosinophilic esophagitis continues to evolve, but it appears to be an allergic response. Males are affected more than females. The history usually includes atopy or food allergy. Symptoms are similar to those seen in gastroesophageal reflux disease (GERD), but are not relieved with acid blockade. Some patients have elevated IgE levels or peripheral eosinophilia (hinted at by their history of eczema and peanut allergy). Endoscopy reveals mucosal furrowing; strictures can develop as well. Biopsy reveals many eosinophils (normal mucosa does not have eosinophils). Treatment includes avoidance of specific food allergens. Steroids may be helpful; using the same steroid metered dose inhaler prescribed for asthmatics, patients are instructed to swallow, rather than inhale, two puffs twice daily; they should not rinse their mouth or eat for 30 minutes after the dose. Fundoplication is a surgical procedure necessary for a patient with reflux, especially if associated with pneumonia or poor growth. Observation would not be helpful in this case.

217. The answer is c. (*Hay et al, pp 49, 638. Kliegman et al, pp 1803-1804. Rudolph et al, pp 1417-1419.*) The plain films demonstrate dilated stomach and proximal loops of bowel. The cross-table upper GI demonstrates a "curly Q" twist of barium as it passes through the malrotated portion of bowel. Malrotation results when incomplete rotation of the intestines occurs during embryologic development. The most common type of malrotation is failure of the cecum to move to its correct location in the right lower quadrant. Most patients present in the first weeks of life with bilious vomiting indicative of bowel obstruction, and/or intermittent abdominal pain. Acute presentation, similar to that in the question, is caused by a volvulus of the intestines. The diagnosis is confirmed by radiographs; barium contrast studies (upper GI and/or enema) demonstrate malposition of the cecum in the vast majority of cases. Treatment is surgical. Appendicitis is rare at this age and presents as an acute, rigid abdomen, and signs of sepsis. Pyloric stenosis usually does not occur until after 3 weeks of life and presents with nonbilious vomiting. If the infant were 6 months or older, intussusception would be higher on the differential, but it is an unusual condition for this age. Jejunal atresia would have been noted on the first day of life, as the patient would not have tolerated any feeds prior to newborn discharge.

218. The answer is b. (*Hay et al, p 49. Kliegman et al, pp 868-869. Rudolph et al, p 1427.*) The radiographs are consistent with meconium ileus, a condition virtually pathognomonic for CF. Approximately 15% of children with CF will present with meconium ileus. Echogenic bowel on prenatal ultrasound can be an early hint. Inspissated meconium obstructs the small bowel, usually at the level of the terminal ileum resulting in clinical findings of delayed stool, distended abdomen and bilious emesis. Radiographs show dilated loops of bowel, and usually reveal a bubbly or granular pattern at the level of obstruction. The enema shows microcolon from disuse. Complications of meconium ileus may include perforation and meconium peritonitis. Meconium ileus should be distinguished from meconium plug, which is a functional obstruction of the colon that can be associated with Hirschsprung disease but not usually with CF. With meconium plug, a water-soluble high osmolality contrast enema may be diagnostic as well as therapeutic. Duodenal atresia would have presented with bilious emesis from the first feed, and infectious gastroenteritis is unlikely in a 1-day old and should not cause bilious emesis.

219. The answer is e. (*Hay et al, pp 665-668. Kliegman et al, pp 1822-1826. Rudolph et al, pp 1460-1467.*) The patient in the vignette has ulcerative colitis, a chronic inflammatory condition usually involving the entire colon; confirmation of the disease is based on biopsy of a colonic lesion which will show polymorphonucleocytes near the base of the crypts. While some genetic predisposition is seen (twin concordance is 16%, while twin concordance for Crohn disease is 36%), inheritance of this condition is not clearly dominant or recessive. Patients usually have intermittent symptoms of bloody diarrhea (leading to iron deficiency anemia as in this case), and can have abdominal pain and growth failure. Perianal disease is uncommon, as are mouth ulcerations. So-called skip areas, portions of the intestine free of disease, are common in Crohn disease, but are not seen in ulcerative colitis. Elevations in inflammatory markers, such as elevated ESR, are found. ASCA is positive in about 55% of those with Crohn disease, but are uncommon in ulcerative colitis; conversely, p-ANCA is positive in about 70% of patients with ulcerative colitis, but in less than 20% of patients with Crohn disease. The most serious complication of ulcerative colitis is toxic megacolon, a medical and surgical emergency in which patients develop fever, tachycardia, dehydration, leukocytosis, and electrolyte abnormalities associated with a markedly dilated colon. This complication comes with a high risk of intestinal perforation; CT scan can assist with making this diagnosis. Patients with ulcerative colitis have a markedly elevated risk of colonic carcinoma; after 10 years of disease, routine colonoscopies are recommended as the annual cumulative risk is 0.5%-1% a year. Strictures are more common in Crohn disease and are unusual in ulcerative colitis.

Lead exposure can cause microcytic anemia, but typically not findings of weight loss, bloody diarrhea, and intermittent fever. Hemolytic uremic syndrome is caused by *E coli* O157:H7 (stool sample cultured on MacConkey media [newer and more rapid enzyme immunoassays (EIA) and nucleic acid amplification tests (NAATs) to identify this organism are available as well]) and presents with acute onset of gastroenteritis, bloody diarrhea, and evidence of acute renal failure. *Clostridium difficile* classically occurs shortly after starting antibiotics as watery diarrhea (rarely contains blood), cramping abdominal pain, and fever.

220. The answer is b. (*Hay et al, pp 643-644. Kliegman et al, pp 1809-1811. Rudolph et al, pp 1436-1437.*) The diagnosis of Hirschsprung disease (congenital aganglionic megacolon) should be suspected in a child with intractable chronic constipation and abdominal distension without fecal soiling (although approximately 3% do have soiling). In contrast, overflow diarrhea caused by leakage of the unformed fecal stream around a rectal impaction is common in functional constipation. A neonatal history of delayed passage of meconium is often obtained (as in this case when the first stool occurred after 24 hours), and the infant can continue to be constipated with bouts of abdominal distention and vomiting. The infant is at risk of developing enterocolitis, a life-threatening consequence of the partial obstruction. Radiologic study by barium enema and rectal manometry are accurate diagnostic tools. Identification of an aganglionic segment of bowel by punch or suction biopsy can establish the diagnosis. Histochemical tissue examination showing increased amounts of acetylcholinesterase in hypertrophic nerve bundles with an absence of ganglia cells is confirmatory. Rectal manometric studies have shown that in aganglionic megacolon, the usual relaxation of the internal rectal sphincter in response to balloon inflation does not occur. Surgery is indicated as soon as the diagnosis is made. Antispasmodic agents and dietary changes are not helpful, and a plain film of the abdomen would not confirm the diagnosis but rather is helpful only if signs of obstruction are noted. Dietary changes would only be helpful with functional constipation.

221. The answer is a. (*Hay et al, pp 633-634. Kliegman et al, pp 1797-1799. Rudolph et al, pp 1420-1421.*) A history of nonbilious vomiting for 10 days in an infant of this age who does not look ill and who has a benign abdominal examination points to infantile hypertrophic pyloric stenosis as the most likely diagnosis; surgical consultation for a likely pyloromyotomy is indicated. The ultrasound in the question demonstrates the thickened pylorus. The incidence of this condition in infants is between one and three per 1000 live infants in the United States, with males affected more often than females. Although there is no specific pattern of inheritance, a familial incidence has been observed in about 15% of patients. Information about predisposing ancestry is conflicting, as are data concerning the assertion of a firstborn predilection. Metabolic alkalosis with low serum potassium and chloride levels is frequently seen in pyloric stenosis as a result of loss of gastric contents from vomiting. Some studies suggest that infants treated with macrolides in the first weeks of life have an elevated risk for pyloric stenosis. A palpable lump, or "olive," is frequently described in the literature; in practice, this finding is difficult to elicit.

An infant with a small-bowel obstruction (who may require an upper GI with small-bowel follow-through to help diagnose the point of obstruction) should develop bilious emesis and should not look well 10 days into the illness; similarly, a child with intussusception (who requires an air contrast enema, which is both diagnostic and perhaps therapeutic) would be markedly ill at this point. Gastroenteritis (IV fluids alone to maintain hydration) does not usually last for 10 days. A brain tumor causing increased intracranial pressure could present with isolated emesis but should result in other symptoms such as irritability, focal neurologic signs, and somnolence.

222. The answer is c. (*Hay et al, pp 701-704. Kliegman et al, pp 1971-1972. Rudolph et al, pp 1531-1534.*) Cholecystitis and cholelithiasis are unusual diseases in children and are almost always associated with predisposing disorders such as hemolytic anemia, pregnancy (as in this case), CF, Crohn disease, obesity, rapid weight loss, or prior ileal resection. Pain in the right upper quadrant, nausea, vomiting, fever, and jaundice are symptoms of acute cholecystitis. The diagnosis is confirmed with an ultrasound of the gallbladder. While some of the other answers listed might result in abnormalities, the findings would be neither sensitive nor specific for cholecystitis. Thus, the diagnostic test of choice is an ultrasound.

223. The answer is a. (*Hay et al, pp 709-711. Kliegman et al, pp 1913-1915. Rudolph et al, pp 1487-1488.*) The child in this question has abdominal trauma, abdominal pain, emesis, fever, and tachycardia; on examination he has a diffusely tender abdomen. While no diagnostic test is completely accurate, an elevated total serum amylase with the correct clinical history and signs and symptoms of pancreatitis as outlined is the best initial diagnostic tool. The causes of pancreatitis in children are varied, with about one-fourth of cases without predisposing etiology and about one-third of cases as a feature of another systemic disease. Traumatic cases are usually due to blunt trauma to the abdomen. Acute pancreatitis is difficult to diagnose; a high index of suspicion is necessary. Common clinical features include severe pain with nausea and vomiting. Tenderness, guarding or rebound pain, abdominal distention, and a paralytic ileus are often seen. Plain films of the abdomen may exclude other diagnoses; ultrasonography of the pancreas can reveal enlargement of the pancreas, gallstones, cysts, and pseudocysts. Supportive care is indicated until the condition resolves.

A hollow viscus injury, such as a duodenal hematoma, is another consideration after blunt abdominal trauma. This injury is classically associated with a fall forward off of a bicycle, with the handlebars hitting the abdomen as the child flips forward. Additionally, blunt force abdominal trauma can result in splenic rupture, classically presenting with left upper quadrant and left shoulder pain. An abdominal CT with intravenous contrast is the imaging modality of choice if these injuries are under consideration and the child is hemodynamically stable. Alternatively, a "focused assessment with sonography for trauma" (FAST) ultrasound examination can demonstrate free intraperitoneal fluid that may require surgical intervention. A child sustaining abdominal trauma with persistent hypotension despite fluid resuscitation should have an emergent exploratory laparotomy.

224. The answer is c. (*Hay et al, p 60. Kliegman et al, pp 1812-1814. Rudolph et al, pp 1428-1429.*) The usual presentation of intussusception is that of an infant between 4 and 10 months of age who has a sudden onset of intermittent colicky abdominal pain (presenting as drawing their legs up in pain as described in the case). The infant can appear normal when the pain abates, but as it recurs with increasing frequency, the child commonly vomits and becomes progressively more obtunded. The passage of stool containing blood and mucus, frequently described as resembling currant jelly, is observed late in the course; the absence of this finding does not preclude the diagnosis of intussusception. Early examination of the abdomen can be unremarkable or can be diffusely tender, but as the problem persists, a sausage-shaped mass in the right upper quadrant is frequently palpated. An air, barium, or saline enema examination under fluoroscopic or ultrasound control can be therapeutic as well as diagnostic when the hydrostatic effects of the contrast serve to reduce the intussusception. Attempted hydrostatic reduction should always be performed with surgical backup, as a complication of attempted reduction is intestinal perforation. Rates of intestinal perforation are lowest with air reduction. Early diagnosis prevents bowel ischemia. The cause of most intussusceptions is unknown, but a Meckel diverticulum or polyp can serve as a lead point; older children with intussusception should be investigated for this. Intussusception is a potential complication of Henoch-Schönlein purpura. None of the other choices would result in a correct diagnosis (and potential therapy) for the child with a classic presentation for intussusception.

225. The answer is d. (*Hay et al, pp 626-628. Kliegman et al, pp 1787-1789. Rudolph et al, pp 1405-1409.*) Gastroesophageal reflux is a common pediatric complaint, often seen in the first 1-2 months of life and resolving by 1-2 years of age. Occasional episodes of gastroesophageal reflux in infancy are physiologic; GERD is the pathologic form, involving respiratory symptoms, esophagitis, related apnea, or weight loss. Sandifer syndrome is the bending or arching of the neck caused by gastroesophageal reflux; this condition may be confused with infantile spasm. About 7% of children have reflux severe enough to require medical attention, and only 2% of that group requires diagnostic investigation. For children who are growing and developing well and do not have respiratory symptoms attributed to reflux, conservative treatment (small feeds, thickened formula, avoiding high-fat meals and overfeeding, etc.) suffices. A small number of cases need pharmacologic therapy. Medications to treat GERD include acid blockade with H2 blockers or proton pump inhibitors, resulting in decreased esophagitis. Prokinetic agents such as bethanechol are occasionally used in conjunction with acid blockade for severe forms of this condition, but have not been consistently shown to decrease symptoms and typically have significant side effects.

Pyloric stenosis presents with nonbilious vomiting in the first weeks of life and not at 12 months of age; confirmation of this condition is made by finding a thickened pyloric muscle on abdominal ultrasound. Similarly, a patient with an obstruction such as partial duodenal atresia would be diagnosed with an upper GI and small-bowel follow-through. These conditions would be noted in the newborn period, likely with bilious vomiting. Hypothyroidism can cause constipation, among other findings, but a presentation with isolated vomiting would be distinctly unusual. A barium swallow might show reflux in this child, but the history already has confirmed that reflux is present. A modified barium swallow is typically used to diagnose swallowing dysfunction; this child has none of those symptoms. Conservative therapy is more appropriate if growth and development are normal as in this case.

226. The answer is c. (*Hay et al, pp 665-668. Kliegman et al, pp 1826-1829. Rudolph et al, pp 1460-1467.*) The presentation of Crohn disease (granulomatous colitis) depends on the location and extent of lesions. Onset of the GI or extraintestinal symptoms can be insidious. The "textbook" presentation is as described in the case, although only 25% of patients have the "triad" of diarrhea, weight loss, and abdominal pain. Crohn disease characteristically is associated with transmural, granulomatous intestinal lesions that are discontinuous and can appear in both the small and large intestines. Although Crohn disease can first appear as a rectal fissure or fistula, the rectum is often spared. Arthritis/arthralgia occurs in a minority of affected children. Other extraintestinal symptoms include erythema nodosum or pyoderma gangrenosum, liver disease, renal calculi, uveitis, anemia, specific nutrient deficiency, and growth failure. Disruption of a previously normal menstrual cycle can point to a chronic inflammatory process. In relation to the general population, the risk of colonic carcinoma in affected persons is increased, but not to the degree associated with ulcerative colitis. This child has no features of chronic appendicitis, chronic pancreatitis, bulimia, or constipation.

227. The answer is e. (*Hay et al, pp 1321-1322. Kliegman et al, pp 1692-1694. Rudolph et al, pp 521-522, 1131-1132.*) Parasites are a common medical problem, found in about 60% of international adoptees, in most cases related to tainted water ingestion. *Giardia* is the most frequent isolate. Patients with *Giardia* infection complain of recurrent abdominal pain, cramping, intermittent diarrhea, bloating, and weight loss (the child in the case has failure to thrive). Although many cases are self-limited, symptoms can recur or become chronic. Identifying *Giardia* cysts or trophozoites makes the diagnosis. Upper endoscopy and microscopic examination of duodenal biopsies can also be diagnostic. Although international adoptees may also have hepatitis, it is much less common than parasitic infection. Most patients with *Giardia* infection have normal CBCs. An upper GI series may reveal nonspecific changes associated with *Giardia* infection, but an ultrasound would not be helpful. An ESR is a nonspecific marker for inflammation, and would not help make the diagnosis. Treatment options in this 4-year old include a single dose of tinidazole, 3 days of BID nitazoxanide, or 5-7 days of TID metronidazole.

228. The answer is c. (*Hay et al, p 641. Kliegman et al, p 891. Rudolph et al, p 1432.*) The infant in the case is a normal infant with normal growth and development. The abdominal examination has a small umbilical hernia with a small underlying defect. Umbilical hernias affect about 15%-20% of children with equal gender distribution. Small for gestational age and premature infants are more commonly affected. The etiology of the defect is persistence of a gap in the abdominal muscular wall where the umbilical vessels entered the umbilicus. Defects less than about 2 cm close by 3 or 4 years of age; parental reassurance is adequate. Those larger than that size or those that fail to close by 3-4 years of age usually require surgical closure. Taping a coin over the defect or use of a "belly" band is common in some cultures, but is not effective. Further testing is unnecessary unless clinical features of hypothyroidism, Down syndrome, Beckwith-Wiedemann syndrome, or mucopolysaccharidosis are noted.

229. The answer is d. (*Hay et al, p 642. Kliegman et al, pp 1804-1805. Rudolph et al, pp 1425-1426.*) The child described has a typical presentation for Meckel diverticulum which can include clinical evidence of blood loss (tachycardia and pallor as noted). The embryonic duct connecting the yolk sac to the intestine can fail to regress completely and persist as a diverticulum attached to the ileum. It is common, occurring in 1.5% of the population; however, it rarely causes symptoms. Children symptomatic with this condition usually present with painless rectal bleeding in the first 2 years of life, but they can have symptoms throughout the first decade. The lining of the Meckel diverticulum usually contains acid-secreting gastric mucosa; the acid can produce ulcerations of the diverticulum itself or the adjacent ileum. Bleeding, perforation, or diverticulitis can occur. More seriously, the diverticulum can lead to volvulus of itself and of the small intestine, and it can also undergo eversion and intussusception. Diagnosis can be made by technetium-99m (^{99m}Tc) pertechnetate scan that labels gastric mucosa; once the diagnosis is made in a child without an acute abdomen as in this case, treatment is surgical excision. Barium studies do not readily reveal the diverticulum, nor do plain films or ultrasound. Stools culture is appropriate for the febrile child with diarrhea; parasites are a rare cause of bloody stools.

230. The answer is b. (*Hay et al, pp 663-664. Kliegman et al, pp 1845, 1876. Rudolph et al, pp 1447-1448.*) This is a normal child who has just added a high concentration of lactose into his diet. Lactase is a disaccharidase localized in the brush border of the intestinal villous cells. It hydrolyzes lactose to its constituent monosaccharides, glucose, and galactose. Intestinal lactase levels are usually normal at birth in all populations, and congenital lactose intolerance is extremely rare. However, lactase deficiency is a common, genetically predetermined condition. Lactase activity is not readily increased by the inclusion of lactose in the diet. The clinical symptoms of lactose malabsorption are due to the presence of osmotically active, undigested lactose, which may act to increase intestinal fluid volume, alter transit time, and produce the symptoms of abdominal cramps, distention, and occasionally, watery diarrhea. Bacterial metabolism of the nonabsorbed carbohydrates in the colon into carbon dioxide and hydrogen may contribute to the clinical symptoms. Acquired lactase deficiency is often associated with conditions of the GI tract that cause intestinal mucosal injury (eg, sprue and regional enteritis). Diagnostic techniques for lactose intolerance include removal of the offending sugar, with a reproduction of symptoms upon reintroduction. Although the ingestion of even small amounts of lactose can be diagnostic if GI symptoms occur, the measurement of breath hydrogen is more specific, as it is not affected by glucose metabolism or gastric emptying. Similarly, an acidic stool pH in the presence of reducing substances would be diagnostic.

231. The answer is b. (*Hay et al, pp 678-682. Kliegman et al, pp 1933-1936. Rudolph et al, pp 1528-1529.*) This is a normal-appearing infant with good growth. Initial laboratory data at birth are compatible with indirect hyperbilirubinemia (elevated total but low direct bilirubin) likely caused by breast-feeding combined with physiologic jaundice. By 4 weeks, however, the laboratory data demonstrate direct hyperbilirubinemia (elevated total and direct bilirubin). Obstructive jaundice (ie, direct-reacting bilirubin > 20% of the total) requires investigation in all infants. Of the many causes of obstructive jaundice in an infant, BA is the most commonly identified at around 30% of all cases. CF and α_1-antitrypsin deficiency should be considered in the diagnostic evaluation of any infant with obstructive jaundice. Other diseases to be excluded are galactosemia, tyrosinemia, choledochal cyst, and urinary tract or other infections (including toxoplasmosis, cytomegalovirus, rubella, syphilis, and herpes virus). Ultrasound examination should be performed early in the evaluation, along with a ^{99m}Tc hepatic iminodiacetic acid (HIDA) scan to assess the patency of the biliary tree. Liver biopsy can assist in the diagnosis by providing a histologic diagnosis (eg, hepatitis, BA), tissue for enzyme activity (ie, inborn error of metabolism), or tissue for microscopic determination of storage diseases. ABO and Rh incompatibility occasionally cause direct hyperbilirubinemia if there were brisk hemolysis at birth, which would then lead to inspissated bile syndrome; this is not possible in this case as the baby is O negative. All of the other causes listed typically lead to indirect hyperbilirubinemia. Note that there is some urgency to making this diagnosis, as children with BA have a demonstrably better outcome when diagnosed early.

232. The answer is d. (*Hay et al, pp 631-632. Kliegman et al, pp 1793-1794. Rudolph et al, pp 1412-1414.*) In patients without respiratory symptoms, observation for 24 hours for some esophageal foreign bodies can be allowed; the foreign body usually passes uneventfully into the stomach. However, button batteries that have lodged in the esophagus, as found on the AP and lateral radiographs shown, may cause corrosive or electrical injury and carry a high risk of esophageal perforation in as little as 1 hour. Batteries must be removed urgently via endoscopy. Patients who have stridor associated with external compression of the airway also need emergent intervention. Some advocate removing esophageal foreign bodies using a balloon catheter (passing the catheter past the foreign body, inflating the balloon, and pulling both the catheter and the object out). However, this does not allow direct visualization of the mucosa to determine the extent of the injury and also carries the risk of aspiration; it should be performed only by experienced personnel.

233. The answer is d. (*Hay et al, pp 665-668. Kliegman et al, pp 1823-1826. Rudolph et al, pp 1460-1467.*) The patient in the vignette likely has ulcerative colitis, a chronic inflammatory condition usually involving the entire colon; confirmation of the disease is based on biopsy of a colonic lesion which will show polymorphonucleocytes near the base of the crypts as outlined in the question. The most serious complication of ulcerative colitis is toxic megacolon, a medical and surgical emergency in which patients develop fever, tachycardia, dehydration, leukocytosis, and electrolyte abnormalities associated with a markedly dilated colon. This complication comes with a high risk of intestinal perforation. While some genetic predisposition is seen (twin concordance is 16%, while twin concordance for Crohn disease is 36%), inheritance of this condition is not clearly dominant or recessive. Patients with ulcerative colitis have a markedly elevated risk of colonic carcinoma; after 10 years of disease, routine colonoscopies are recommended as the annual cumulative risk is 0.5%-1% a year. Strictures and skipped lesions are more common in Crohn disease and are unusual in ulcerative colitis.

234. The answer is b. (*Hay et al, pp 719-722. Kliegman et al, pp 390-391. Rudolph et al, pp 1681-1682.*) The description is that of an infant with hypernatremic dehydration (in this case, the infant's sodium was 170 mEq/dL); the "doughy" skin is often seen in this type of dehydration. The extracellular fluid and circulating blood volumes tend to be preserved with hypernatremic dehydration at the expense of the intracellular volume. Therefore, hypotension may not be observed, nor may the other signs of circulatory inadequacy that are typical of isotonic or hypotonic dehydration. Signs suggesting involvement of the central nervous system (such as irritability or lethargy) are characteristic of both hypotonic and hypertonic dehydration. Isotonic saline is the best fluid for an initial bolus in a patient such as the one described in the question.

The use of one-fourth normal saline (38.5 mEq sodium/L) or D10 water (100 g glucose/L) in this dehydrated infant would not expand the intravascular space and its hyponatremic nature might lead to cerebral edema. The infant in the question is hypernatremic, so 3% saline (513 mEq sodium/L) would only exacerbate the problem; its use in dehydration might be considered for some patients with severe hyponatremia with neurologic symptoms. Fresh-frozen plasma can be used in the situation described, but it is generally not rapidly available, is more expensive, can be associated with infectious agents, and offers no advantage to saline.

235. The answer is a. (*Hay et al, pp 748-749. Kliegman et al, pp 248-249. Rudolph et al, pp 1681-1682.*) The infant in the question has had an emergency line placed for dehydration and has hypernatremic dehydration (high sodium, with elevated creatinine and low bicarbonate on the electrolyte panel). Initial bolus therapy in the emergency center should have been with isotonic fluid such as normal saline or lactated Ringer's solution. Slow correction of this hypernatremia (0.5 mEq/L per hour over several days) prevents significant fluid shifts in the brain that may result in increased intracranial pressure and herniation. Hyperglycemia may be seen in hypernatremic dehydration because of decreased insulin secretion and cell sensitivity to insulin; this is particularly important to recognize because an increased serum glucose can cause the serum sodium lab result to be falsely decreased. Blood products such as fresh-frozen plasma are not indicated, and rapid infusion of hypotonic solutions such as D10W and one-fourth normal saline could cause rapid fluid shifts resulting in cerebral edema and death. Hypertonic (3%) saline is used only in the event of seizures caused by rapid rehydration (or in children with hyponatremic dehydration and associated central nervous system symptoms), along with other emergent measures typically used to reduce cerebral edema.

236. The answer is a. (*Hay et al, pp 469-470. Kliegman et al, p 1768. Rudolph et al, pp 1350-1351.*) In general, mandibular teeth erupt before maxillary teeth; teeth tend to erupt in girls before they do in boys. The first teeth to erupt usually are the mandibular central incisors at 5-7 months, followed by the maxillary central incisors at 6-8 months. Lateral incisors (mandibular then maxillary) erupt next at 7-11 months, followed by the first molars (10-16 months), the cuspids (16-20 months), and the second molars (20-30 months). Note that the "normal" time of initial eruption can vary widely; the mandibular incisors can erupt as late as 16-18 months of age. Further delay, while rare, warrants investigation.

237. The answer is d. (*Hay et al, pp 660-661. Kliegman et al, pp 1884-1887. Rudolph et al, pp 1377-1381.*) Recurrent abdominal pain (more currently called functional abdominal pain, part of "functional gastrointestinal disorders," or FGIDs) is a common complaint occurring in at least 10% of school-age children. In children older than 2 years, less than 10% of cases have an identifiable organic cause. In the case presented the pain occurs only in school, the examination is normal, growth parameters are not concerning, and baseline laboratory data are normal. Management of these children is difficult and frustrating for the physician and the family. Excessive testing and treatments are not typically useful. A thorough history and physical examination, including growth parameters, are frequently helpful in separating organic from nonorganic causes of abdominal pain. Any signs or symptoms of organic causes, such as growth failure, should be pursued. If nothing in the history or physical examination is found, as is likely in the case described, reassurance of the children and family members is indicated. Close follow-up for new or changing symptoms as well as further reassurance to the family is important.

238. The answer is d. (*Hay et al, pp 471-473. Kliegman et al, pp 1773-1775. Rudolph et al, pp 1343-1344.*) The pattern of dental disease found with the use of bottles that contain high concentrations of sugars, which promotes dental disease, includes extensive maxillary decay (especially frontal) and posterior maxillary and mandibular decay, but essentially normal mandibular frontal teeth. Prevention of this disease is possible through counseling families to avoid the use of fruit juices in bottles or sweetened pacifiers. In addition, children should never be permitted to take a bottle to bed with them; weaning from the bottle should be discussed with the parents toward the end of the first year of life. Genetic predisposition seems to play a role as well.

239. The answer is a. (*Hay et al, pp 640-641. Kliegman et al, pp 1903-1904. Rudolph et al, pp 1429-1432.*) A congenital indirect inguinal hernia is the result of incomplete closure of the processus vaginalis. This is in contrast to the less commonly acquired direct inguinal hernia, caused by weakness in the musculature of the inguinal canal. Inguinal hernias are commonly seen in premature infants (16%-25%). Incarceration is common; elective repair is often considered prior to hospital discharge. Transillumination, while frequently mentioned as a method to distinguish hydrocele from hernia, can be misleading. The diagnosis of congenital indirect inguinal hernia in a preterm infant is so common that diagnostic tests are performed infrequently; when there is diagnostic uncertainty, a scrotal ultrasound may be performed.

240. The answer is b. (*Hay et al, p 344. Kliegman et al, pp 463-464. Rudolph et al, p 466.*) Endoscopic examination of the esophagus and stomach is a diagnostic method of determining the extent of the mucosal injury, as significant esophageal injury may be present even in the absence of oral burns.

This is true of accidental ingestions of both bases (eg, drain cleaner) and acids (eg, toilet bowl cleaner). The most severe cases present with shock after perforation somewhere along the GI tract. Vomiting is contraindicated as it would expose the mucosal surfaces to the caustic agent a second time. The child can be given small amounts of milk or water, but large amounts, which might cause vomiting, are unwise. Neutralization of the caustic liquid can result in an exothermic reaction and produce a thermal burn. The use of steroids after endoscopy in second-degree chemical burns of the esophagus has been effective in diminishing the inflammatory response in some patients. Optimal treatment is still controversial and requires expert consultation or review of the most current literature. Charcoal, however, does not absorb the alkaline agent in drain cleaner. Esophageal strictures are the primary long-term complication of caustic ingestion.

241. The answer is d. (*Hay et al, p 336. Kliegman et al, pp 454-464. Rudolph et al, p 457.*) The absorption of certain toxins from the GI tract is diminished by the use of activated charcoal administered during the first few hours after the ingestion. The typical dose is 1 g/kg, or 10-30 g for a child or 30-100 g for an adult. Activated charcoal exerts its effect by adsorbing particles of toxin on its surface. Compounds not adsorbed include alcohols, acids (such as toilet cleaners), ferrous sulfate, strong bases (such as drain cleaners and oven cleaners), cyanide, lithium, and potassium. For drugs with an enterohepatic circulation (eg, phenobarbital and tricyclic antidepressants), or those with prolonged absorption (eg, sustained-release theophylline), the use of multiple-dose activated charcoal can be effective in decreasing the half-life and increasing the total body clearance of the toxic substance.

242 to 246. The answers are 242-c, 243-a, 244-h, 245-f, 246-b. (*Hay et al, pp 41-42, 634-635, 1273-1275. Kliegman et al, pp 870-871, 1816-1817, 1854-1864. Rudolph et al, pp 246-249, 1389, 1454-1460.*) Swallowed maternal blood can be differentiated from neonatal hemorrhage by the Apt (or Apt-Downey, or alkali denaturation) test, which distinguishes fetal hemoglobin from adult hemoglobin based on the specimen's reaction to alkali (fetal hemoglobin is unchanged, whereas adult hemoglobin changes to hematin). Infants may swallow blood during delivery or from a cracked nipple during breast-feeding.

Necrotizing enterocolitis (NEC) is a life-threatening condition seen mostly in premature infants. Although the precise etiology is unknown, contributing factors include GI tract ischemia, impaired host immunity, the presence of bacterial or viral pathogens, and the presence of breast milk or formula in the gut. Findings include bloody stools, abdominal distension, hypoxia, acidosis, and emesis. The initial diagnostic test of choice is plain film radiographs. The characteristic radiographic finding in NEC is pneumatosis intestinalis; free air in the peritoneum may also be seen. Perforation is a surgical emergency; otherwise, observation, gastric decompression, and antibiotics are indicated.

Enterohemorrhagic *Escherichia coli* are Shiga-like toxin-producing pathogens found in poorly cooked beef, and some have been responsible for outbreaks of bloody diarrhea that were well-publicized in the media. Other sources include exposure to exotic animals or to nursing home patients. These organisms secrete Shiga toxin. Routine stool cultures do not distinguish this particular pathogen from other *E coli*; the laboratory must use sorbitol-MacConkey agar to isolate the bacteria. Enzyme assays for Shiga toxin are available as well.

Forceful emesis can result in small tears in the esophagus, termed Mallory-Weiss syndrome. This is usually a benign condition, only occasionally resulting in significant blood loss. In a patient who is otherwise stable, diagnostic procedures are not indicated.

Peptic ulcer disease can result in hematemesis and melena, along with the typically epigastric abdominal pain. Children can have both chronic and acute blood loss associated with ulceration; pallor may be a clinical finding as in the case presented. Fiberoptic endoscopy is the diagnostic method of choice. An upper GI series can sometimes reveal an ulcer as well. While *H pylori* serum assays are available, they have limited usefulness in children.

247 to 251. The answers are 247-c, 248-j, 249-h, 250-e, 251-f. (*Hay et al, pp 284-292. Kliegman et al, pp 317-369. Rudolph et al, pp 92-94, 1546-1548.*) Treatment for tuberculosis usually includes the medication isoniazid (INH), and INH competitively inhibits pyridoxine utilization. In most children, this does not result in clinical manifestations, but in individuals with a poor dietary intake of pyridoxine (eg, teenagers, vegetarians, and exclusively breast-fed infants), numbness and tingling of the hands and feet may develop. Treatment is replacement of pyridoxine.

Cow's milk contains an insufficient quantity of iron to sustain normal RBC production. Therefore, infants whose primary caloric source is cow's milk are likely to develop iron-deficiency anemia, characterized by microcytosis and hypochromia on the peripheral smear. In the question presented, the child has pallor and tachycardia.

Hemorrhagic disease of the newborn is now rare, as the vast majority of newborns receive a vitamin K injection shortly after birth. Classic disease presents within the first week of life and is characterized by hematemesis, hematuria, umbilical stump and circumcision oozing, and purpura. Parents who refuse vitamin K for their newborns should be vigorously educated about the potentially devastating consequences of this condition.

Vitamin C deficiency impairs wound healing. In its severe form, also termed *scurvy*, children can have diffuse tenderness, which is worse in the legs; evidence of hemorrhage; irritability; low-grade fever; swelling; tachypnea; and poor appetite. Diagnosis is based on clinical picture and radiographic findings; if laboratory studies are desired, a plasma ascorbate level less than 0.2 mg/dL suggests deficiency.

Vitamin D deficiency leads to rickets, a failure of bone mineralization, and the clinical picture described in the question. Rickets is unusual in the developed parts of the world, but still occurs; the American Academy of Pediatrics recommends all breast-fed infants receive vitamin D supplementation until weaned on to vitamin D containing infant formula, or whole milk after 1 year of age. In addition to nutritional rickets, there are congenital forms of rickets; despite vitamin D supplementation, these children can have permanent bony disfigurement.

The Urinary Tract

Questions

252. You are seeing a 5-year-old girl for a routine checkup. The mother reports the child to be in good health overall, but does report that she has a 4-day history of foul-smelling, purulent vaginal discharge. She has no significant medical history. She lives with her parents and does not attend day care. On physical examination she has normal vital signs and no remarkable findings other than a foul-smelling, purulent vaginal discharge. Hymen is intact, and neither vaginal nor rectal trauma is noted. Which of the following is the most appropriate next step in managing this child?

a. Refer to pediatric surgery for examination under anesthesia.
b. Place patient in knee-chest position and examine vagina with nasal speculum.
c. Apply topical hydrocortisone cream for a week.
d. Refer to social services for possible sexual abuse.
e. Apply topical estrogen cream daily for 6 weeks.

253. At the 2-week checkup of a term female neonate, the mother reports a grayish and occasionally blood-tinged vaginal discharge since birth. The neonate's mother and grandmother are the only caretakers. Examination of the external genitalia reveals an intact hymen with a thin grayish mucous discharge. Which of the following is the most appropriate next step?

a. Parental reassurance
b. MRI of the brain with attention to the pituitary gland
c. Ultrasound of the abdomen
d. Gonorrhea and chlamydial swabs
e. Genital examination under anesthesia

254. A 25-year-old woman who has had no prenatal care delivers a 3000 g boy. The neonate (Photograph) is noted to have undescended testes, clubfeet, and to be in respiratory distress. Which of the following test findings would have assisted in prenatal diagnosis?

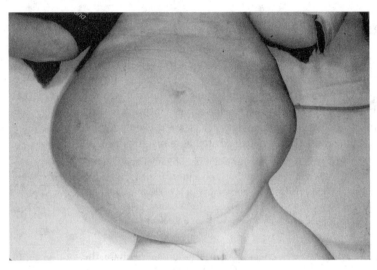

(Used with permission from Michael L. Ritchey, MD.)

a. Reduced levels of amniotic phosphatidylinositol (lecithin)
b. Prenatal ultrasound showing excessive neck fold thickness and edematous hands and feet
c. Prenatal ultrasound demonstrating oligohydramnios and dysplastic kidneys
d. Abnormal chromosome analysis on Chorionic villus sampling
e. Measurement of low maternal folate levels

255. A 7-year old presents to your office for puffy eyes. Her past history is significant for attention-deficit/hyperactivity disorder (ADHD) for which she takes a stimulant medicine, and an upper respiratory tract infection that resolved the previous week. Her blood pressure is 97/57 mm Hg, heart rate is 90 beats per minute, and respiratory rate is 18 breaths per minute. A careful physical examination reveals bilateral orbital, labial, and ankle edema. Her examination is otherwise normal. You obtain a urinalysis that reveals 4+ protein, without leukocytes or blood, and her serum creatinine is 0.2 mg/dL. Which of the following is the most likely diagnosis?

a. Postinfectious glomerulonephritis
b. Henoch-Schönlein purpura (HSP) nephritis
c. Systemic lupus erythematosus (SLE) nephritis
d. Nephrotic syndrome due to minimal change disease
e. Hemolytic uremic syndrome (HUS)

256. A 1-year-old child is seen in the pediatric clinic for excessive thirst and is constantly crying for his sippy cup. The parents also note frequent wet diaper changes that persist even when they limit his liquid intake. They report three previous hospital admissions in the first 6 months of life for dehydration, only once associated with vomiting or diarrhea. The child is awake, alert, active, and in no distress. Length and head circumference are at the 10th percentile, weight is less than the 3rd percentile. The examination is normal. Which of the following is most appropriate next step?

a. Admission for a 3-day calorie count with high calorie nutritional supplements
b. Measurement of serum and urine glucose levels and serum hemoglobin A1C
c. Repeated measurement of serum sodium and urine-specific gravity levels during a controlled fluid restriction challenge
d. Obtain skeletal survey, an ophthalmologic evaluation, and call child protective services
e. Measurement of serum protein, cholesterol, and triglyceride levels as well as 24-hour urine protein excretion measurement

257. A 6-month-old infant has poor weight gain, vomiting, episodic fevers, and chronic constipation. Laboratory studies reveal:

Serum electrolytes:
  Sodium: 139 mEq/L
  Potassium: 4.5 mEq/L
  Chloride: 135 mEq/L
  Bicarbonate: 14 mEq/L
  Glucose: 100 mg/dL
  Calcium: 7.9 mg/dL (normal: 8.5-10.2 mg/dL)
  Phosphorus: 3.1 mg/dL (normal: 2.5-4.5 mg/dL)
  Protein: 7 mg/dL (normal: 6-8 mg/dL)
  Albumin: 4 mg/dL (normal: 3.5-5 mg/dL)
  Urine: pH of 8.0, specific gravity of 1.010, 1+ glucose, 1+ protein, anion gap is normal. What is the best diagnosis to explain these findings?

a. Hypertrophic pyloric stenosis
b. Congenital hypothyroidism
c. Renal tubular acidosis (RTA) type 4
d. Hereditary Fanconi syndrome
e. Congenital nephrotic syndrome

258. A 14-year-old Asian boy arrives via ambulance to your emergency room from the local international airport. About half-way through his 12-hour flight he developed severe, intermittent abdominal pain that radiates into his scrotum. He denies fever, but does report dysuria and red colored urine. Of the following, which is the most appropriate next step in the management of this child?

a. Order an air contrast enema.
b. Obtain an emergency ultrasound with Doppler flow studies of his testes.
c. Order a noncontrast spiral CT of the abdomen and pelvis.
d. Administer a dose of ceftriaxone intramuscularly and begin a 10-day course of doxycycline.
e. Send stool for ova, cysts, and parasites.

259. A 9-month-old boy is seen for fever. His mother reports that he has been cranky and having decreased interest in eating his normal food but has been drinking well. She reports that his urine has a "strong smell". He has been in good health otherwise; he has had no previous serious illnesses. Vital signs include a temperature of 38.5°C (101.1°F), heart rate 90 beats per minute, respiratory rate of 18 breaths per minute, and a blood pressure of 90/75 mm Hg. He is awake, alert, and fussy but calms easily. The rest of his examination is normal. Which of the following is the most appropriate next step in his management?

a. Bladder catheterization for urinalysis and culture
b. Bag urine for culture
c. Referral for renal ultrasound
d. Complete blood count and differential
e. Initiation of broad-spectrum antibiotics

260. Physical examination of an infant boy shortly after birth reveals a large bladder and palpable kidneys. The nurses note that he produces a weak urinary stream. A voiding cystourethrogram (VCUG) is shown in the photograph. He appears to be otherwise normal. Which of the following is the most likely diagnosis?

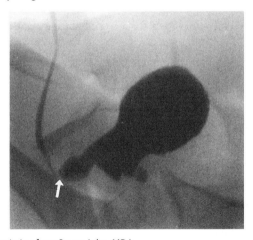

(Used with permission from Susan John, MD.)

a. Ureteropelvic junction obstruction
b. Posterior urethral valve
c. Prune belly syndrome
d. Duplication of the collecting system
e. Horseshoe kidney

261. An 18-year-old girl is seen in the emergency center with the complaint of generalized weakness, muscle tenderness, and cola-colored urine. She had been in good health until finishing track practice 2 hours earlier. Vital signs include a temperature of 38.5°C (101.1°F), heart rate 120 beats per minute, respiratory rate of 18 breaths per minute, and a blood pressure of 110/75 mm Hg. On physical examination she has generalized muscle tenderness, especially in her legs. Laboratory data show:

Hemoglobin: 13.5%
Hematocrit: 41%
WBC: 11,000/mm³
Platelet count: 175,000/mm³
Urine: pH of 6.5, specific gravity of 1.025, 1+ protein, 2+ heme, no RBC

Which of the following is the most appropriate next step in the management of this patient?

a. Encourage increased oral liquid intake for future track practice.
b. Measure serum antistreptolysin O levels.
c. Begin intravenous normal saline at two to three times maintenance.
d. Initiate hemodialysis.
e. Admit for renal biopsy.

262. A 4-year-old boy is seen for a well-child check. He has been in good health and appears to be developing normally, although the family is concerned with his occasional nocturnal enuresis. Vital signs include a temperature of 36.7°C (98°F), heart rate of 100 beats per minute, respiratory rate of 18 breaths per minute, and a blood pressure of 95/59 mm Hg. Height and weight are at the 50th percentile for age. Urinalysis shows a pH of 7.0, specific gravity of 1.010, 3+ protein, and negative for heme, RBCs, nitrite, nitrate, and glucose. Which of the following is the most likely condition affecting this child?

a. Orthostatic (postural) proteinuria
b. Poststreptococcal glomerulonephritis
c. Berger disease (IgA nephropathy)
d. Alport syndrome
e. Nephrotic syndrome

263. The 1-year-old boy in the photograph, who recently had a circumcision, requires an additional operation on his genitalia that will probably eliminate his risk of which of the following?

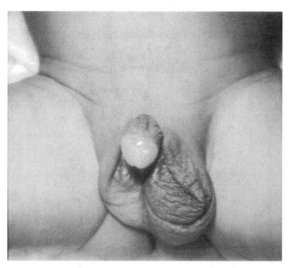

(Used with permission from Michael L. Ritchey, MD.)

a. Testicular malignancy
b. Decreased sperm count
c. Torsion of testes
d. UTI
e. Epididymitis

264. A newborn in the low-risk nursery of the hospital is noted to have the genital finding noted in the photograph. He was born at term after an uneventful pregnancy. His examination is otherwise normal. Which of the following is the most appropriate next step in his management?

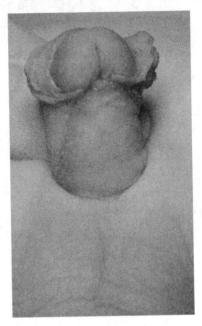

(Used with permission from Eric Jones, MD.)

a. Circumcision
b. Initiation of prophylactic antibiotics
c. Chromosome analysis
d. Referral to urologist
e. Renal ultrasound

265. A 4-year-old African American child has returned home from visiting his grandmother in a rural area. He spent most of his time outside swimming, playing in the yard, helping in the gardens, and chasing his grandmother's chihuahua. He was noted 2 weeks ago to have "infected mosquito bites" on his neck and chin for which the local doctor had him scrub with soap and apply over-the-counter topical antibiotic cream; a few lesions remain and are shown in the photograph. His mother brings him into the office with the complaint of dark urine, swelling around his eyes, and shortness of breath. Vital signs include a temperature of 36.7°C (98°F), heart rate 120 beats per minute, respiratory rate of 28 breaths per minute, and a blood pressure of 120/80 mm Hg. On physical examination the child has the pictured lesions and mild periorbital edema. He has tachycardia, a few rales on chest examination, and a mildly enlarged liver. Which of the following is the most appropriate next step?

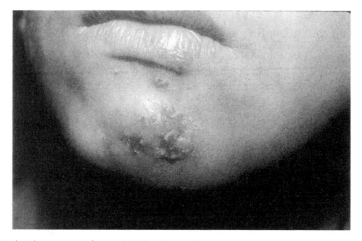

(Used with permission from Adelaide Hebert, MD.)

a. Renal biopsy and measurement of serum compliment levels
b. Oral cephalosporin, close monitoring of blood pressure, and potential fluid restriction
c. Measurement of serum and urine calcium levels
d. Intravenous ceftazidime, VCUG, and renal ultrasound
e. Intramuscular ceftriaxone followed by 10 days of oral doxycycline

266. A 4-year-old boy and his family recently had a family reunion in the local park. Several of the family members developed "gastroenteritis" with fever and diarrhea, but the 4-year-old boy's stool was slightly different, as it contained blood. His mother reports that in the past 24 hours he developed pallor and lethargy; she relates that his face looks swollen and that he has been urinating very little. Laboratory evaluation reveals a hematocrit of 28% and a platelet count of 72,000/μL. He has blood and protein in the urine. Which of the following immediate therapies is likely to result in a reduction in mortality associated with this condition?

a. Begin immediately a 10-day course of intravenous ceftriaxone.
b. Immediate renal biopsy and initiation of steroids.
c. Stat air contrast enema.
d. Stat technetium-99m (^{99m}Tc) pertechnetate scan of the abdomen.
e. Supportive care with control of hypertension and attention to fluid, electrolyte, and nutritional status.

267. A 16-year-old boy with known sickle cell disease calls you on Saturday evening with the complaint of a painful, unwanted erection for the previous 4 hours. He denies fever, pain elsewhere, and recent sexual activity. Which of the following is the most appropriate next step in the management of his condition?

a. Warm shower and short aerobic exercise
b. Oral pain medication and increase fluid intake
c. Admission for partial exchange transfusion
d. Referral to emergency room for corpora cavernosa irrigation
e. Initiation of an oral adrenergic (pseudoephedrine)

268. A 15-year-old girl is seen with the history of 2 months of intermittent fever, malaise, and weight loss. Recently she has developed swollen hands, wrists, and ankles, the pain of which seems out of proportion to the clinical findings. She also complains of cold extremities and has some ulceration of her distal digits. Which of the following laboratory tests is most likely to assist in the diagnosis of this condition?

a. Antibodies to nDNA and Sm nuclear antigens
b. Throat culture for group A β-hemolytic streptococcus
c. Simultaneously acquired urine and serum bicarbonate levels
d. Urine microscopy for casts
e. Erythrocyte sedimentation rate

269. A 12-year-old boy comes to the ED at midnight with a complaint of acute and severe scrotal pain since 7 PM. He has no history of trauma, but he does complain of nausea and vomiting. Which of the following is the most appropriate first step in management?

a. Order a surgical consult immediately.
b. Order a radioisotope scan as an emergency.
c. Order a urinalysis and Gram stain for bacteria.
d. Arrange for an ultrasound examination.
e. Order a Doppler examination.

270. The mother of a 2-year-old girl reports that her daughter complains of burning when she urinates and that she has foul-smelling discharge from her vagina. She has some slight staining on the front of her underwear, but denies fever, nausea, vomiting, or other constitutional signs. The child does not attend day care, and she has demonstrated no change in behavior. The physical examination is normal with an intact hymen, but the child's vulva is reddened and a malodorous scent is noted. Her urinalysis and culture are normal. Management of this condition includes which of the following?

a. Complete genitourinary (GU) examination under general anesthesia
b. Progesterone cream to the affected area for a week
c. Advise to stop taking prolonged bubble baths
d. Mebendazole to eradicate pinworm infestation
e. Referral to social services for possible sexual abuse

271. A 7-year-old boy has cramping abdominal pain and the rash shown in the photograph, distributed on the back of his legs and buttocks as well as on the extensor surfaces of his forearms. Urinalysis shows a pH of 7.0, specific gravity of 1.020, 2+ protein, 2+ RBCs, and no glucose. In addition to his rash and abdominal pain, what other finding is he likely to have?

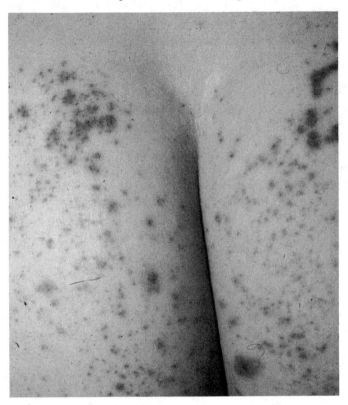

a. Chronic renal failure
b. Arthritis or arthralgia
c. Seizures
d. Unilateral lymphadenopathy
e. Bulbar nonpurulent conjunctivitis

272. A 13-year-old boy's scrotum is shown in the photograph. He complains of several months of swelling but no pain just above his left testicle. He is sexually active with two partners and states that he usually uses condoms. On physical examination, the area in question feels like a "bag of worms." Which of the following is the most appropriate management for this condition?

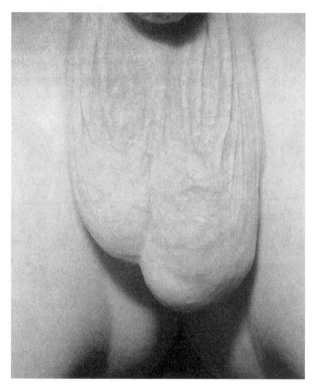

(Used with permission from Michael L. Ritchey, MD.)

a. Doppler flow study of testes
b. Radionuclide scan of testes
c. Urinalysis and culture
d. Ceftriaxone intramuscularly and doxycycline orally
e. Reassurance and education only

273. A 3-day-old neonate's scrotum is shown in the photograph. Palpation reveals a tense, fluid-filled area surrounding the right testicle. The scrotum transilluminates well and the amount of fluid does not vary with mild pressure. Which of the following is the most appropriate approach to this condition?

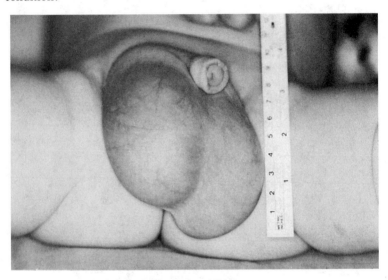

(Used with permission from Michael L. Ritchey, MD.)

a. Request a surgical consultation
b. Incision and drainage
c. Administer prophylactic antibiotics
d. Observe only
e. Perform a chromosome determination

274. A 2-year-old girl arrives late to your office with her father. He is very apologetic and tells you through the sign language interpreter that he had car trouble at his dialysis center and thus was late picking up the child from day care. The father is concerned about his child having intermittent red, bloody-looking urine, especially after an upper respiratory infection. A gross inspection of the child's urine in your office looks normal, but the dipstick demonstrates 3+ blood. Which of the following is the most likely to assist in the diagnosis of this child's condition?

a. Ophthalmologic evaluation
b. Renal ultrasound with renal vein Doppler flow studies
c. Disseminated intravascular coagulation screen
d. Measurement of serum PT, PTT, and levels of factors VII, IX, and XI
e. Evaluation of sputum for evidence of blood or hemosiderin-laden macrophages

275. A 9-year-old boy is brought to the office by his grandmother for a preparticipation physical examination for summer camp. She reports that the boy's parents complain that they often find his urine-soaked underwear hidden under his bed in the morning. The grandmother reports that her son (the child's father) had similar challenges at that age but that after a few years of adjusting his diet his symptoms resolved. In light of the boy's upcoming camp trip, his grandmother asks what dietary changes will help. In response, you suggest which of the following about this child's condition?

a. A thorough family history would likely determine that the condition affects most of the boys on both sides of the family.
b. A psychiatric evaluation is warranted.
c. Dietary changes are unnecessary in the child.
d. That the father faced similar challenges as a boy is likely coincidental.
e. Short courses of desmopressin acetate (DDAVP) lead to permanent cure in 80% of cases.

276. A 21-year-old woman presents to the emergency room in active labor. She has had no prenatal care, but her last menstrual period was approximately 9 months prior. Her membranes are artificially ruptured, yielding no amniotic fluid. She delivers an 1800-g (4 lb) term infant who develops significant respiratory distress immediately at birth. The first chest radiograph on this neonate is shown in the photograph. After stabilization, the most appropriate next step for this neonate is which of the following?

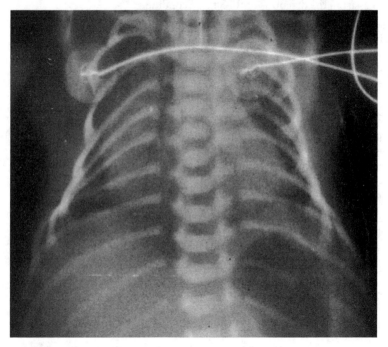

a. Cardiac catheterization
b. Renal ultrasound
c. VCUG
d. Liver and spleen scan
e. Technetium-99m (^{99m}Tc) renal scan

Questions 277 to 280

For each condition listed as under, match the category to which it belongs. Each lettered option may be used once, more than once, or not at all.

a. Nephrotic syndrome
b. HSP nephritis
c. Alport syndrome
d. Acute glomerulonephritis
e. Sickle cell nephropathy
f. Idiopathic hypercalciuria
g. Beeturia
h. Urolithiasis
i. Urinary tract infection
j. Goodpasture disease
k. HUS
l. IgA nephropathy (Berger nephropathy)
m. Chlamydial urethritis
n. SLE
o. Bartter syndrome
p. Renal medullary carcinoma

277. An 18-year-old black man has gross hematuria, back pain, and unexplained weight loss. His past history is positive for sickle trait disease.

278. A 6-year-old girl with a 1-day complaint of "bloody urine"; her vital signs, physical examination, and urinalysis is completely normal.

279. Elevated levels of cholesterol and triglycerides found in a 6-year-old boy whose mother reports that he has been awakening with puffy eyes each morning. On your physical examination, you determine that he has had unexpected weight gain and has scrotal edema.

280. A 12-month-old girl whose height and weight are less than the fifth percentile; she has had several bouts of constipation and two previous admissions for dehydration. She is again admitted for dehydration and is noted to have serum potassium of 2.7 mEq/L.

The Urinary Tract

Answers

252. The answer is b. (*Kliegman et al, pp 2607-2613.*) The patient very well may have a vaginal foreign body. The offending object may have been intentionally placed by the child, who did not tell her parents, or may be something such as a wad of toilet paper in a child who is undergoing toilet training. The first step in identification of the problem is a visual inspection. An attempt at placing the cooperative child in a knee-chest position and visualization with a nasal speculum may identify the offending object. If an object is identified and is unable to be removed, or if no object is identified and suspicion for foreign body remains high, an examination under anesthesia is the next most appropriate step. Child sexual abuse must always be on the differential; without vaginal or rectal findings referral to social services as the first step would be premature. Labial adhesion (also called labial agglutination) is a usually benign condition in which the labia minora are fused. Treatment for asymptomatic girls can be merely observation, as the condition often resolves with the estrogenization that occurs with puberty. Alternatively, nightly application of an estrogen cream with or without betamethasone for 6 weeks resolves this condition in the majority of patients.

253. The answer is a. (*Hay et al, p 15. Kliegman et al, pp 1869-1870. Rudolph et al, p 179.*). This patient has a physiologic discharge related to estrogen withdrawal; greyish mucous that becomes blood-tinged is common and normal. Examination can exclude vaginal trauma and foreign body, and the history makes sexual abuse unlikely. Neither imaging nor examination under anesthesia is indicated at this point. Parents should be reassured that it will resolve in a few weeks.

254. The answer is c. (*Hay et al, p 757. Kliegman et al, pp 2572-2573. Rudolph et al, pp 1743-1744.*) The child in the photo has prune belly syndrome (also known as Eagle-Barrett syndrome), a condition almost always found in males. Prenatal ultrasound findings include oligohydramnios, an abnormal urinary tract including dysfunction and dysplasia, and intra-abdominal testicular tissue. Postnatal findings include a lax, wrinkled abdominal wall, pulmonary hypoplasia and respiratory distress, congenital hip dislocation, clubfeet, and intestinal malrotation with secondary volvulus. Although medical and surgical care has improved, the perinatal death rate is around 30%. Current research suggests prune belly syndrome may have an autosomal recessive inheritance, but the exact chromosome abnormality (which could be obtained prenatally via Chorionic villus sampling) has not been identified.

Reduced levels of amniotic lecithin levels are found in premature infants with surfactant deficiency. Excessive neck fold thickness and edematous hands and feet are seen in infants with Turner syndrome. Low maternal folate consumption during pregnancy is associated with an increased incidence of neural tube defects.

255. The answer is d. (*Hay et al, pp 760-761. Kliegman et al, pp 2521-2528. Rudolph et al, pp 1722-1727*). Nephrotic syndrome is a constellation of findings that can be seen in glomerular disease. The classic triad of symptoms includes hypoalbuminemia, edema, and hyperlipidemia, all related to the underlying problem of large urinary loses of protein. "Nephrotic-range" proteinuria is defined as more than 40 mg/m^2/h or a protein-to-creatinine ratio of more than 2:1. While there are many causes of nephrotic syndrome (including malignancy, malaria, drugs, infections, and metabolic conditions), children most commonly have primary, or idiopathic, nephrotic syndrome. Minimal change disease is the most common glomerular lesion associated with idiopathic nephrotic syndrome, and 90% of children with minimal change disease respond well to steroids.

The glomerulonephritides present with edema and proteinuria, but also with hypertension, hematuria, and renal insufficiency. HUS usually presents after diarrhea caused by a toxin producing strain of *Escherichia coli*.

256. The answer is c. (*Hay et al, p. 772. Kliegman et al, pp 2644-2646. Rudolph et al, pp 2026-2027.*) The case is that of a failure to thrive child with classic congenital nephrogenic diabetes insipidus, a hereditary disorder in which the urine is hypotonic and produced in large volumes because the distal tubule and collecting duct of the kidneys fail to respond to antidiuretic hormone (vasopressin). Males are primarily affected through an X-linked recessive inheritance; autosomal dominant and recessive forms are also known. Although the condition is present at birth, the diagnosis is often not made until several months later, when excessive thirst, frequent voiding of large volumes of dilute urine, dehydration, and failure to thrive due to excessive water ingestion become obvious. The diagnosis can be confirmed in the hospital during a fluid-deprivation test which will show rising serum sodium levels with continued dilute urine specific gravity.

A 3-day calorie count often is utilized to determine protein-calorie malnutrition, but the episodes of dehydration and the remarkable family history would be unexpected. Diabetes mellitus rarely presents with a protracted course in such a young child; it is usually a more acute illness and often with vomiting. Child abuse would be unlikely, especially with a family history as noted. Nephrotic syndrome can be diagnosed as in the final option of the answers but would be expected to present with other signs such as edema and proteinuria.

257. The answer is d. (*Hay et al, pp 936-937. Kliegman et al, pp 2529-2532. Rudolph et al, pp 1732-1733.*) The nonspecific findings of anorexia, polydipsia and polyuria, vomiting, and unexplained fevers, along with the more specific laboratory abnormalities of glucosuria but normal blood sugar, abnormally high urine pH in the face of mild or moderate serum hyperchloremic metabolic acidosis, and mild albuminuria in the presence of normal serum protein and albumin, suggest Fanconi syndrome (also called global proximal tubular dysfunction). Fanconi syndrome can be hereditary or acquired; hereditary forms are usually secondary to a genetic abnormality such as cystinosis, galactosemia, Wilson disease, and some mitochondrial abnormalities. A number of agents can cause Fanconi syndrome, including gentamicin (or other aminoglycosides), outdated tetracycline, cephalothin, cidofovir, valproic acid, streptozocin, 6-mercaptopurine, azathioprine, cisplatin, ifosfamide, heavy metals (eg, lead, mercury, cadmium, uranium, and platinum), paraquat, maleic acid, and toluene (from sniffing glue). The mechanism of action of these agents is through acute tubular necrosis, alteration of renal blood flow, intratubular obstruction, or allergic reactions within the kidney itself. Many of these toxic effects are reduced or eliminated with removal of the offending agent.

Hypertrophic pyloric stenosis typically begins after the first three weeks of life and before the fifth month of life. Nonbilious, progressive, and classically projectile vomiting are presenting signs. Ultimately hypovolemia and hypochloremic metabolic alkalosis develops. Congenital hypothyroidism is rare where mandatory screening at birth occurs. Presenting signs might include low muscle tone, prolonged hyperbilirubinemia, umbilical hernia, macroglossia, large fontanels, poor feeding, and coarse cry. Urine abnormalities are not an expected feature. Renal tubular acidosis (RTA) type 4 is a distal RTA occurring as a result of impaired aldosterone production or renal response to aldosterone; presenting findings of growth failure, polyuria, and dehydration are seen. Laboratory tests of these children show a hyperkalemic non-anion gap metabolic acidosis. The urine may be alkaline or acidic; the urine has elevated levels of sodium with inappropriately low levels of potassium. Congenital nephrotic syndrome is a rare version of nephrotic syndrome, characterized by edema early in infancy, with hypoalbuminemia due to excessive urine loss of protein but normal urine glucose levels.

258. The answer is c. (*Hay et al, pp 772-773. Kliegman et al, pp 2600-2604. Rudolph et al, pp 1738-1741.*) The child in the case likely has urolithiasis. While renal stones in children are relatively uncommon in the United States, their incidence is increasing due to obesity and changes in dietary habits (increase in sodium and fructose with decreased calcium and water intake). In the United States stones are more commonly related to metabolic abnormalities (where they are twice as common in boys). In southeast Asia stones are endemic and related to diet. A stone in the renal pelvis, calyx, or ureter causes obstruction and the symptoms are as presented in the case. A stone in the distal ureter results in symptoms of dysuria, urgency, and frequency. Once in the bladder, the stone is asymptomatic unless it moves into the urethra, then dysuria and voiding difficulties may arise. While some stones may be visible via plain abdominal radiograph, the noncontrast spiral CT scan will accurately diagnose the number and location of the stone(s) as well as assist in confirming if the affected kidney is hydronephrotic. Once the child's condition has stabilized (the stone passed or retrieved), a metabolic evaluation is undertaken in an attempt to identify the cause of the stone.

An air contrast enema would be diagnostic and therapeutic for a patient with suspected intussusception. While both urolithiasis and intussusception cause intermittent abdominal pain, the presentation of intussusception in an adolescent (as opposed to a child in the first 2 years of life) would be distinctly unusual. Ultrasonography with Doppler flow studies of the testes would diagnose a testicular torsion, but the pain from torsion would be expected to arise from the affected testis and radiate to the abdomen. The antibiotic regimen outlined might be used for an adolescent suspected of having a sexually transmitted disease; the clinical presentation would likely include more dysuria and less abdominal pain, but would not necessarily include a urethral discharge. Without diarrhea or other change in stools, parasitic disease would be unlikely to assist as an initial test for this child with severe abdominal pain.

259. The answer is a. (*Hay et al, pp 773-775. Kliegman et al, pp 2559-2562. Rudolph et al, pp 950-956.*) The child in the question has a febrile illness but is not toxic. The "foul smelling urine" suggests urinary tract infection as a possible cause of the fever. To confirm the diagnosis of UTI a urinalysis must suggest infection (pyuria and/or bacteriuria). At least 50,000 colony-forming units per mL of a uropathogen cultured from a urine specimen obtained through bladder catheterization, or any growth from a suprapubic bladder aspiration, is required. Antibiotics are started only after the gathering of appropriate cultures. An ultrasound is typically performed after the first UTI in a child, but a VCUG is not necessary after the first UTI if the ultrasound is normal. Blood work (culture, CBC, or serum electrolytes) are not required in the nontoxic appearing child. A bag urine culture will frequently be positive for multiple pathogens including skin and gut flora; urine obtained in this manner is not appropriate for culture.

260. The answer is b. (*Hay et al, p. 757. Kliegman, pp 1845-1846. Rudolph, p 1743.*) The findings described point to posterior urethral valves; the radiograph shows an area of obstruction and proximal dilatation of the bladder. Posterior urethral valves are the most common form of urinary tract obstruction in newborn boys, caused by obstructing leaflets of tissue in the prostatic urethra. The condition occurs in 1:5000-8000 boy infants; girls are not affected. The clinical picture of posterior valves ranges from that described in the question to severe renal obstruction with renal failure and pulmonary hypoplasia. UTIs are common complications in older children, and sepsis occasionally can be the presenting sign in afflicted newborns. Despite early recognition and correction of the obstruction, the prognosis in these children for normal renal function is guarded. Prenatal diagnosis is often accomplished because of widespread use of ultrasound.

Ureteropelvic junction obstruction, a common urinary obstruction in children that results in isolated hydronephrosis, can be found either on a prenatal ultrasound or after birth when the child is noted to have a mass, pain, or infection. Serial ultrasounds of the kidney assist in following the associated hydronephrosis. Prune belly syndrome occurs almost exclusively in boys; it is diagnosed in an infant with absent abdominal muscular tone, undescended testes, and urinary tract anomalies including hydronephrosis and dilated ureters and bladder. Duplication of the collecting system is often asymptomatic, but can present with symptoms of obstruction and reflux. Horseshoe kidney is often an asymptomatic condition, and results when both kidneys are joined at the lower pole by a fibrous band of tissue or by renal parenchyma; symptoms may arise resulting from obstruction and/or reflux.

261. The answer is c. (*Hay et al, p 1072. Kliegman, pp 773-775.*) The patient in the question likely has rhabdomyolysis caused by excessive physical exertion, especially in hot weather. Aggressive hydration will result in improved glomerular filtration rate, oxygen delivery to damaged muscle, and dilution of myoglobin and other renal-damaging toxins that are being released from the damaged muscle. Screening laboratory data will demonstrate elevated creatine kinase and urine that is positive for heme but has few or no red blood cells. Additional laboratory data are needed to guide ultimate therapy of this patient. Abnormalities such as hyperkalemia, hyperphosphatemia, hypocalcemia, hyperuricemia, and acidosis may be found early on and would require specific treatment approaches. Progression to renal failure is a possibility; dialysis may ultimately be required should the renal damage be severe. Increased fluid intake for future training sessions may help prevent future illness, but acute treatment is required for the ongoing rhabdomyolysis to prevent acute renal injury.

Dark urine can be a result of Group A poststreptococcal infection, and measurement of ASO titers may assist in the diagnosis if the streptococcal culture is negative. The urine in such cases, however, is positive for blood. A renal biopsy would be indicated for a patient with renal failure of unknown etiology.

262. The answer is a. (*Hay, p 755. Kliegman, p 2519. Rudolph, pp 1691-1692.*) The patient in the question is a normally developing child with normal vital signs. Occasional enuresis at 4 years of age is normal, but the isolated proteinuria suggests another diagnosis. The most common cause of persistent proteinuria in up to 60% of children is postural proteinuria. The diagnosis can be confirmed most easily by obtaining the first void for three consecutive mornings (after ensuring the bladder has been fully emptied the night before) which should demonstrate a lack of proteinuria and a normal urinary protein to urinary creatinine of less than 0.2. No treatment is required; parental reassurance is indicated. Poststreptococcal glomerulonephritis results in cola-colored urine that is positive for blood, and can be associated with hypertension and edema. Berger disease, or IgA nephropathy, causes episodic gross hematuria associated with an upper respiratory

Pediatrics

tract infection. Nephrotic syndrome may have isolated but persistent proteinuria; associated findings include hypertension and orbital and scrotal edema, as well as serum findings of hypoalbuminemia and hyperlipidemia. Patients with Alport syndrome have microscopic hematuria, possible episodes of gross hematuria, and frequently hearing loss depending on the genetic mutation.

263. The answer is c. (*Hay et al, p 1086. Kliegman et al, pp 2592-2593. Rudolph et al, p 1747.*) The child in the photograph has an undescended testis, or cryptorchidism. By 6 months of life, 0.8% of boys born at term still have cryptorchidism. In adults with cryptorchidism, the risk of testicular malignancy is much higher than in unaffected men. Orchiopexy does not eliminate this risk, but repositioning the testes makes them accessible for periodic examinations. Whether the testes are brought into the scrotum or not, the sperm count can be reduced. The failure of the testes to develop, and their subsequent atrophy, can be detected by 6 months of age. Torsion of the testis is a potential risk because of the excessive mobility of the undescended testis. Orchiopexy helps eliminate this problem by anchoring the testis to the scrotal wall. The incidence of UTI and epididymitis is not affected by the position of the testes.

264. The answer is d. (*Kliegman et al, pp 2586-2588. Rudolph et al, pp 1745-1746.*) The patient in the question has isolated hypospadias with chordee, a condition that is frequently encountered in the newborn nursery affecting about 1 in 250 newborn males. Treatment is surgical correction at 6-12 months of age with use of the foreskin in some cases (thus circumcision is contraindicated). Isolated hypospadias is not associated with an increased risk of infection or renal conditions. The condition is increased in conditions of disordered sex differentiation, anorectal malformations, and congenital heart disease, none of which are noted in this otherwise normal child.

265. The answer is b. (*Hay et al, pp 757-758. Kliegman et al, pp 2498-2501. Rudolph et al, pp 1711-1715.*) The child in the case likely has acute poststreptococcal glomerulonephritis (PSGN) following his skin infection (impetigo) as shown in the photograph. PSGN can also be seen following pharyngitis caused by certain nephritogenic strains of group A β-hemolytic streptococci. Hematuria often colors the urine dark, and decreased urinary output can result in circulatory congestion from volume overload with pulmonary edema, periorbital edema, tachycardia, and hepatomegaly; these complications are avoided by fluid restriction. Acute hypertension is common and can be associated with headache, vomiting, and encephalopathy with seizures. Treatment with antibiotics does not alter the course of the glomerulonephritis, but will treat the impetigo and will eliminate carriage of the nephritogenic strain of GABHS and decrease the risk of passing it to a close contact. In general, patients with PSGN do well without long-term sequelae, but close follow-up is required to demonstrate resolution of urine abnormalities.

It should be noted that while "rheumatogenic" strains of group A streptococci are only associated with pharyngitis, "nephritogenic" strains can be associated with either pharyngeal or skin infections. Also note that some sources refer to this condition more broadly as postinfectious glomerulonephritis (PIGN), to reflect the fact that other types of infection can result in nephritis.

Pyelonephritis (intravenous antibiotics, VCUG, and renal ultrasound) and sexually transmitted diseases (intramuscular ceftriaxone and oral doxycycline) can cause blood in the urine, but rarely present with impetigo and the other signs in the case. IgA nephropathy (complement level measurement and renal biopsy) is rare in African American children and rarely presents with hypertension. Idiopathic hypercalciuria, which can be diagnosed with measurement of serum and urine calcium levels, presents with blood and renal stones, but the other findings in the case are distinctly unusual.

266. The answer is e. (*Hay et al, pp 762-763. Kliegman et al, pp 2507-2510. Rudolph et al, pp 1727-1729.*) HUS is most common in children younger than 4 years of age and is characterized by an acute microangiopathic hemolytic anemia, thrombocytopenia from increased platelet utilization, and renal insufficiency from vascular endothelial injury and local fibrin deposition. Ischemic changes result in renal cortical necrosis and damage to other organs such as the colon, liver, heart, brain, and adrenal glands. Laboratory findings associated with HUS include low hemoglobin level, decreased platelet count, hypoalbuminemia, and evidence of hemolysis on peripheral smear (burr cells, helmet cells, schistocytes). Urinalysis reveals hematuria and proteinuria. A marked reduction of renal function leads to oliguria and rising levels of blood urea nitrogen (BUN) and creatinine. Gastrointestinal bleeding and obstruction, ascites, and central nervous system findings such as somnolence, convulsions, and coma can occur.

Infection by the Shiga toxin-producing *E coli* 0157:H7 has been implicated as the cause of over 90% of cases of HUS. This organism is epizootic in cattle. Outbreaks associated with undercooked contaminated hamburgers, roast beef, cow's milk, and fresh apple cider have been seen. The Coombs test is not positive in this type of hemolytic anemia. Antibiotic therapy in a patient actively infected with Shiga-toxin-producing *E coli* may worsen the risk of HUS. Rather, meticulous detail to fluid and electrolyte management is warranted and has resulted in dramatic decreases in the previously reported mortality associated with this disease.

Steroids and renal biopsy might be indicated for other forms of renal disease but are not indicated for a patient with HUS. Intussusception is seen in children of this age, but the lack of episodic colicky abdominal pain or emesis makes this diagnosis unlikely and the air contrast enema a poor choice. Meckel diverticulum causes painless bloody stool without fever or other associated symptoms, and it does not cause anuria; a ^{99m}Tc test is not warranted in this case.

267. The answer is d. (*Hay et al, pp 950-952. Kliegman et al, pp 2336-2345. Rudolph et al, pp 1556-1561.*) The young man in the question has had 4 hours of priapism due to this sickle cell disease; his condition is now a medical emergency. The optimal therapy for this condition is unknown, but initial therapies such as warm shower, improved hydration, oral pain medications, and oral adrenergic agents such as pseudoephedrine might be started when the priapism begins. For episodes lasting about 2-4 or more hours, more aggressive therapy such as aspiration of the corpora cavernosa and irrigation with dilute phenylephrine or epinephrine is appropriate. Simple blood transfusion or partial exchange transfusion is recommended by some, especially if the irrigation fails, but the detumescence does not occur as quickly.

268. The answer is a. (*Hay et al, p 759. Kliegman, pp 1176-1180. Rudolph, pp 814-817, 1719-1720.*) The fever, malaise, and weight loss as well as the arthritis involving mainly small joints are common findings of SLE. Raynaud phenomenon resulting in digital ulceration and gangrene in a few patients may also be seen. Not described in this patient is the oft-seen malar rash in a butterfly distribution across the bridge of the nose and the cheeks.

Simultaneous urine and serum electrolytes for bicarbonate determination hint at RTA, which often presents with failure to thrive and unexplained acidosis, sometimes with repeated episodes of dehydration and anorexia. Poststreptococcal glomerulonephritis can present with red cell casts, but the symptoms usually develop 8-14 days after an acute throat or skin infection. UTIs, especially of the upper collecting system, can result in casts, but they would be expected to consist of white rather than red cells.

Elevation of the erythrocyte sedimentation rate may be found in SLE, but this is a nonspecific finding noted in many other chronic and acute inflammatory conditions; its diagnostic usefulness in this situation is limited.

269. The answer is a. (*Kliegman et al, pp 1861-1862. Rudolph et al, pp 1746-1747.*) The majority of cases of acute scrotal pain and swelling in boys 12 years of age and older are caused by testicular torsion. If surgical exploration occurs within 4-6 hours, the testes can be saved 90% of the time. Too often, delay caused by scheduling imaging and laboratory tests, such as those outlined in the question, results in an unsalvageable gonad. Physical examination findings include an edematous, erythematous, tender testis that may be slightly elevated and lying horizontally. The cremasteric reflex, which is the elevation of the testis in response to stroking the inner upper thigh, is almost always absent. Typically the elevation of the affected testis (Prehn sign) does not improve, and sometimes worsens, the pain, but this sign is not specific enough to make the diagnosis.

One of the more important diagnoses in the differential is epididymitis. It is often gradual in onset, and the physical examination usually will reveal the testicle to be in its normal vertical position and to be of equal size to its counterpart. Epididymitis usually presents with redness, warmth, and scrotal swelling (but normal cremasteric reflex); the pain is posterior (over the epididymis). Pain relief on elevation of the testicle is typical and may be helpful to diagnose epididymitis although it is not specific.

270. The answer is c. (*Hay et al, p 1244. Kliegman et al, pp 1366-1367.*) The symptoms listed are those of vulvovaginitis, with nonspecific (or chemical) vulvovaginitis accounting for 70% of all pediatric vulvovaginitis cases. The discharge in nonspecific vulvovaginitis is usually brown or green and with a fetid odor. The burning with urination occurs because of contact between raw skin and urine. Further history in this case might reveal use of tight-fitting clothing (including swimsuits or dance outfits), nylon undergarments, prolonged bubble baths with contamination of the vagina with soap products, use of perfumed lotions in the vaginal area, or improper toilet habits (wiping of fecal material toward rather than away from vagina). Attention to these causative conditions usually results in resolution of the symptoms. The finding of a normal hymen, the history of a single caretaker, and the absence of behavioral changes all point away from, but do not completely exclude, sexual abuse. A vaginal examination under general anesthesia is usually required when a vaginal foreign body is suspected. Pinworms can infest the vagina, but symptoms usually include significant itching of the rectum and vagina. Estrogen cream, as well as antibiotic creams, is sometimes helpful in reducing the discomfort of vaginitis. In a sexually active adolescent (or in a sexually abused younger child), a variety of infectious agents, such as candida, *Chlamydia trachomatis*, *Trichomonas vaginalis*, *Gardnerella vaginalis*, and *Neisseria gonorrhoeae*, would be higher on the differential.

271. The answer is b. (*Hay et al, p 759. Kliegman et al, pp 1215-1218. Rudolph et al, pp 810-812, 1720-1721.*) HSP, or anaphylactoid purpura, is a systemic IgA-mediated vasculitis. The condition is typically a disease of childhood, with the peak incidence between 4 and 6 years of age. The rash appears much like that in the photograph of this child's buttocks and most often involves extensor surfaces of the extremities; the face, soles, palms, and trunk are less often affected. Other significant symptoms include edema, arthralgia or arthritis, colicky abdominal pain with GI bleeding, acute scrotal pain, and renal abnormalities ranging from proteinuria and microscopic hematuria to acute renal failure. Intussusception is the most common complication in the GI tract. As HSP is a systemic vasculitis, any organ system can be affected. The prognosis, however, is excellent, with only a small percentage of children going on to end-stage renal failure.

Treatment is generally supportive, focusing on hydration and pain control. Depending on the presentation and likelihood of follow-up, some children with HSP can be managed at home. Steroids are occasionally used for severe cases of abdominal pain, but there is no strong evidence that suggests steroids affect the disease course.

Seizures are an uncommon complication of CNS involvement; more commonly, patients will complain of headache and will have behavioral changes. Unilateral lymphadenopathy and nonpurulent conjunctivitis are not typical of HSP (but are criteria for Kawasaki disease, another pediatric vasculitis).

272. The answer is e. (*Kliegman et al, pp 2596-2597. McMillan et al, pp 1832-1833. Rudolph et al, pp 1747-1748.*) Varicocele, a common condition seen after 10 years of age, occurs in about 15% of adult males. It results from the dilatation of the pampiniform venous plexus (usually on the left side) due to valvular incompetence of the spermatic vein. Reduced sperm counts are possible with this condition; surgery may ultimately be indicated for infertility problems. Typically, this condition is not painful, but the affected testis can become tender with strenuous exercise. The typical "bag of worms" appearance on palpation makes the diagnosis apparent in most cases. For a 13-year-old boy, reassurance and education seem appropriate.

A Doppler flow study of testes or a radionuclide scan might be indicated if the area was painful and the diagnosis of testicular torsion was being entertained. The child does not have evidence of a UTI (dysuria or fever), so a urinalysis and culture are unlikely to be helpful. If this sexually active child had painful testes and the diagnosis of epididymitis was likely, then ceftriaxone intramuscularly and doxycycline orally might be considered.

273. The answer is d. (*Kliegman et al, pp 1904-1905. Rudolph et al, pp 1429-1432.*) The description is that of a hydrocele, an accumulation of fluid in the tunica vaginalis. Small hydroceles usually resolve spontaneously in the first year of life. Larger ones or those that have a variable fluid level with time will likely need surgical repair. This is a common condition affecting 2% of males; thus, chromosomes are not indicated. Incision and drainage and antibiotics are not indicated for this developmental condition.

274. The answer is a. (*Hay et al, p 759. Kliegman et al, pp 2497-2498. Rudolph et al, pp 1729-1730.*) The most common type of hereditary nephritis is Alport syndrome. Clinically, patients present with asymptomatic microscopic hematuria, but gross hematuria is also possible, especially after an upper respiratory infection. Hearing loss, eventually leading to deafness, is associated with Alport syndrome in up to 75% of cases. End-stage renal disease, as hinted in the vignette with the father going to a dialysis center, is common by the second or third decade of life. This syndrome is mostly commonly an X-linked dominant disorder, which explains the more severe course in males. Other findings include ocular abnormalities (30%-40%) and, rarely, leiomyomatosis of the esophagus or respiratory tree.

An otherwise healthy child is unlikely to have disseminated intravascular coagulation. Renal vein Doppler flow studies might be helpful to diagnose renal vein thrombosis, but the intermittent nature of this child's hematuria makes that diagnosis unlikely. Measurement of factors VII, IX, and XI would assist in the diagnosis of hemophilia, a condition much more likely to present with bruising, soft-tissue bleeding, and hemarthrosis and not solely with intermittent hematuria. Goodpasture syndrome results in pulmonary hemorrhages in addition to the signs and symptoms of glomerulonephritis; it is a rare disease in children.

275. The answer is c. (*Hay et al, pp 94-95. Kliegman et al, pp 2585-2586. Rudolph et al, pp 1694-1696.*) Nocturnal enuresis is involuntary voiding at night at an age when control of micturition is expected. Nocturnal enuresis can be split into two categories: primary nocturnal enuresis, when the child has never been dry at night; and secondary nocturnal enuresis, when the child has had a few months of dry nights before developing enuresis. By 5 years of age, most children (90%-95%) are completely dry during the day, and 80%-85% are dry during the night. Over the years, the incidence of nocturnal enuresis decreases, dropping to 7% at 7-8 years of age, and down to 1% at 14 years of age. A careful history and physical examination will usually identify any potential organic causes. In most cases, no etiology is found. A family history is common. Minimal laboratory testing beyond screening urinalysis is indicated. The condition is more common in boys than in girls. Therapy is aimed at reassurance to the parents that the condition is self-limited, avoidance of punitive and consideration of purchasing a bed-wetting alarm. Spontaneous cure rates are high regardless of therapy. Short courses of desmopressin (a synthetic analog of antidiuretic hormone) lead to control in 60%-75% of cases while the patient takes the medication, and would be appropriate to consider in this boy and in other situations in which patients need episodic control of their enuresis (eg, summer camp or sleep-overs). However, desmopressin is not a cure, and episodes frequently return when the medication is stopped.

276. The answer is b. (*Hay et al, p 1166. Kliegman et al, p 2554. Rudolph et al, p 1699.*) Oligohydramnios can cause a number of serious problems in the neonate, including constraint deformities (such as clubfoot) and pulmonary hypoplasia, as shown in the photograph, which shows essentially no lung development. These neonates have usually experienced intrauterine growth retardation and frequently have an associated serious renal abnormality. Ultrasound of the kidneys is important to rule out renal involvement as a cause of the oligohydramnios. None of the other testing would be expected to identify an etiology for the oligohydramnios and pulmonary hypoplasia, although this neonate's ultimate clinical course might necessitate additional testing. The finding of bilateral renal agenesis is termed Potter sequence; almost all affected neonates die shortly after birth from respiratory failure.

277-280. The answers are 277-p, 278-g, 279-a, 280-o. (*Hay et al, pp 757-762, 771-775, 930-932, 950-952, 1412, 2468, 2511-2512. Kliegman et al, pp 358-359, 1176-1180, 1216-1218, 1493-1496, 2087-2088, 2121, 2342, 2468, 2496-2501, 2507-2512, 2521-2528, 2556-2562, 2600-2604. Rudolph et al, pp 928-929, 950-956, 1560, 1644-1647, 1710-1711, 1716-1717, 1719-1724, 1727-1730, 1736-1741.*) Renal medullary carcinoma is found almost exclusively in black patients with sickle cell trait, and less commonly in patients with sickle cell disease or sickle C disease. This aggressive tumor presents with gross hematuria, flank pain, weight loss, and abdominal pain.

In a small number of individuals, absorption of betalain, a component of beets, results in red urine in the absence of myoglobin, heme, or red blood cells (aka 'beeturia").

Elevated levels of cholesterol and triglycerides are common in nephrotic syndrome because of increased generalized protein synthesis in the liver (including lipoproteins) and because of a decrease in lipid metabolism due to reduced plasma lipoprotein lipase levels. In the nephrotic syndrome, albumin is lost in the urine and, despite increased hepatic synthesis, serum levels drop. The upper limit of protein excretion in healthy children is 0.15 g/24 h; in nephrotic syndrome, proteinuria can exceed 2.0 g/24 h. When the serum protein level drops low enough, the oncotic pressure of the plasma becomes too low to balance the hydrostatic pressure. Plasma volume, therefore, decreases as edema occurs. Periorbital edema in the morning and scrotal edema in boys during the day are commonly reported. Endocrine and renal mechanisms then partially compensate by retaining water and salt. Overzealous monitoring and restriction of water and salt intake usually are not required.

Hypertension commonly accompanies glomerulonephritis, but only occasionally accompanies nephrotic syndrome. Diuretics are sometimes used in both nephrotic syndrome and glomerulonephritis with temporary effect, but are not curative. A combination of albumin infusions followed by a diuretic also has been used to temporarily decrease the edema in patients with severe nephrotic syndrome. Because both illnesses are usually self-limited, temporary measures are important. In all cases, blood pressure must be evaluated for the age of the child (eg, the 6-year-old girl with a blood pressure of 120/80 mm Hg is significantly hypertensive).

Bartter syndrome (also known as juxtaglomerular hyperplasia) is an autosomal recessive condition that causes hypokalemia, hypercalciuria, alkalosis, hyperaldosteronism, and hyperreninemia; blood pressure is usually normal. Clinical presentations occurring frequently between 6 and

12 months of age include failure to thrive with constipation, weakness, vomiting, polyuria, and polydipsia. Treatment is aimed at preventing dehydration, providing nutritional support, and returning the potassium level to normal.

HSP nephritis presents with a purpuric rash, arthritis, and abdominal pain, and has an associated glomerulonephritis that can cause gross or microscopic hematuria.

IgA (Berger) nephropathy is the most common chronic glomerulonephritis. Initially thought to be benign, it is now known to progress over decades to chronic renal failure in many afflicted patients. IgA is found in the mesangium, but this occurs with other disease processes as well. The most common clinical finding is episodic gross hematuria frequently associated with a febrile illness.

Typical findings of Alport syndrome include microscopic hematuria, possible episodes of gross hematuria, a positive family history (depending on genetic mutation) and progressive hearing loss.

With acute glomerulonephritis, oliguria (often presenting with dark, cola-colored urine) frequently occurs as a direct consequence of the disease process itself; on occasion, it can be profound, with virtual anuria for several days. During this period of time, it is vital to monitor and restrict fluid intake lest massive edema, hypervolemia, and even pulmonary edema and death occur.

Sickle cell nephropathy is a chronic, progressive condition likely the cumulative effects of sickled cells in the kidney resulting in ischemia, papillary necrosis, and interstitial fibrosis. Myriad renal conditions are found in patients with sickle cell disease including proteinuria reaching nephrotic syndrome levels, glomerulosclerosis and glomerulonephritis, RTA, acute kidney, and progressive renal failure requiring dialysis and transplantation.

Idiopathic hypercalciuria causes recurrent gross hematuria, persistent microscopic hematuria, and complaints of dysuria or abdominal pain without initial stone formation. Over time, however, stones may form in 15% of cases.

Urolithiasis classically presents with flank pain and hematuria, although many children less than about six have stones identified as incidental findings upon imaging for other reasons. Urine in children with stones may have crystals found in the sediment.

Urinary tract infection classically presents with frequency, urgency, dysuria, possible fever, and urine containing white blood cells and bacteria.

Goodpasture disease classically presents with several days or weeks history of cough, fatigue, and hemoptysis (or bloody emesis in small children due to swallowed blood). Urine will show hematuria and proteinuria. Blood testing will identify the antiglomerular basement membrane (GBM) antibodies, anemia, elevated blood urea nitrogen, and increased creatinine.

HUS, most common in children younger than 4 years of age, is characterized by hemolytic anemia, thrombocytopenia, and renal insufficiency. Urinalysis reveals hematuria and proteinuria.

Chlamydial urethritis is classically described in the sexually active adolescent or adult with a mucoid urethral discharge although a huge reservoir of asymptomatic carriers, especially in women, is seen. In children, chlamydial urethritis would be suggestive of child sexual abuse.

SLE classically is described as chronic fever, malaise, and weight loss in a patient with a malar rash in a butterfly distribution across the bridge of the nose and cheeks. Arthritis involving mainly small joints with pain in excess of clinical findings is common. Raynaud phenomenon resulting in digital ulceration and gangrene can be seen. Urine in these patients will have persistent, significant proteinuria and cellular casts.

The Neuromuscular System

Questions

281. An 8-year-old boy is noted by his teachers in the first week of school to have become disruptive in class. His teachers report that several times a day he grunts loudly as if he is clearing his throat and then twitches his head to the left, much to the amusement and laughter of his classmates. They also report that a reward system, timeouts, and trips to the principal's office have not improved his behavior. His parents report that after being off his attention-deficit/hyperactivity disorder (ADHD) medications for the summer they restarted his methylphenidate at the same dose. He was seen by his pediatrician about 1 month prior and was found to be normal; he was started on nasal steroids for "seasonal allergies" which were felt to be causing him to have intermittent cough. Which of the following is the most likely explanation for his condition?

a. Attention deficit disorder
b. Simple motor tic
c. Tourette syndrome
d. Side effect of methylphenidate
e. Dystonic reaction to the nasal steroids

282. A 7-year-old boy is seen in the emergency department (ED) after suffering a 3-minute long left-sided tonic-clonic seizure. His mother reports that he had an upper respiratory infection about 2 weeks prior from which he had completely recovered, but earlier in the day he developed fever, ataxia, weakness, headache, and emesis. He has been a healthy child without serious illness. On physical examination the temperature is 38.5°C (101.1°F), heart rate is 110 beats per minute, respiratory rate is 22 breaths per minute, and blood pressure is 100/69 mm Hg. He is confused as to person and place. Head is without trauma. Neck is somewhat stiff. The mucous membranes are pink, moist, and without lesions. Extraocular eye movement and fundoscopic examinations are normal. The chest is clear. Heart has a normal S1 and S2 without murmur. The abdomen is soft and nontender. No hepatosplenomegaly or adenopathy is noted. Muscles are weak, toes are upgoing, and lower extremity reflexes are reduced. Gait is unsteady. A rapid magnetic resonance imaging (MRI) with contrast of the brain is shown in the photograph. Which of the following therapies is most appropriate for his condition?

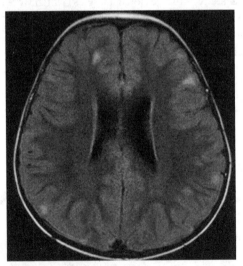

(Used with permission from Susan John, MD.)

a. Initiation of daily subcutaneous glatiramer acetate (Copaxone)
b. Infusion of high-dose corticosteroids
c. Biopsy of the lesion
d. Initiation of broad-spectrum antibiotics
e. Begin course of albendazole

283. A 4-year-old child is seen by the pediatrician for well-child evaluation. The family reports that the child is in good health. Past medical history is unknown as the family adopted the child from another country only 2 weeks prior. On physical examination vital signs are normal. She is awake, alert, and is happily running around the room showing off her favorite doll. Cranial nerves are normal. No focal neurologic findings are noted. The examination of child's back is shown in the photograph. Which of the following statements about this child's condition is true?

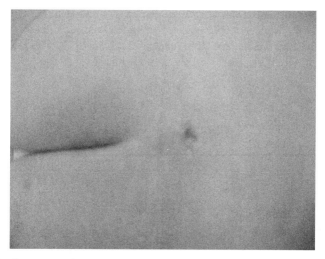

(Used with permission from David I. Sandberg, MD.)

a. Symptoms are more likely to be seen in younger children and resolve as the child grows older.
b. Pes planus (flat foot) is commonly seen in adolescents with this condition.
c. Hypertrophy of the lower extremity muscles on one or both sides is associated with a better prognosis.
d. Hyperreflexia of the lower extremities is diagnostic at all ages.
e. Frequent urinary tract infections are commonly found.

284. A 6-month-old infant is seen in the ED for the acute onset of inability to move the right side of his body. The family reports that he had been in his normal state of good health until the event occurred about 1 hour previously. They deny fever, vomiting, change in behavior, or trauma. His medical records show that he was born term, vaginally and was discharged after a 48-hour hospital stay. Birth growth parameters were at the 50th percentile at birth for length, weight, and head circumference. A review of his most recent outpatient visit on the electronic medical record show his developmental assessment to include an ability to roll from stomach to back occasionally but not very well from back to stomach. He could bear weight on his legs but would not sit without assistance. His weight was the 25th percentile at 2 months, 10th percentile at 4 months, and is now at the 5th percentile. Which of the following is most likely to explain this infant's condition?

a. Phenylketonuria (PKU)
b. Homocystinuria
c. Cystathioninuria
d. Maple syrup urine disease
e. Histidinemia

CDC Growth Charts: United States

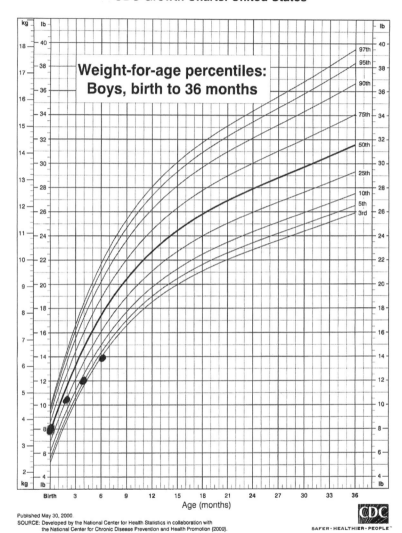

Weight-for-age percentiles: Boys, birth to 36 months

Published May 30, 2000.
SOURCE: Developed by the National Center for Health Statistics in collaboration with the National Center for Chronic Disease Prevention and Health Promotion (2000).

(Reproduced with permission from the National Center for Health Statistics in collaboration with the National Center for Chronic Disease Prevention and Health Promotion [2000].)

285. A 6-month-old infant is seen by the pediatric nurse practitioner for a well-child visit. The mother reports no problems. The infant was born by cesarean section for cephalopelvic disproportion to a 20-year-old woman whose pregnancy was complicated by gestational hypertension. Discharge was at 72 hours of life. The infant has been breast-feeding well in the interim period. On physical examination vital signs are normal. Weight, length, and head circumference are at the 50th percentile. She is awake, alert, and in no distress. Head shape is shown in the photograph. Cranial nerves are normal. No focal neurologic findings are noted. Which of the following is the most appropriate next step in management?

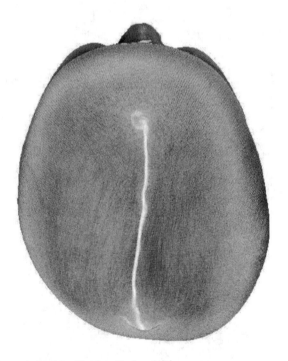

(Used with permission from Matthew Greives, MD.)

a. Obtain chromosomes.
b. Cranial CT scan with three-dimensional reconstruction.
c. Measure serum vitamin D levels.
d. Consult a neurosurgeon.
e. Instruct the family to provide frequent "tummy time".

286. A 9-year-old child is seen by the pediatrician with the complaint of weakness. The mother reports that for the previous several weeks the child appears to be normal in the morning, but by mid to late afternoon seems to be more tired and wants to sit and rest more than normal. She notes that by early evening he is unable to keep his eyes open. To see properly, he must hold open his eyelids with his fingers. He was a normal, term delivery and has been developing well. He takes no medications other than daily multi-vitamins. Review of systems is negative other than some recent gagging of food when he eats. On physical examination vital signs are normal. He is awake, alert, and in no distress. His face is somewhat droopy, appearing to be sad, although he laughs easily. Head is without trauma. Pupils are equal and reactive. Mild ptosis is noted. The mucous membranes are moist and without lesions. The chest is clear. Heart has a normal S1 and S2 without murmur. Abdomen is soft and without hepatosplenomegaly. Cranial nerves are normal. No focal neurologic findings are noted. Which of the following is most likely to aid in the diagnosis?

a. Identification of scattered degenerating and regenerating myofibers on muscle biopsy
b. Finding of elevations of creatine phosphokinase (CPK)
c. Effect of a test dose of edrophonium
d. Findings of enlarged thymus on chest x-ray
e. Documentation of antinuclear antibodies (ANAs)

287. A 14-year-old girl with a long-standing history of seizures controlled by valproic acid is seen by the pediatric hospitalist. She was admitted from the ED 36 hours prior after requiring a dose of diazepam to control a tonic-clonic episode with moaning and crying. After admission she has had several similar episodes of tonic-clonic activity not associated with loss of bowel or bladder control; none required additional acute antiepileptic medication intervention. Between the episodes she is sleepy but oriented. On physical examination vital signs are normal. She is sleepy but arousable, and is oriented to person and place. Head is without trauma. Pupils are equal and reactive. Fundoscopic examination is normal. The mucous membranes are moist and without lesions. The chest is clear. Heart has a normal S1 and S2 without murmur. Abdomen is soft and without hepatosplenomegaly. Cranial nerves are normal. No focal neurologic findings are noted.

Laboratory data show:
Urine drug screen: negative
Valproic acid level: 75 µg/mL (normal 50-125 µg/mL)
24-hour video EEG in the epilepsy monitoring unit shows:
Multiple episodes of tonic and clonic motor activity with moaning and crying
Excessive muscle artifact but no epileptiform discharges
No loss of bladder or bowel control

Which of the following treatments is the most appropriate for this condition?

a. Add a scheduled benzodiazepine for her muscular symptoms.
b. Add carbamazepine to her current seizure medication.
c. Increase her dose of valproic acid.
d. Withdraw all seizure medications.
e. Request a psychiatric evaluation.

288. A previously healthy 7-year-old child is seen in the ED minutes after suddenly complaining of a headache and falling to the floor at school. No family member has yet arrived, but the staff member who accompanied him reports that they know of no trauma prior to the event, that he has been in good health, takes only occasional β-agonist for wheezing, and is not known to have any chronic illness other than mild asthma which flares briefly with season changes. On physical examination vital signs are normal. He is lethargic and somewhat arousable. Head is without trauma. Left central facial muscles are weak. Pupils are equal and reactive. Fundoscopic examination is normal. The mucous membranes are moist and without lesions. The chest is clear. Heart has a normal S1 and S2 without murmur. Abdomen is soft and without hepatosplenomegaly. Left arm and leg are weak. Cranial nerve examination shows conjugate ocular deviation to the right. Which of the following is the most likely diagnosis?

a. Hemiplegic migraine
b. Supratentorial tumor
c. Todd paralysis
d. Acute subdural hematoma
e. Acute infantile hemiplegia

289. A 7-month-old infant is seen in the pediatric office for a new, well-child visit. The mother reports the pregnancy to be uncomplicated other than a seizure disorder well-controlled with levetiracetam (Keppra). Birth was vaginal, and the infant was discharged home after 48 hours. Family history is positive for myocardial infarction in the paternal grandfather at age 85, and a seizure disorder in both of the mother's sisters. She reports that he rolled at about 4 months, sits without help, and is trying to pull himself to standing. On physical examination his weight, length, and head circumference are at the 50th percentile. Head is normal in size and shape. Pupils are equal and reactive. Mouth is moist without teeth or lesions. Chest is clear. Heart has normal rhythm and no murmur. Abdomen is soft without hepatosplenomegaly. Neurologic examination is normal. Skin demonstrates numerous 8-10 mm hyperpigmented lesions scattered over the back and chest. Which of the following conditions is most likely to be diagnosed in this child?

a. Peutz-Jeghers syndrome
b. Noonan syndrome with multiple lentigines
c. Neurofibromatosis type 1
d. Legius syndrome
e. Carney complex

290. A 4-year-old boy is seen by the pediatrician for follow-up of a recent ED visit. The child was seen 10 days prior for abdominal pain, and while appendicitis was ruled out and the child's abdomen has returned to normal the ED physician noted an incidental finding of an elevated serum creatine kinase. He was born at term and has had no serious illness. The family notes that he began to walk independently at about 18 months of age, that he is more clumsy than their daughter was at the same age (especially when trying to hold onto small objects), and that he seems to be somewhat sluggish when he runs, climbs stairs, rises from the ground after he sits, and rides his tricycle. Further history and physical examination are likely to reveal which of the following?

a. Hirsutism
b. Past seizure activity
c. Proximal muscle atrophy
d. Cataracts
e. Enlarged gonads

291. A 9-year-old girl is seen by the pediatrician for headaches for the past several months, one of which resulted in her going to the ER. The child reports the headache to be diffuse, throbbing, and to last several hours. She denies vomiting or other symptoms. She reports that she cannot tell a headache is about to begin; after taking a nap the headache typically resolves. The headaches occur several times a week, and on all days of the week. She was a term infant born vaginally and has had no other serious illnesses and takes no medications. The child lives with the mother and pet Chihuahua. Her school performance is excellent. Family history is positive for diabetes on the mother's side, and possible headaches on the father's side (he has not been involved since the birth of the child). On physical examination vital signs are normal. She is awake, alert, and in no distress. The mucous membranes are moist and without lesions. Eyes have some cobble stoning of the conjunctivae. Nasal turbinates are somewhat enlarged and boggy but without nasal discharge. The chest is clear. Heart has a normal S1 and S2 without murmur. Abdomen is soft and without hepatosplenomegaly. Cranial nerves are normal. No focal neurologic findings are noted. Which of the following is the most appropriate next step in the diagnosis and management of this child's likely condition?

a. Initiation of ibuprofen immediately at the onset of symptoms
b. Trial of oral loratadine and nasal fluticasone
c. MRI of the brain
d. Computed tomographic (CT) scan of the sinuses and initiation of oral antibiotics
e. Lumbar puncture opening pressure, cell count and protein levels

292. An 8-year-old child is seen in the ED for fever and altered mental status. The family reports that over the previous several days the child has had low-grade fevers without other symptoms, but now seems to be less alert and less oriented. They report she was difficult to arouse that morning. They deny trauma, exposure to medications or drugs, or other illnesses. Past medical history is negative. On physical examination the temperature is 38.5°C (101.1°F), heart rate is 110 beats per minute, respiratory rate is 22 breaths per minute, and blood pressure is 100/69 mm Hg. She is somewhat difficult to arouse. Head is without trauma. Neck is stiff. The mucous membranes are pink, moist, and without lesions. Extraocular eye movement and fundoscopic examinations are normal. The chest is clear. Heart has a normal S1 and S2 without murmur. The abdomen is soft and nontender. No hepatosplenomegaly or adenopathy is noted. Generalized weakness but no focal neurologic abnormalities are noted.

CT scan with contrast of the brain:
Enhancement of the basal cisterns by the contrast material.
Spinal fluid analysis shows:
Glucose: 15 mg/dL (normal: 45-80 mg/dL)
Protein: 150 mg/dL (normal: 15-45 mg/dL)
WBC: 85/µL (normal: 0-5/µL)
Lymphocytes: 100% (normal: 0-10/µL)
RBC: 2/µL (normal: 0-10/µL)
Gram stain negative

Which of the following is the most appropriate next step in her therapy?
a. Initiation of rapamycin (mTOR inhibitors) therapy
b. Administration of isoniazid, rifampin, pyrazinamide, and streptomycin or ethambutol
c. Intravenous heparin and subcutaneous enoxaparin (Lovenox)
d. Intravenous ceftriaxone and vancomycin
e. Administration of acetazolamide (Diamox)

293. An irritable 6-year-old child has a somewhat unsteady but nonspecific gait. Physical examination reveals very mild left facial weakness, brisk stretch reflexes in all four extremities, bilateral extensor plantar responses (Babinski reflex), and mild hypertonicity of the left upper and lower extremities; no peripheral muscular weakness is found. Which of the following is the most likely diagnosis?

a. Pontine glioma
b. Cerebellar astrocytoma
c. Tumor of the right cerebral hemisphere
d. Subacute sclerosing panencephalitis (SSPE)
e. Progressive multifocal leukoencephalopathy

294. A 4-year-old boy is seen by the pediatrician with the complaint of 2 weeks of fever unresponsive to the antibiotics given for chronic otitis media, worsening headache for 2 days, and new-onset ataxia in the last 12 hours. On physical examination the temperature is 38.5°C (101.1°F), heart rate is 112 beats per minute, respiratory rate is 22 breaths per minute, and blood pressure is 102/71 mm Hg. He is arousable and complains of head pain. Head is without trauma. Neck is supple. Ears have dull tympanic membranes. Extraocular eye movement shows nystagmus and fundoscopic examination reveals papilledema. There is a harsh systolic ejection murmur over the pulmonic area and left sternal border with a single second heart sound. He is ataxic when tries to walk. Which of the following would be the most appropriate first test to order?

a. Urine drug screen
b. Blood culture
c. Lumbar puncture
d. MRI of the brain
e. Stat echocardiogram

295. A 6-year-old child in the observation unit of a hospital develops unilateral pupillary dilatation, focal seizures, depressed consciousness, and hemiplegia. He was seen in the ED about 12 hours prior after a short period of unconsciousness associated with a fall from a playground swing. His examination in the ED was normal other than the bruise over the right temporal region. He was made NPO, given a dose of pain medication for the headache and placed in observation. Which of the following is the most likely mechanism for his condition?

a. Infection of the meninges
b. Collection of intracranial blood
c. Dehydration and electrolyte disturbance
d. Overdose of pain medication
e. Ingestion of a drug

296. A 6-year-old boy is seen in the office for evaluation of polyuria. His mother also reports several months of headache and occasional emesis. She denies change in behavior, medications, or other illnesses. Your physical examination reveals a child who is less than 5th percentile for weight. He has mild papilledema. His serum glucose is 98 mg/dL, and his first urine void specific gravity after a night without liquids is 1.005 g/mL. Which of the following is the most likely associated finding?

a. Sixth nerve palsy
b. Unilateral cerebellar ataxia
c. Unilateral pupillary dilatation
d. Unilateral anosmia
e. Bitemporal hemianopsia

297. A 6-year-old boy is seen in the ED for acute onset of ataxia. His mother reports that he had been in his normal state of good health until a few hours prior when he developed difficulty in walking, falling and inability to maintain his balance. He has had no fever, nausea, vomiting, or recent illnesses. Past medical history is positive for varicella infection 2 months previously, but otherwise he has had occasional upper respiratory infections only. He takes no medications, his school performance is good, and his mother denies any untended medications in the home. On physical examination vital signs are normal. He is awake, alert, and in no distress. Head is without trauma. Neck is supple. The mucous membranes are pink, moist, and without lesions. Extraocular eye movement and fundoscopic examinations are normal. The chest is clear. Heart has no murmur and normal S1 and S2. The abdomen is soft and nontender. No hepatosplenomegaly or adenopathy is noted. He is somewhat ataxic upon standing but sits relatively well. He has no focal neurologic findings. Skin is normal. Which of the following is the most appropriate next step?

a. Obtain urine drug screen
b. MRI to evaluate his corpus callosum
c. Close scrutiny of his skin for telangiectasia
d. Perform a muscle biopsy of the gastrocnemius muscle
e. Identification of a triplet repeat expansion on chromosome 9

298. A 9-year-old boy has developed headaches that are more frequent in the morning and are followed by vomiting. Over the previous few months, his family has noted a change in his behavior (generally more irritable than usual) and his school performance has begun to drop. Imaging of this child is most likely to reveal a finding in which of the following regions?

a. Subtentorial brain
b. Supratentorial brain
c. Intraventricular brain
d. C1-C2 spinal canal
e. Peripheral nervous system

299. A 3-week-old neonate is seen by the pediatric ED attending for a possible "rule out sepsis" evaluation. The neonate was born vaginally at term to a 20-year-old woman whose pregnancy was uncomplicated. He was seen at 2 weeks of age, had regained birth weight, and had a complaint at that time of "constipation" being treated with home remedies recommended by the great grandmother. New symptoms necessitating his visit to the ER include worsening constipation, lethargy, weak cry, gagging when he eats, and overall decreased movement. On physical examination the temperature is 37°C (98.5°F), heart rate is 122 beats per minute, respiratory rate is 30 breaths per minute, and blood pressure is 98/69 mm Hg. He is arousable but rather sleepy. Head is normocephalic. He has ptosis and diminished corneal reflexes. Suck is poor with drooling from his mouth; gag is poor. Neck is supple but head control is poor. The abdomen is soft, somewhat distended, nontender, and has decreased bowel sounds. No hepatosplenomegaly or adenopathy is noted. His lumbar puncture attempt must be aborted after the collection of the first tube of fluid is gathered due to his developing respiratory distress during the procedure. Which of the following is likely to confirm your suspicions about his diagnosis?

a. Results of the spinal fluid HSV PCR
b. Examination of both parents for electromyographic depiction of myotonic discharges
c. Resolution of his hypotonia upon administration of edrophonium
d. Finding of a tick buried in the hair on his scalp
e. Identification of botulinum toxin in the neonate's serum

300. A 6-month-old infant is seen by the pediatrician for a routine checkup. He was born by repeat cesarean section at term to a 24-year-old woman whose pregnancy was complicated by mild preeclampsia. Prenatal laboratories were negative. The neonate did well in the hospital, breast-fed normally, and was discharged at 48 hours of age. The infant was seen at 5 days, 2 weeks, and 2 months of age and appeared to be doing well. The family lost their insurance and missed their 4 month visit but report no illnesses. They are concerned that he is no longer interested in rolling from stomach to back and that he seems to overreact each time their Chihuahua barks. On examination he has poor head control, generalized weakness, and an inability to sit or roll. He has an enlarged liver and spleen, macroglossia, coarse facial features, and a cherry-red spot noted in the center of the macula on retinal examination. Which of the following is the most likely mechanism of disease?

a. Defect in copper absorption
b. Reduced activity of α-galactosidase
c. Defective gene (*MECP2)* on the X chromosome
d. Reduced activity of β-hexosaminidase A
e. Deficient activity of galactosyl-3-sulfateceramide sulfatase

301. A 2-year-old girl is brought to the emergency center by her parents with the complaint that she has had a seizure. They report her to have been in good health until the seizure occurred. She has had no hospitalizations, has had no serious illnesses, and vaccines are current. Family history is positive for the father having seizures as a child. On physical examination the temperature is 39°C (102.2°F), heart rate is 122 beats per minute, respiratory rate is 30 breaths per minute, and blood pressure is 100/70 mm Hg. She is fussy but easily consoled. Head is normocephalic and neck is supple. Chest is clear. Heart is without murmur. She has no hepatosplenomegaly. Neurologic examination is nonfocal. Thirty minutes after receiving acetaminophen she is running around the examination room. Which part of the story would suggest the best outcome in this condition?

a. A CSF white count of 100/μL.
b. Otitis media on examination.
c. The seizure lasted 30 minutes.
d. The child was born prematurely with an intraventricular hemorrhage.
e. The family reports the child to have had right-sided tonic-clonic activity only.

302. A previously healthy 12-year-old boy is seen for weakness. His mother reports that about 3 days prior he complained of weakness in his legs, and over the ensuing period he began to have difficulty walking. He has had no fever, vomiting, or diarrhea. He had a mild upper respiratory infection about 2 weeks prior that resolved quickly. Past medical history is positive for attention-deficit/hyperactivity disorder for which he takes a stimulant medication. School performance is good, and he had participated actively in sports until the current illness. He denies alcohol, smoking, or other drug use. On physical examination vital signs are normal. He is awake, alert, and in no distress. Head is without trauma. Neck is supple. The mucous membranes are pink, moist, and without lesions. Extraocular eye movements and fundoscopic examinations are normal. The chest is clear. Heart has no murmur and normal S1 and S2. The abdomen is soft and nontender. No hepatosplenomegaly or adenopathy is noted. Overall lower extremity muscle strength is reduced; deep tendon reflexes at the knee and ankle are absent. He has no muscle atrophy or muscle pain. Laboratory data show:

CBC:
    Hemoglobin: 14.2 g/dL
    Hematocrit: 41.5%
    WBC: 7,500/mm^3
        Segmented neutrophils: 49%
        Band forms: 0%
        Lymphocytes: 51%
    Platelet count: 138,000/mm^3
Serum electrolytes:
    Sodium: 139 mEq/L
    Potassium: 4.5 mEq/L
    Chloride: 110 mEq/L
    Bicarbonate: 22 mEq/L
    Glucose: 100 mg/dL
    Creatinine: 0.9 mEq/L
    Blood urea nitrogen (BUN): 10 mEq/L
Spinal fluid analysis:
    Glucose: 79 mg/dL(normal: 45-80 mg/dL)
    Protein: 350 mg/dL (normal: 15-45 mg/dL)
    WBC: 0 (normal: 0-5/μL)
    RBC: 0 (normal: 0-10/μL)
    Gram stain negative

Which of the following is the most likely diagnosis in this patient?

a. Bell palsy
b. Muscular dystrophy
c. Guillain-Barré syndrome
d. Charcot-Marie-Tooth disease
e. Werdnig-Hoffmann disease

303. A 6-month-old infant is seen for a routine visit. The mother reports the child cannot hold his head up, roll, nor sit. He was born vaginally at term after what seemed to be an uncomplicated pregnancy. His birth weight and length were at the 25th percentile, and head circumference at the 5th percentile. His neonatal course was complicated by hepatosplenomegaly, prolonged neonatal jaundice, and purpura. On physical examination today the weight and length are at the 10th percentile, and the head circumference is less than the 5th percentile. The calcific densities in the skull imaging shown are likely the result of which of the following?

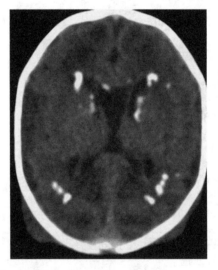

(Used with permission from Susan John, MD.)

a. Congenital cytomegalovirus (CMV) infection
b. Congenital toxoplasmosis infection
c. Congenital syphilis infection
d. Tuberculous meningitis
e. Craniopharyngioma

304. The infant pictured develops infantile spasms. Which of the following is most likely to be an associated finding?

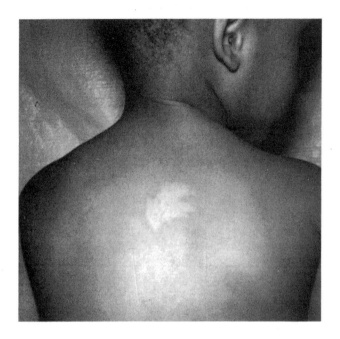

a. Lisch nodules
b. Renal angiomyolipoma
c. Hypodontia with conical or pegged teeth
d. Distribution of lesions along skin tension lines
e. Koebner phenomenon

305. A neonate in the NICU is evaluated by the neonatologist. The 37-week-gestation infant was born by cesarean section for decreased fetal movement to a 20-year-old woman. Immediately after birth the neonate had an increased respiratory rate and difficulty feeding necessitating transfer from the level I to level III nursery. The mother denies any complications during the pregnancy, although she received no prenatal care. She took only prenatal vitamins and denies smoking, alcohol, or other drug use. On physical examination the temperature is 37°C (98.5°F), heart rate is 155 beats per minute, respiratory rate is 60 breaths per minute, and blood pressure is 70/50 mm Hg. Weight, length, and head circumference are 50th percentile. He is arousable but rather sleepy and in mild respiratory distress. Head is normocephalic with flat fontanels. Pupils are equally reactive and round. Mucous membranes are moist. Suck is poor with drooling from his mouth; gag is poor. Tongue fasciculations are noted. Neck is supple. The chest is clear with shallow respirations. Heart has no murmur and normal S1 and S2. The abdomen is soft, nontender, and without masses. No hepatosplenomegaly or adenopathy is noted. Extremities demonstrate twitching of the fingers and toes, and generalized hypotonia. Deep tendon reflexes are absent. Laboratory data show:

CBC:
    Hemoglobin: 15.2 g/dL
    Hematocrit: 45.5%
    WBC: 22,500/mm^3
        Segmented neutrophils: 60%
        Band forms: 0%
        Lymphocytes: 40%
    Platelet count: 175,000/mm^3
Serum electrolytes:
    Sodium: 139 mEq/L
    Potassium: 4.5 mEq/L
    Chloride: 110 mEq/L
    Bicarbonate: 22 mEq/L
    Glucose: 100 mg/dL
    Creatinine: 0.9 mEq/L
    Blood urea nitrogen (BUN): 10 mEq/L
Spinal fluid analysis:
    Glucose: 78 mg/dL (normal: 45-80 mg/dL)
    Protein: 16 mg/dL (normal: 15-45 mg/dL)

WBC: 0 (normal: 0-5/μL)
RBC: 0 (normal: 0-10/μL)
Gram stain negative

Which of the following is the most likely mechanism of disease?

a. Absence of the muscle cytoskeletal protein dystrophin
b. Degeneration of anterior horn cells in the spinal cord
c. Antibody production that binds the acetylcholine receptor at the postsynaptic muscle membrane
d. Progressive autoimmune demyelination
e. Birth trauma with accumulation of blood in the subdural space

306. A 3-year-old boy is seen by the pediatrician for well-child visit. His parents report that he has been doing well but has developed difficulty walking. They state that over the previous several months they have noticed an increased curvature of the lower spine as he walks and that his gait has become "waddling" in nature. His past medical history is positive for occasional upper respiratory tract infections and two bouts of otitis media. He rolled at 4 months, sat alone at 6 months, and first stood holding to furniture at about 9 months. He took his first steps at about 13 months of age. On physical examination vital signs are normal. Growth is at the 75th percentile for height and weight, and 50th percentile for head circumference. He is a happy, alert child in no distress. Head is normocephalic. Pupils are equally round and reactive. Mucous membranes are moist. Dentition is good. Neck is supple. The chest is clear. Heart has no murmur and normal S1 and S2. The abdomen is soft, nontender, and without masses. No hepatosplenomegaly or adenopathy is noted. Spine is intact without dimples or hair tufts. The lower spine has inward curvature. Extremities have full range of motion, deep tendon reflexes are normal, and the muscles of the calves are enlarged. Which of the following is the most appropriate next step in management?

a. Obtain an ultrasound of the lower spine.
b. Measure serum creatinine phosphokinase (CPK) levels.
c. Schedule an MRI of the brain.
d. Arrange for lumbar puncture and nerve conduction studies.
e. Measure serum botulinum titers.

307. Your 6-year-old son awakens at 1:00 AM screaming. You note that he is hyperventilating, is tachycardic, and has dilated pupils. He cannot be consoled, does not respond, and is unaware of his environment. After a few minutes, he returns to normal sleep. He recalls nothing the following morning. Which of the following is the most appropriate next step in his management?

a. Obtain an EEG.
b. Observation only.
c. Urine toxicology screen.
d. Psychiatric evaluation.
e. Trial of ergotamine containing nonsteroidal anti-inflammatory medications.

308. A 16-year-old girl is seen in the emergency center for a "falling out" spell at a local restaurant. Her friends report that she was about to order her food, said she felt faint, and then fell to the floor. They report that she lost consciousness for about 30 seconds, had no tonic-clonic activity, but did have some irregular twitching of her arms. Emergency medical services were called, and in the interim 5 minutes she returned to her normal baseline. Past medical history is positive for occasional upper respiratory infections and streptococcal pharyngitis 6 months prior. Her menstrual cycles began at age 13, are regular, and the last period ended about 2 weeks ago. She describes them as light and without significant pain. She denies taking any medications, alcohol use, smoking, or taking other drugs. She denies sexual activity. She is an honors student in the tenth grade. On physical examination the temperature is 37°C (98.5°F), heart rate is 90 beats per minute, respiratory rate is 18 breaths per minute, and blood pressure is 110/75 mm Hg. Weight and height are at the 50th percentile for age. She is awake, alert, and in no distress. Head is normocephalic without trauma. Pupils are equally round and reactive. Mucous membranes are moist. Neck is supple. The chest is clear. Heart has no murmur and normal S1 and S2. The abdomen is soft, nontender, and without masses. No hepatosplenomegaly or adenopathy is noted. Neurologic examination is normal. Electrocardiogram (ECG) is normal. Which of the following is the most appropriate next step in her management?

a. Obtain an EEG.
b. Refer to a child psychiatrist.
c. Begin β-blocker therapy.
d. Encourage adequate fluid and salt intake.
e. Obtain serum and urine drug screens.

Questions 309 to 311

Children who report pain in their head often is a concerning symptom to parents, but usually can be explained with a careful history and physical examination. Choose the cause of head pain associated with the clinical presentation listed later. Each lettered option may be used once, more than once, or not at all.

a. Tension headache
b. Hypervitaminosis A
c. Factitious headache
d. Hypertension
e. Vascular headache (migraine)
f. Tuberculous meningitis
g. Hemiplegic migraine
h. Berry aneurysm
i. Acute subarachnoid hemorrhage
j. Increased intracranial pressure
k. Systemic lupus erythematosus
l. Multiple sclerosis (MS)

309. A 15-year-old girl has an acute, recurrent, pulsatile headache localized behind the eyes that tends to occur more frequently around menses. She has no symptoms that occur prior to the headache; her neurologic examination is normal.

310. A 7-year-old boy has chronic, worsening headache without preceding symptoms. He complains of emesis in the morning before breakfast for the last 2 weeks.

311. A 12-year-old boy has frequent headaches that worsen during the school day, especially during tests. These headaches are not associated with nausea or emesis, and he does not have any symptoms prior to the headache.

Questions 312 to 314

For each description, select the most likely diagnosis. Each lettered option may be used once, more than once, or not at all.

a. Rett syndrome
b. Transient tic disorder of childhood
c. Fragile X syndrome
d. Tourette syndrome
e. Sydenham chorea
f. Smith-Magenis syndrome
g. Lesch-Nyhan syndrome
h. Dystonia
i. Cerebral palsy
j. Cornelia de Lange syndrome

312. An otherwise healthy 8-year-old boy has frequent eye blinking and throat-clearing noises.

313. A 6-year-old girl has emotional lability, outburst of dysarthric speech, and new poor school performance. On examination she has frequent episodes of flinging her hair and milkmaid's grip (irregular contractions of the hand muscles when squeezing the examiner's fingers).

314. An 8-year-old hospitalized boy has unusual "spasms" of his neck and arms shortly after receiving promethazine (Phenergan) for nausea caused by his chemotherapy.

The Neuromuscular System

Answers

281. **The answer is c.** (*Hay et al, pp 830-832. Kliegman et al, pp 140-143. Rudolph et al, pp 2221-2222.*) The most likely explanation is Tourette since the child has both motor (neck twitching) and vocal (grunting) findings. Other common motor findings include eye blinking, grimacing, lip smacking, and shrugging of one or both shoulders. Common verbal findings include clearing of the throat, sniffing or snorting, and cough-like noises. In addition to the motor and vocal findings, comorbidities frequently seen include ADHD, obsessive-compulsive disorder, and impulse control problems. Oft-described coprolalia and echolalia are relatively infrequent. Simple motor tic are isolated, nonrhythmic, spasmodic, involuntary, stereotypical behaviors that involve any muscle group such as eye blinking, facial movements, or throat clearing lasting for weeks to about a year. Exacerbation of simple motor tics (but not Tourette's) with the initiation of stimulant medications for ADHD was once felt to be common; this relationship is likely overstated. Dystonic reactions are sometimes seen in patients receiving phenothiazine medications. Affected patients have unusual neck, arm, or leg muscle twitches that are sometimes confused with seizure activity. Diphenhydramine, infused intravenously, usually rapidly reverses this relatively common idiosyncratic drug reaction. The "postnasal drip" being treated by steroids in the child in this case likely represented a tic (cough).

282. **The answer is b.** (*Hay et al, p 825. Kliegman et al, pp 2924-2925. Rudolph et al, p 920.*) Acute disseminated encephalomyelitis (ADEM) is an autoimmune demyelinating disease seen in children younger than 10 years of age. It may follow many different types of infections, including upper respiratory tract infections, varicella, mycoplasma, herpes simplex virus, rubella, rubeola, and mumps; it may also follow immunizations. The MRI presented in the question shows multiple "white" plaques scattered across the brain representing areas of demyelination. The history and physical examination findings of ADEM are similar to multiple sclerosis (MS); differences include age of onset (ADEM is usually seen in < 10-year olds), the presence of systemic findings like fever and emesis, and the lack of progression in the lesions once identified. Mortality is high, with 10%-30% of affected patients dying. Treatment for ADEM is high-dose corticosteroids. One therapy for MS is subcutaneous glatiramer acetate. Meningitis is treated with broad-spectrum antibiotics until the pathogen is isolated, and then the spectrum restricted based on sensitivities. Malignancies require biopsy or excision of the lesion, and albendazole may be used for infections such as neurocysticercosis (CNS infection by the tapeworm *Taenia solium*). None of these three later lesions have MRI findings as demonstrated.

283. The answer is e. (*Kliegman et al, pp 2803-2804. Rudolph et al, pp 2154-2155.*) The child in the photograph has a pit over the spine which may represent a dermal sinus; virtually any abnormality (except Mongolian spots) over the lower spine points to the possibility of occult spinal dysraphism. This designation includes a number of spinal cord and vertebral anomalies that due to tethering of the spinal cord may produce loss of neurologic function, particularly in the region of the back, the lower extremities (hypotonia and muscle atrophy), and the urinary system (leading to urinary tract infections). Examples of these abnormalities are tufts of hair, subcutaneous lipomeningomyelocele, diastematomyelia, hamartoma, lipoma, tight filum terminale, tethered cord, dermal and epidermal cysts, neurenteric canals, and angiomas. Occasionally, the loss of neurologic function from such anomalies is mild and, as a result, easily overlooked or may develop only as the child gets older. Recurrent meningitis of unknown etiology may be presenting sign of a dermal sinus tract. Prompt evaluation of these lesions, probably by MRI, is indicated.

284. The answer is b. (*Hay et al, pp 1118-1119. Kliegman et al, pp 644-646. Rudolph et al, p 569.*) The growth curve shown demonstrates poor growth over the 6 months of this infant's life. Homocystinuria is an autosomal recessive metabolic disease caused by deficiencies of cystathionine β-synthase, methylenetetrahydrofolate reductase, or the coenzyme for N_5-methyltetrahydrofolate methyltransferase, which result in an accumulation of homocysteine and its metabolites. Manifestations include poor growth, arachnodactyly, osteoporosis, dislocated lenses, and intellectual disability. In addition, thromboembolic phenomena may be seen in the pulmonary and systemic arteries and particularly in the cerebral vasculature; vascular occlusive disease is, in turn, one of the many causes of acute infantile hemiplegia. None of the other disorders listed in the question are associated with acute hemiplegia. Phenylketonuria (phenylalanine hydroxylase deficiency) causes intellectual disability and, on occasion, seizures. Maple syrup urine disease, an abnormality of the metabolism of branch chain amino acids leucine, isoleucine, and valine, leads to seizures and rapid deterioration of the CNS in newborns. Most states now include these diseases in their newborn screening programs.

Histidinemia (deficiency of histidase) and cystathioninuria (defect in cystathionine gamma-lyase) are most likely benign aminoacidurias with no effect on the CNS.

285. The answer is e. (*Hay et al, pp 812-814. Kliegman et al, pp 2819-2823. Rudolph et al, pp 710-713.*) The infant in the question, who is completely healthy otherwise, appears to have positional plagiocephaly, an asymmetrical flattening of the scalp often caused by consistently sleeping on the same area of the head. An unintended consequence of the AAP's Back to Sleep campaign to reduce the incidence of sudden infant death syndrome by supine sleeping has been insufficient "tummy time" when the child is awake; babies who are always on their backs can develop positional plagiocephaly. Treatment in most children who are otherwise normal, that is, do not have conditions such as congenital torticollis, is "tummy time" at least three times per day and alternating the sleep position such that the deformed side is no longer resting on the mattress. Severe or unresponsive cases may require physical therapy and molding (helmet) therapy. A variety of syndromes result in abnormal head shapes, but chromosome analysis would be reserved for cases in which other features such as limb, heart, or facial abnormalities are also found. Palpable ridges over suture lines suggest craniosynostosis. A neurosurgical evaluation is warranted, and in these cases if repair is being considered the neurosurgeon may request a cranial CT scan with three-dimensional reconstruction. Exclusively breast-fed infants are at risk for vitamin D deficiency and, thus, are supplemented with vitamin D. Nutritional rickets would present with abnormal long-bone shape or fractures but not skull-shape abnormalities.

286. The answer is c. (*Hay et al, pp 853-854. Kliegman et al, pp 2991-2996. Rudolph et al, pp 2235-2240.*) Myasthenia gravis is an autoimmune disorder in which circulating acetylcholine receptor-binding antibodies result in neuromuscular blockade. The earliest signs of myasthenia gravis are ptosis and weakness of the extraocular muscles, followed by dysphagia and facial muscle weakness. The distinguishing hallmark of this disease is rapid fatiguing of the involved muscles. In children older than about 2 years, the clinical test for myasthenia gravis is the administration of edrophonium chloride which should result in improvement of the ptosis and ophthalmoplegia in a few seconds, and improvement in fatigability of other muscles as well. This drug is avoided in younger children as cardiac arrhythmias may result and the improvement in muscle strength is too fleeting for objective measurement; in these children a longer acting agent (neostigmine) would be used instead. Alternatively, the conduction velocity of the motor nerve typically is normal in this condition. When the involved muscle is repetitively stimulated for diagnostic purposes, the electromyogram (EMG) shows a decremental response, which can be reversed by the administration of cholinesterase inhibitors as described above. Cholinesterase inhibitors are the primary therapeutic agents. Other therapeutic modalities for myasthenia gravis include immunosuppression, plasmapheresis, thymectomy (an enlarged thymus is frequently seen on chest x-ray but is not diagnostic), and treatment of hypothyroidism. CPK should be normal. Muscle biopsy has little place in the evaluation for myasthenia gravis. Degenerating and regenerating myofibers on biopsy would be diagnostic of muscular dystrophy. Circulating acetylcholine receptor-binding antibodies levels may be increased; serum ANAs are normal.

287. The answer is e. (*Hay et al, pp 786-800. Kliegman et al, p 2862. Rudolph et al, p 2224.*) Seizure-like activity with no epileptiform activity on EEG is consistent with pseudoseizure. These episodes may be very convincing for seizures and may include unusual posturing and sounds, but typically do not involve loss of bowel or bladder control. In addition, the patient usually will not cause self-injury, and pupillary response to light is normal. These episodes can be deliberate or part of a conversion disorder, and do not require treatment with antiepileptic or other medications. However, many patients with pseudoseizures also have true epileptic seizures, so withdrawal of antiepileptic medication would be inappropriate at this point. Psychiatric or psychologic evaluation is the best way to begin managing pseudoseizures.

288. The answer is e. (*Hay et al, pp 806-809. Kliegman et al, pp 2925-2929. Rudolph et al, pp 2165-2168.*) The abrupt onset of a hemisyndrome, especially with the eyes looking away from the paralyzed side, strongly indicates a diagnosis of acute infantile hemiplegia. Most frequently, this represents a thromboembolic occlusion of the middle cerebral artery or one of its major branches. CNS infection is another potential cause, presenting as an acute syndrome of fever and partial seizure with resulting hemiparesis. Childhood stroke can result from trauma, infection, a hypercoagulable state, arteritis, and congenital structural or metabolic disorders.

Hemiplegic migraine commonly occurs in children with a history of migraine and during a headache episode. Todd paralysis follows after a focal or Jacksonian seizure and generally does not last more than 24-48 hours. The clinical onset of supratentorial brain tumor is subacute, with repeated headaches and gradually developing weakness. A history of trauma usually precedes the signs of an acute subdural hematoma. Clinical signs of other diseases can appear fairly rapidly, but not often with the abruptness of occlusive vascular disease as described in the case.

289. The answer is c. (*Hay et al, p 820. Kliegman et al, pp 2874-2877. Rudolph et al, pp 728-730.*) Neurofibromatosis type 1 (NF1) is a progressive neurocutaneous syndrome that results from a defect in neural crest differentiation and migration during the early stages of development. It has an autosomal dominant pattern of inheritance; the gene locus has been identified on chromosome 17. Any organ or system can be affected, neurologic complications are frequent, and patients are at high risk of developing malignant neoplasms of various types. The presence of any two of the following findings confirms the diagnosis of NF1: (1) five or more café au lait spots over 5 mm in diameter in prepubertal patients; six or more over 15 mm in diameter in postpubertal patients; (2) axillary freckling; (3) two or more Lisch nodules (hamartomas of the iris); (4) two or more neurofibromas, typically involving the skin and appearing during adolescence or pregnancy, or one plexiform neuroma involving a nerve track present at birth; (5) bony lesions leading to pathologic fracture and kyphoscoliosis; (6) optic glioma; (7) NF1 in a first-degree relative. The child in the question has the required café au lait spots, and the family history of seizures, which occur in about 8% of NF1 patients, hints at NF1 in a first-degree relative.

All of the other choices may have café au lait spots as well. Cardinal features of Peutz-Jeghers syndrome include hyperpigmented lesions on the lips, around the mouth, and around the anus. Affected patients subsequently develop gastrointestinal polyps and are at increased risk for developing various cancers. Noonan syndrome with multiple lentigines is a rare, autosomal dominant disease that, in addition to café au lait lesions, includes findings of hypertelorism, pulmonary stenosis, cryptorchidism, deafness, and delayed growth over the first year of life. Legius syndrome is an autosomal dominant condition which visually may appear similar to NF although it is much rarer and macrocephaly is common. Genetic testing, if necessary, will differentiate the two. Carney complex is a rare autosomal dominantly inherited condition that has in addition to café au lait spots around the lips, eyes, and genitalia the finding of myxomas (especially of the heart) as a prominent feature.

290. The answer is d. (*Hay et al, pp 1160, 1162. Kliegman et al, pp 2980-2983. Rudolph et al, pp 2244-2245.*) The child in the question appears to have myotonic muscular dystrophy. An elevated creatinine kinase (especially in the preclinical phase) often is found, and psychomotor retardation can be the presenting complaint (but may be identified only in retrospect). Ptosis, baldness, hypogonadism, facial immobility with distal muscle wasting (in older children), and neonatal respiratory distress (in the newborn period) are major features of this disorder. Cataracts are commonly seen, presenting either congenitally or at any point during childhood. The prominence of distal muscle weakness in this disease is in contrast to the proximal muscle weakness seen in most other forms of myopathies. The diagnosis is confirmed by a molecular blood test. Seizures are not a feature of myotonic dystrophy. Enlarged gonads are associated with fragile X syndrome, and hirsutism is found (among other things) in children with congenital adrenal hyperplasia.

291. The answer is a. (*Hay et al, pp 801-804. Kliegman et al, pp 2863-2873. Rudolph et al, pp 2216-2219.*) In contrast to adults, children with migraine most often have "common" migraine: bifrontal headache without an aura or diffuse throbbing headache of only a few hours' duration. As with adults, the headaches can be terminated with vomiting or sleep. Abortive medications such as appropriate doses of ibuprofen taken less than 30 minutes after the onset of symptoms can be highly effective. Family history is frequently positive. Tension headaches are possible, but the severity of this child's headache and the throbbing nature suggests migraine. One always considers the possibility of brain tumor in children with headaches, but the duration of this headache, lack of findings on clinical examination, and lack of changes in behavior or school performance suggest this is not likely. Allergic rhinitis can cause nasal congestion and headache, and the treatment would be oral antihistamines and nasal steroids; this child's symptoms and clinical findings do not suggest this as the cause. Sinusitis is likely to cause symptoms including nasal discharge and persistent pain over the sinuses. Meningitis or pseudotumor cerebri are unlikely to be this indolent.

292. The answer is b. (*Hay et al, pp 835-840. Kliegman et al, pp 1452-1453. Rudolph et al, pp 1049-1057.*) The clinical data show enhancement of the basal cisterns, low CSF glucose, dramatically elevated CSF protein, and an increased number of WBCs in spinal fluid (all of which are lymphocytes). Included among those processes that can cause the clinical picture are viral meningitis, tuberculous meningitis, meningeal leukemia, and medulloblastoma, all of which can cause pleocytosis as well as elevated protein and lowered glucose concentrations in CSF. Of the four diseases (and the likely diagnosis of this patient), tuberculous meningitis is associated with the lowest glucose levels in CSF. The CT scan with contrast can be an excellent clue for diagnosing tuberculous meningitis. Exudate in the basal cisterns that shows enhancement by contrast material is typical; tuberculomas, ringed lucencies, edema, and infarction can be apparent; and hydrocephalus can develop. Confirmation with culture is mandatory. The x-ray of the chest will be likely to show signs of pulmonary tuberculosis. A high index of suspicion is necessary to diagnose tuberculous meningitis early. Treatment for tuberculous meningitis is with the drugs listed in the answer.

In pseudotumor cerebri (sometimes treated with acetazolamide) a high opening pressure is found, but the constituents of CSF are generally normal except for low-protein content in some instances. Acute bacterial disease must be considered for this patient, but typically causes polymorphonuclear cells and positive Gram stains; it is treated with systemic intravenous ceftriaxone and vancomycin as described. Neither tuberous sclerosis (sometimes treated with rapamycin) nor stroke typically causes these findings on CSF examination.

293. The answer is a. (*Hay et al, pp 997-1001. Kliegman et al, pp 2453-2460. Rudolph et al, pp 1656-1660.*) A child who has a subacute disorder of the CNS that produces cranial nerve abnormalities (especially of cranial nerve VII and the lower bulbar nerves), long-tract signs, unsteady gait secondary to spasticity, and some behavioral changes is most likely to have a pontine glioma. These diffuse tumors are difficult to treat. Tumors of the cerebellar hemispheres can, in later stages, produce upper motor neuron signs, but the gait disturbance would be ataxia. Dysmetria and nystagmus also would be present. Supratentorial tumors are quite common in 6-year-old children; headache and vomiting likely would be the presenting symptoms and papilledema a finding on physical examination. SSPE is a rare disorder seen in children having experienced an episode of measles; extremely rare cases of SSPE can be associated with the vaccine. The patients have insidious behavior changes, deterioration in schoolwork, and finally dementia. No other findings are usually seen. Progressive multifocal leukoencephalopathy, caused by a chronic polyomavirus infection, is usually found in patients with immune deficiencies; although still rare, it has become more common as the incidence of AIDS increased.

294. The answer is d. (*Hay et al, pp 835-840. Kliegman et al, pp 2949-2950. Rudolph et al, pp 916-918.*) The patient in the question has a brain abscess, a condition that presents more indolently than does meningitis. A typical patient has nonspecific, low-grade fevers, headache, and lethargy that may result in the administration of oral antibiotics, especially if findings of otitis media, sinusitis, or other common pediatric illness are found. Severe headache, vomiting, seizures, papilledema, and neurologic findings develop later. A high index of suspicion is required to make the diagnosis. The diagnostic tool of choice is MRI, but CT with contrast is also acceptable. Lumbar puncture would be contraindicated in this patient until after imaging (the patient is at risk for brain herniation) and the CSF (and blood) cultures are usually negative. The child has a heart murmur, and brain abscesses are more commonly seen in children with right-to-left shunts such as in transposition of the great vessels or tetralogy of Fallot, but an echocardiogram is not indicated immediately. If the patient has negative imaging of the brain, then a urine drug screen might be indicated, but not as a test of first choice.

295. The answer is b. (*Hay et al, pp 409-413. Kliegman et al, pp 507-512. Rudolph et al, pp 2163-2164.*) Compression of cranial nerve III and distortion of the brain stem, resulting in unilateral pupillary dilatation, hemiplegia, focal seizures, and depressed consciousness, suggests a progressively enlarging mass, most likely an epidural hematoma. Such a hematoma displaces the temporal lobe into the tentorial notch and presses on the ipsilateral cranial nerve III. Brain stem compression by this additional tissue mass leads to progressive deterioration of consciousness. Rising blood pressure, irregular respiration, and falling pulse rate (Cushing triad) are characteristic of increasing intracranial pressure. The most urgent test to diagnose this condition is a CT scan.

Meningitis results from an infection of the meninges; presenting signs and symptoms include fever, headache, nausea/vomiting, stiff neck, and progressive altered mental status. While this child was playing outside, dehydration and electrolyte disturbances typically are seen after prolonged play in especially hot weather, or in the child with a history of acute illness associated with vomiting and/or diarrhea. An overdose of pain medications would be expected to cause bilateral pin-point pupils and respiratory depression. Ingestion of an unknown drug would be expected to cause bilateral pupillary response (dilation or miosis) depending on the drug.

296. The answer is e. (*Hay et al, p 999. Kliegman et al, pp 2459-2460. Rudolph et al, p 1660.*) The findings of poor growth, diabetes insipidus, and papilledema could be explained by a craniopharyngioma. This tumor is one of the most common supratentorial tumors in children, often causing growth failure through disruption of pituitary excretions such as growth hormone. Upward growth of a craniopharyngioma results in compression of the optic chiasm. Particularly affected are the fibers derived from the nasal portions of both retinas (ie, from those parts of the eyes receiving stimulation from the temporal visual field). Early in the growth of a craniopharyngioma, a unilateral superior quadrantanopsic defect can develop, and an irregularly growing tumor can impinge upon the optic tract and cause homonymous hemianopia. Treatment is surgical excision and may include radiation therapy for large lesions. However, significant morbidity is associated with these tumors and their removal, including vision loss, growth failure, and panhypopituitarism.

297. The answer is a. (*Hay et al, pp 824-829. Kliegman et al, pp 250-254. Rudolph et al, pp 2197-2198.*) Cerebellar ataxia in childhood can occur in association with infection, metabolic abnormalities, ingestion of toxins, hydrocephalus, cerebellar lesions, MS, labyrinthitis, polyradiculopathy, and neuroblastoma. Although a muscle biopsy might help identify muscular dystrophy, the finding of a triplet repeat expansion on chromosome 9 might identify Friedreich ataxia, and finding skin telangiectasia might help identify ataxia telangiectasia, none of these would be expected to cause acute ataxia but rather more chronic symptoms. Ingestion (intentional or accidental) of barbiturates, phenytoin, alcohol, and other drugs also must be considered; the first step for management of this child is to rule out ingestion. Agenesis of the corpus callosum is usually diagnosed by imaging studies; however, it does not cause acute ataxia. Acute cerebellar ataxia related to his recent bout with varicella should be in the differential. Findings with this, however, include truncal ataxia (challenges with sitting and walking), vomiting, horizontal nystagmus, and dysarthria.

298. The answer is a. (*Hay et al, pp 997-1001. Kliegman et al, pp 1656-1660. Rudolph et al, pp 1771-1775.*) Brain tumors are the most common solid tumor in childhood, and account for 25%-30% of all pediatric malignancies. While supratentorial tumors are predominate in the first year of life (including choroid plexus tumors and teratomas), brain tumors in children 1-10 years old are more frequently infratentorial (posterior fossa) and include cerebellar and brain stem tumors such as medulloblastoma or cerebellar astrocytoma. After 10 years of age, supratentorial tumors (eg, diffuse astrocytoma) are again more common.

299. The answer is e. (*Hay et al, pp 1308-1310. Kliegman et al, pp 1428-1431. Rudolph et al, p 2240.*) Botulism has been associated with the ingestion of raw honey (which was one of the "home remedies" recommended by the grandmother in the question) as well as exposure to clothing of family members who are outside gardeners or construction workers; in young children, it often presents with constipation before the development of the other symptoms listed. Constipation is an unusual presenting feature in the other disorders listed in the question.

Constipation in a young infant is a common complaint of parents, and potentially is unrelated to this neonate's problem. Some of the other diagnostic considerations listed in the question are possibilities if the constipation is coincidental. Neonatal HSV infection is a serious, potentially life-threatening condition that can have neurologic symptoms but usually has prominent findings associated with sepsis. Neonatal myasthenia gravis, although uncommon, must be considered in a newborn infant who has the symptoms described in the question; it seems less likely in this instance since the mother was asymptomatic and the congenital (autosomal dominant) form is rare. The symptoms presented (excepting prominent constipation) also could represent tick paralysis but this seems highly unlikely in this aged child. Myotonic dystrophy can be inherited but findings at birth or earlier than 3 weeks would be expected.

300. The answer is d. (*Hay et al, p 820. Kliegman et al, pp 706-708. Rudolph et al, pp 2250-2255.*) β-Hexosaminidase A deficiency (GM$_2$ gangliosidosis, type 1 or Tay-Sachs disease) presents as psychomotor retardation and hypotonia beginning at about 6-12 months of age; the children are usually normal at birth. A pronounced startle reflex and severe hyperacusis, seizures, loss of vision (with cherry-red macular spots), and macrocephaly are seen. The cherry-red spot represents the center of a normal retinal macula that is surrounded by ganglion cells in which an abnormal accumulation of lipid has occurred, thus altering the surrounding retinal color so that it is yellowish or grayish white; it is also seen in GM_1 generalized gangliosidosis type 1, Sandhoff disease, and Niemann-Pick disease type A.

Menkes disease is an X-linked condition in which defects in copper absorption result in growth retardation, infantile spasms or status epilepticus, developmental delay, and twisted, split, and easily broken hairs; the optic disk examination shows pallor. Reduced activity of α-galactosidase (Fabry disease) presents in older children as acroparesthesia (numbness or tingling in one or more extremities), intermittent painful crises of the extremities or the abdomen, frequently low-grade fevers, and sometimes cataracts. Patients with Rett syndrome (defective gene called *MECP2* on the X chromosome) present as normal girls at birth, but then have a rapid decline in motor and cognitive functions beginning between 6 and 18 months of age. Affected girls demonstrate loss in the use of their hands and loss in their ability to communicate and socialize.

Metachromatic leukodystrophy (deficient activity of galactosyl-3-sulfateceramide sulfatase) has its onset between 1 and 2 years of age and is notable for progressive ataxia, weakness, and peripheral neuropathy. In this disorder, gray macular lesions can be seen that look somewhat similar to cherry-red spots.

301. The answer is b. (*Hay et al, pp 798-799. Kliegman et al, pp 2829-2831. Rudolph et al, pp 2204-2206.*) The child in the question likely had an illness-associated (febrile) seizure. Febrile seizures usually occur in children between the ages of 9 months and 5 years, generally in association with upper respiratory illness, roseola, shigellosis, or gastroenteritis. A family history is often found. The generalized seizures are mostly brief (2-5 minutes), and the CSF is normal. Since other more serious processes cause seizure and fever, each child must be carefully evaluated. Children younger than about 12-18 months have unreliable neck examination for meningismus; lumbar punctures are done for those less than 6 months of age and are optional in unvaccinated children between 6 to 12 months of age. In a simple febrile seizure, EEG and CNS imaging usually are not necessary. Infants who have seizures that are prolonged (longer than 15 minutes), focal or lateralized, or who had neurologic problems before the febrile seizure (including intraventricular hemorrhage), are at a higher risk of developing an afebrile seizure disorder during the subsequent 5-7 years. CSF is usually normal after a seizure, so a pleocytosis requires evaluation for meningitis or encephalitis.

302. The answer is c. (*Hay et al, pp 842-843. Kliegman et al, pp 3010-3012. Rudolph et al, pp 2232-2233.*) The laboratory data shown include a normal CBC and electrolyte panel. The spinal fluid has isolated elevation of the CSF protein level. The paralysis of Guillain-Barré often occurs about 10 days after a nonspecific viral illness. Weakness is gradual over days or weeks, beginning in the lower extremities and progressing toward the trunk. Later, the upper limbs and the bulbar muscles can become involved. Involvement of the respiratory muscles is life-threatening. The syndrome seems to be caused by a demyelination in the motor nerves and, occasionally, the sensory nerves. Measurement of spinal fluid protein is helpful in the diagnosis; protein levels are increased to more than twice normal, while glucose and cell counts are normal. Hospitalization for observation is indicated. Treatment can consist of observation alone, intravenous immunoglobulin, steroids, or plasmapheresis. Recovery is not always complete.

Bell palsy usually follows a mild upper respiratory infection, resulting in the rapid development of unilateral weakness of the face. Muscular dystrophy encompasses a number of entities that include weakness over months. Charcot-Marie-Tooth disease has a clinical onset including peroneal and intrinsic foot muscle atrophy, later extending to the intrinsic hand muscles and proximal legs. Werdnig-Hoffmann disease is an anterior horn disorder that presents either *in utero* (in about one-third of cases) or by the first 6 months of life with hypotonia, weakness, and delayed developmental motor milestones.

303. The answer is a. (*Hay et al, pp 1250-1253. Kliegman et al, pp 1590-1594. Rudolph et al, pp 1152-1154.*) Periventricular calcifications are a characteristic finding in infants who have congenital CMV infection. The encephalitic process especially affects the subependymal tissue around the lateral ventricles and thus results in the periventricular deposition of calcium. Calcified tuberculomas, if visible radiographically, are not particularly periventricular; congenital tuberculosis presenting such as the patient described would be extraordinarily unusual. Granulomatous encephalitis caused by congenital toxoplasmosis is associated with scattered and soft-appearing intracranial calcification, and suprasellar calcifications are typical of craniopharyngiomas. Congenital syphilis does not produce intracranial calcifications. The unscientific, but sometimes useful, way of keeping intracranial calcifications caused by CMV differentiated from those caused by toxoplasmosis is to remember that "CMV" has a V in it, as does "periventricular"; "toxoplasmosis" has an X in it, and the lesions associated with it typically are scattered throughout the "cortex," which also has an X in it.

304. The answer is b. (*Hay et al, pp 816-817. Kliegman et al, pp 2877-2879. Rudolph et al, pp 730-731.*) In infants, hypomelanotic skin patches (also called ash leaf spots), especially in association with infantile spasms, are characteristic of tuberous sclerosis, an autosomal dominantly acquired condition. Other dermal abnormalities (adenoma sebaceum and subungual fibromata) associated with this disorder appear later in childhood. Children with this condition may present with infantile spasms, and a Wood lamp evaluation of their skin may assist in the identification of the hypopigmented, "ash-leaf" lesions. Renal angiomyolipoma is one of the "major" criteria for diagnosis. CT scan of the brain may demonstrate calcified tubers, but these may not be evident until 3-4 years of age.

Although children who have neurofibromatosis may have a few hypomelanotic patches, the identifying dermal lesions are café au lait spots. Children with neurofibromatosis classically are described as having Lisch nodules found on ophthalmologic evaluation. Incontinentia pigmenti also is associated with seizures; the skin lesions typical of this disorder begin as bullous eruptions that later become hyperpigmented lesions. Associated findings with this condition are hypodontia with conical or pegged teeth. Pityriasis rosea begins with a single "herald patch" with later spread of the rash along skin tension lines, especially on the trunk resulting in a "Christmas tree" pattern. Psoriasis, lichen planus, and Darier disease (keratosis follicularis) are classically described as resulting in Koebner phenomenon (skin lesions that appear along lines of trauma).

305. The answer is b. (*Hay et al, pp 851-852, 1160. Kliegman et al, pp 2996-2998. Rudolph et al, pp 1997-1998, 2228-2229.*) The laboratory data presented are normal, including the CSF examination. The neonate described has spinal muscular atrophy (SMA) type I, also referred to as

Werdnig-Hoffman disease, or infantile progressive SMA. The defect is found in the survivor motor neuron (SMN) gene that stops apoptosis of motor neuroblasts. During development, an excess of motor neuroblasts is noted, and through apoptosis only about half survive in the normal newborn; the SMN gene regulates this natural destruction. A defect in the SMN gene results in a continuation of apoptosis, resulting in progressive destruction of motor neurons in the brain stem and spinal cord. In 2016 the FDA approved nusinersen (Spinraza) to treat this condition; the drug appears to increase the expression of the surviving motor neuron proteins which are deficient in SMA. More recently, in May of 2019 the FDA approved the first gene therapy for SMA. Without treatment infants with SMA I usually die of respiratory complications by the second or third year of life. Three other types of SMA have been described: SMA 0, a rare severe form that is fatal in the perinatal period; SMA II, in which infants may suck normally and despite progressive weakness may survive into the school-aged years; and SMA III, which usually presents later and with a better prognosis. Intelligence is normal, and the heart is not affected.

Absence of dystrophin is seen in muscular dystrophy. Antibodies binding to the acetylcholine (ACh) receptor at the postsynaptic membrane are the underlying cause of myasthenia gravis. Progressive postinfectious autoimmune demyelination is the underlying problem in Guillain-Barré syndrome. Birth trauma may cause CNS bleeding, which would be expected to result in seizures, but not generalized weakness. It should be noted that congenital Guillain-Barré syndrome rarely has been described, but in those cases, CSF protein is elevated. In addition, congenital myasthenia gravis has been described in patients born to mothers with myasthenia.

306. The answer is b. (*Hay et al, pp 1160-1161. Kliegman et al, pp 2975-2979. Rudolph et al, pp 2240-2243.*) The most common form of muscular dystrophy is Duchenne muscular dystrophy. It is inherited as an X-linked recessive trait. Male infants are rarely diagnosed at birth or early infancy since they often reach gross milestones at the expected age. Soon after beginning to walk, however, the features of this disease become more evident. While these children walk at the appropriate age, the hip girdle weakness is seen by the age of 2 years. Increased lordosis, while standing, is evidence of gluteal weakness. Gower sign (use of the hands to "climb up" the legs in order to assume the upright position) is seen by 3-5 years of age, as is the hip waddle gait. Ambulation ability remains through about 7-12 years of age, after which use of a wheelchair is common. Associated features include mental impairment and cardiomyopathy. Death caused by respiratory failure, heart failure, pneumonia, or aspiration is common by early adulthood. An elevation of the serum CPK level would be expected. An ultrasound of the lower spine would detect an occult spina bifida. MRI of the brain would be helpful to identify intracranial abnormalities such as brain tumor. Lumbar puncture with elevated protein and abnormal nerve conduction studies might suggest Guillain-Barré syndrome, and elevated serum botulinum titers suggest botulism.

307. The answer is b. (*Hay et al, pp 100, 792. Kliegman et al, p 2863. Rudolph et al, p 1942.*) The case is a classic description of night terrors for which intervention is neither required nor appropriate. Night terrors are most common in children between the ages of 5 and 7 years. Children awaken suddenly, appear frightened and unaware of their surroundings, and have the clinical signs outlined in the question. The child cannot be consoled by the parents. After a few minutes, sleep returns, and the patient cannot recall the event in the morning. Sleepwalking is common in these children. Exploring the family dynamics for emotional disorders may be helpful; usually pharmacologic therapy is not required, and family reassurance is indicated.

308. The answer is d. (*Hay et al, pp 650, 802. Kliegman et al, pp 2857-2863. Rudolph et al, pp 1851-1852.*) Simple syncope occurs following an alteration in brain blood flow, possibly as a result of hypotension. The majority of syncopal episodes are vasovagal. Other considerations include cardiac causes (such as prolonged QTc, arrhythmia, or outflow obstruction), migraine, seizure, hypoglycemia, hyperventilation, and vertigo. Ischemia of the higher cortical levels results in neuronal discharges from the reticular formation (which is no longer influenced by the cortical level) producing brief tonic contractions of muscles of the upper extremities, trunk, and face. The sequence of events described in the question probably resulted from vasovagal stimulation, often precipitated by pain, fear, excitement, or standing for long periods. This condition is common in adolescent girls. After a careful history and physical examination and a normal ECG, an organic cause of this fainting episode is unlikely to be identified; reassurance is usually all that is required. Counseling on proper diet and fluid intake is appropriate; patients should also increase their salt intake. Occasionally, patients with recurrent vasovagal syncope may be managed using β-blockers or fludrocortisone.

309 to 311. The answers are 309-e, 310-j, 311-a. (*Hay et al, pp 801-804. Kliegman et al, pp 2863-2874. Rudolph et al, pp 424-425, 2216-2219.*) Headaches are a common pediatric complaint and can be quite concerning to parents. Vascular (migraine) headaches can occur in all ages, and patients usually have a family history of migraine. Migraine without aura is the most common form in both children and adults. Triggers might include menstrual periods, inadequate sleep and skipped meals. A nonspecific prodrome may include a change in mood, temperament, or appetite.

Worsening headaches with nausea and emesis (particularly early morning emesis) are concerning for increased intracranial pressure from a mass lesion. Other associated findings may be decreased school performance, behavioral changes, or focal neurologic deficits. Papilledema may be present. Imaging would be necessary with this presentation.

Tension headaches are common in the older child and adolescent. They will worsen during the day, and may worsen with stressful situations such as tests. They are typically described as squeezing, but are not usually pulsatile. Nausea and vomiting are not typical.

Factitious headache, as with any factitious diagnosis, should be one of exclusion. Hemiplegic migraine is descriptive of a typical aura that involves unilateral sensory or motor signs with a migraine headache. Patients can have unilateral weakness, numbness, and aphasia. These signs may resolve quickly or may last for days. This particular type of migraine is more common in children than in adults. Hypervitaminosis A requires ingestion of high amounts of the vitamin over a prolonged period of time. Headache can be a finding, but other findings would include dry skin, fatigue, change in behavior, and hepatomegaly. Headache associated with hypertension classically also presents with retinal hemorrhages or exudates along with altered mental status and likely seizures. Patients with tuberculous meningitis are most commonly 6 months to 4 years of age with rapid progression of disease more common in the younger age group. Initial signs and symptoms include fever, headache, and change in sensorium. Later, nuchal rigidity and focal neurologic findings are seen. Berry aneurysm typically are asymptomatic in children unless they rupture, but might present with localized headache, pupillary dilation, blurred vision, and dysarthria. Acute subarachnoid hemorrhage, from ruptured berry aneurysm or otherwise, result in symptoms such as sudden headache, change in consciousness, nausea and vomiting, nuchal rigidity, change in vision, weakness, and dysarthria. Headache associated with systemic lupus erythematosus would be only one of a variety of complaints including such features as fever, weight loss, arthritis, rash, hemolytic anemia, proteinuria, and hepatosplenomegaly. MS often presents with hemiparesis or paraparesis, focal sensory loss, ataxia and optic neuritis; headache is not a prominent isolated feature.

312 to 314. The answers are 312-b, 313-e, 314-h. (*Hay et al, pp 463, 830-832. Kliegman et al, pp 140-143. Rudolph et al, pp 872-873, 2178-2181, 2143-2146, 2220-2222.*) Tics are commonly seen in a pediatric practice. All have in common the nonrhythmic, spasmodic, involuntary, stereotypical behaviors that involve any muscle group. Transient tic disorder is the most common and is seen more often in boys; a family history is often noted. In this condition, the patient has eye blinking, facial movements, or throat clearing lasting for weeks to about a year. No medications are needed. Chronic motor tics persist throughout life and can incorporate motor movements involving up to three muscle groups.

Gilles de la Tourette syndrome is a lifelong condition that is characterized by motor and vocal tics, obsessive-compulsive behavior, and a high incidence of attention-deficit/hyperactivity disorder (ADHD). Therapy for the ADHD is helpful, as is medication to control the motor or vocal tics. Multiple psychosocial problems exist with these children; a multidisciplinary approach is helpful.

The term "chorea" describes involuntary uncoordinated jerks of the arms and legs. Sydenham chorea is the most commonly acquired chorea of childhood, is seen after infections with group A β-hemolytic streptococci, and is associated with rheumatic heart disease and arthritis. In addition to the motor symptoms, patients may be hypotonic, emotionally labile, and have a "milkmaid" grip with sequential grip tightening and relaxing. Other findings include a darting tongue and "spooning" of an extended hand (flexion at the wrist and extension of the fingers).

Dystonic reactions are sometimes seen in patients receiving phenothiazine medications. They have unusual neck, arm, or leg muscle twitches that are sometimes confused with seizure activity. Diphenhydramine, infused intravenously, usually rapidly reverses this relatively common idiosyncratic drug reaction.

Cerebral palsy is a static condition of movement and posture disorders frequently associated with epilepsy and abnormalities of vision, speech, and intellect. A defect in the developing brain is felt to be the cause. No significant change in the incidence of cerebral palsy has been noted in the past few decades despite drastically improved obstetric and neonatal care.

No treatment for cerebral palsy is available; a multidisciplinary approach to manage the many medical problems associated with the condition is helpful.

Rett, fragile X, Smith-Magenis, Lesch-Nyhan, and Cornelia de Lange syndromes all have stereotypic movements as features of their condition. Girls with Rett syndrome (defective gene called *MECP2* on the X chromosome) present as normal girls at birth, but then have a rapid decline in motor and cognitive functions beginning between 6 and 18 months of age. Affected girls demonstrate repetitive hand-wringing and loss in the use of their hands to communicate and socialize. Patients with fragile X syndrome have intellectual disability, autistic behavior with various stereotypic movements, macroorchidism (notable especially after puberty), characteristic facial features (large ears, elongated face, and high arched palate), gait ataxia, and intention tremor. Patients with Smith-Magenis syndrome have intellectual disability, delayed development of speech and language, and distinctive facial features (deeply set eyes, full cheeks, prominent jaw, flattened nasal bridge, and broad-square face) that becomes prominent as the child ages. Stereotypic behaviors in these patients include self-hugging, biting, hitting, head banging, and skin picking. The cause is a deletion on the short arm of chromosome 17. Lesch-Nyhan syndrome patients are normal at birth, but after several months develop hypotonia, vomiting, and challenges handling secretions. Further developmental delay and intellectual disability becomes apparent as the child ages. By about 8 to 12 months dystonic movements are noted; self-injurious behavior can begin as early as 1 year of age. These patients have an abnormal HPRT gene that has been localized to the long arm of the X chromosome. Cornelia de Lange syndrome includes poor growth, distinctive facies (arched brows that meet, long eyelashes, low seat ears, upturned nose), microcephaly, hypertrichosis, intellectual disabilities, and tendency toward autistic and self-destructive behaviors.

Infectious Diseases and Immunology

Questions

315. A 13-year-old boy is seen in the emergency department (ED) with a 3-day history of fever, muscular pain (especially in the neck), headache, and malaise. He reports that drinking sour liquids causes much pain in the affected area. He denies sick exposures, travel, or intake of medications. His past medical history is positive for occasional upper respiratory infections, but no serious illnesses. He has had one sexual encounter and reports condom use; he denies smoking, alcohol, and other drugs. On physical examination the temperature is 38.5°C (101.1°F), heart rate is 88 beats per minute, respiratory rate is 14 breaths per minute, and blood pressure is 100/69 mm Hg. He is awake, alert, and in no distress. Head is without trauma. Neck is supple with the area on the right side from the back of the mandible toward the mastoid space being full and tender. The earlobe on that side is protuberant. The mucous membranes are pink, moist, and without lesions. Extraocular eye movement and fundoscopic examinations are normal. The chest is clear. Heart has a normal S1 and S2 without murmur. The abdomen is soft and nontender. No hepatosplenomegaly or adenopathy is noted. GU examination is Tanner 3 with tender testicles but no mass. Neurologic examination is nonfocal. Which of the following vaccines would have prevented this condition?

a. Measles-mumps-rubella (MMR)
b. Varicella
c. Human papilloma virus (HPV)
d. Conjugated meningococcal
e. Tetanus toxoid, reduced diphtheria toxoid, and acellular pertussis vaccine adsorbed

316. A 1-hour-old male infant is seen in the normal newborn nursery. The delivery was by repeat cesarean section to a 23-year-old woman whose pregnancy was complicated by HIV. The mother was diagnosed with HIV 2 years prior; she has been on antiretroviral (ARV) medication since diagnosis. She was followed by the high-risk obstetrics clinic and was compliant in taking her antiretrovirals and prenatal vitamins. Her latest HIV viral load was undetectable. She was given ARV medications in the intrapartum period. Which of the following should be considered for this infant?

a. Encourage breast-feeding.
b. Begin immediately single drug therapy with zidovudine.
c. Initiate prophylaxis against *Pneumocystis jirovecii* (previously *P carinii*).
d. Begin immediately triple drug therapy (zidovudine, lamivudine, and nelfinavir).
e. Avoid circumcision.

317. A mother reports that her 4-year-old son was seen in the emergency room 1 week prior with a 3-day history of cough, congestion, and fever. His influenza A testing was positive and he was treated successfully with a 5-day course of antiviral therapy. He appears to be essentially back to his baseline. Past medical history is positive for Kawasaki disease. Current medications include long-term aspirin therapy. In counseling of this mother, which of the following initial new symptoms would suggest a complication to his recent illness?

a. Development of pinpoint pupils
b. Profound lethargy
c. Generalized seizures
d. Diarrhea
e. Abrupt onset of significant vomiting

318. An 18-month-old child is seen by the emergency room physician after having had a brief, generalized tonic-clonic seizure. His father reports that he had been in good health until a few hours prior when he developed malaise, was warm to touch, and seemed to have abdominal pain. On physical examination the temperature is 40°C (104°F), heart rate is 125 beats per minute, respiratory rate is 24 breaths per minute, and blood pressure is 90/50 mm Hg. He is asleep and appears to be postictal. Head is without trauma. Neck is supple. The mucous membranes are pink, moist, and without lesions. Pupils are equally round and reactive. The chest is clear. Heart has a normal S1 and S2 without murmur. The abdomen is soft and nontender. No organomegaly is found. Neurologic examination is postictal. During the lumbar puncture he has a large, watery stool that has both blood and mucus in it. Laboratory data show:

CBC:
  Hemoglobin: 14.2 g/dL
  Hematocrit: 41.5%
  WBC: 12,500/mm^3
    Segmented neutrophils: 49%
    Band forms: 20%
    Lymphocytes: 31%
  Platelet count: 175,000/mm^3
Serum electrolytes:
  Sodium: 137 mEq/L
  Potassium: 4.5 mEq/L
  Chloride: 110 mEq/L
  Bicarbonate: 20 mEq/L
  Glucose: 100 mg/dL
  Creatinine: 0.9 mEq/L
  Blood urea nitrogen (BUN): 10 mEq/L
Spinal fluid analysis:
  Glucose: 85 mg/dL
  Protein: 10 mg/dL
  WBC: 0
  RBC: 0
  Grams stain negative

Which of the following is the most likely diagnosis in this patient?

a. *Salmonella*
b. Enterovirus
c. Rotavirus
d. *Campylobacter*
e. *Shigella*

319. An 8-month-old boy is admitted to the hospital with pneumonia that proves to be *P jiroveci*. He was born vaginally at term after an unremarkable pregnancy. At birth he was noted to have distinctive features that included a short philtrum of the upper lip, a bifid uvula with cleft palate, hypertelorism, a small jaw, and low-set ears. He was moved to the neonatal intensive care unit after he developed seizures related to hypocalcemia where he was also found to have an interrupted aortic arch. Which of the following immunologic patterns is likely to be found in this condition?

Serum IgG	Serum IgA	Serum IgM	T-Cell Function	Parathyroid Function
a. Normal	Normal	Normal	Decreased	Decreased
b. Low	Low	Low	Normal	Normal
c. Low	Low	Low	Decreased	Normal
d. Normal	High	Low	Decreased	Normal
e. Normal	Normal	Normal	Normal	Normal

320. A 4-year-old African-American boy is seen by the pediatrician for hair loss. The mother reports that the lesion began as a small spot that has enlarged, now becoming squishy. She has tried a variety of topical over-the-counter and home remedies that have not helped with the condition. His past medical history is positive for occasional upper respiratory infections, but no hospitalizations. He takes no medications. Family history is negative. On physical examination vital signs are normal. Growth parameters show height and weight to be in the 75th percentile. Head is normocephalic with the lesion noted in the photograph; the lesion is boggy, has tiny pinpoint black dots throughout, and does not fluoresce with a Wood lamp. Neck is supple with some shoddy adenopathy on the right side. The mucous membranes are pink, moist, and without lesions. Pupils are equally round and reactive. The chest is clear. Heart has a normal S1 and S2 without murmur. The abdomen is soft and nontender. No organomegaly is found. Neurologic examination is normal. Which of the following is the most likely diagnosis?

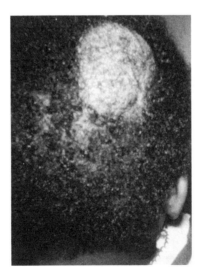

a. Traction alopecia
b. Tinea capitis
c. Seborrheic dermatitis
d. Biotin deficiency
e. Hypothyroidism

321. An 8-year-old girl arrives to the emergency center in respiratory distress. Her mother reports that over the previous several days she has become increasingly tired and pale. The mother denies fever, nausea, vomiting, or change in behavior other than fatigue. No one else in the home is sick. Past medical history is positive for sickle cell disease. Medications include daily folate and penicillin. On physical examination the temperature is 37°C (98.5°F), heart rate 120 beats per minute, respiratory rate is 24 breaths per minute, and blood pressure is 90/56 mm Hg. She is awake and alert. Head is without trauma. Neck is supple. The mucous membranes are pale, slightly icteric, moist, and without lesions. Pupils are equally round and reactive. The chest is clear. Heart has a normal S1 and S2 with a 2/6 blowing SEM at the left lower sternal boarder. The abdomen is soft and nontender. No organomegaly is found. Neurologic examination is nonfocal. Laboratory data show:

CBC:
   Hemoglobin: 3.2 g/dL
   Hematocrit: 9.5%
   WBC: 12,500/mm^3
      Segmented neutrophils: 10%
      Band forms: 0%
      Lymphocytes: 90%
   Platelet count: 175,000/mm^3
   Retic: 0%

Which of the following is the most likely mechanism of disease?

a. Infection with human herpes virus 6
b. Infection with parvovirus B19
c. Infection with coxsackie A16
d. Sequestration of blood in the spleen
e. Replacement of bone marrow with leukemic cells

322. A 6-year-old boy is seen for a 1-day history of achy pain in his anterior right thigh and a limp. His mother reports that he has been healthy since a mild upper respiratory infection resolved about 10 days ago. On physical examination he is awake, alert, and in no distress while sitting on the examination table. He is afebrile. The mucous membranes are moist and pink. The abdomen is soft, nontender, and without organomegaly. Skin is without bruising. The right hip is held in slight abduction and is externally rotated; moderate pain and mild range of motion limitation is noted with manipulation. His thighs and hips are without pain. Laboratory data show:

CBC:
   Hemoglobin: 14 g/dL
   Hematocrit: 42%
   WBC: 7500/mm^3
      Segmented neutrophils: 65%
      Band forms: 0%
      Lymphocytes: 35%
   Platelet count: 175,000/mm^3
   Erythrocyte sedimentation rate (ESR): 3 mm/h (normal: < 20 mm/h)
   C-reactive protein (CRP): <1 mg/dL (normal: > 1 mg/dL)

Which of the following is the most appropriate next step in his management?

a. MRI of the hip
b. Aspiration of the hip joint
c. Ibuprofen every 6 hours
d. Initiation of antistaphylococcal antibiotics
e. Bone marrow aspiration

323. An 8-year-old boy is seen by the pediatrician for a 3-week history of low-grade fever of unknown source, fatigue, weight loss, myalgia, and headaches. On repeated examinations during this time, he is found to have developed a heart murmur, petechiae, and mild splenomegaly. Which of the following is the most appropriate next step in the diagnosis of this child's condition?

a. Measurement of antistreptolysin antibodies.
b. Serial measurement of platelet count and initiation of aspirin therapy.
c. Obtain a rapid streptococcal test.
d. Obtain an echocardiogram.
e. Order a chest radiograph and placement of a purified protein derivative (PPD).

324. A 15-month-old boy is seen by the emergency room physician for a worsening fever and new-onset rash. His mother reports that he was healthy until about 24 hours prior when he developed ear pain. He was seen by his primary-care physician about 6 hours prior, was diagnosed with otitis media, and was given amoxicillin. His mother reports that he no longer is interested in eating and that the rash is spreading rapidly. She denies other medications or sick exposures. His health is generally been good with occasional upper respiratory infections and a case of bronchiolitis the prior winter. On physical examination the temperature is 40°C (104°F), heart rate is 126 beats per minute, respiratory rate is 24 breaths per minute, and blood pressure is 80/50 mm Hg. He is asleep but arousable and then quite irritable. Head is without trauma. Ears have normal pinna and canals. The right tympanic membrane is red, does not move with insufflation, and has fluid behind it; the left ear examination is normal. Neck is supple. The mucous membranes are pink, moist, and without lesions. Pupils are equally round and reactive. The chest is clear. Heart has a normal S1 and S2 without murmur. The abdomen is soft and nontender. No organomegaly is found. Neurologic examination shows him to be irritable. Skin has erythematous and purple lesions of various sizes on his face, trunk, and extremities, some of which do not blanch on pressure. Which of the following is the most appropriate next step in management?

a. Begin administration of IV ampicillin.
b. Begin diphenhydramine and topical steroid cream.
c. Discontinue administration of oral ampicillin and begin trimethoprim with sulfamethoxazole.
d. Perform a right-sided myringotomy with culture of the fluid.
e. Perform a lumbar puncture.

325. A 5-year-old boy is seen for discharge from his left ear. A review of his medical records from his previous provider shows that beginning at about 6 months of age he has had almost monthly episodes of otitis media, a bout of meningitis due to *Streptococcus pneumoniae* at 14 months, frequent episodes of bullous impetigo, and several visits for pneumonia that required prolonged courses of antibiotics. On physical examination the temperature is 38.5°C (101.1°F), heart rate is 88 beats per minute, respiratory rate is 14 breaths per minute, and blood pressure is 100/69 mm Hg. Height is 25th percentile, weight 10th percentile, and head circumference 45th percentile. He is awake, alert, and in no distress. Head is without trauma. The pinnae are normal. The right tympanic membrane is scared with cloudy fluid visible behind it. There is pus in the left ear canal; the left tympanic membrane is not visible. Neck is supple. The mucous membranes are pink, moist, and without lesions. Extraocular eye movement and fundoscopic examinations are normal. Tonsils are small without exudate. The chest is clear. Heart has a normal S1 and S2 without murmur. The abdomen is soft and nontender. Liver and spleen are not enlarged. Lymph nodes are palpable but not enlarged. Neurologic examination is nonfocal. Laboratory data show:

CBC:
  Hemoglobin: 11 g/dL
  Hematocrit: 33%
  WBC: 8500/mm^3
    Segmented neutrophils: 35%
    Band forms: 5%
    Lymphocytes: 13%
    Monocytes: 40%
  Platelet count: 175,000/mm^3
Serum IgM undetectable
Serum IgA undetectable
Serum IgG less than 10th percentile for age
Serum IgE less than 25th percentile for age

Which of the following is the most likely diagnosis?

a. Severe combined immune deficiency
b. DiGeorge syndrome
c. Wiskott-Aldrich syndrome
d. Bruton agammaglobulinemia
e. X-linked lymphoproliferative syndrome

326. A 14-year-old boy is seen by the emergency room physician for a 3-week history of fever between 38.3°C and 38.9°C (101°F and 102°F), lethargy, and a 2.7-kg (6-lb) weight loss. He denies cough, vomiting, or abdominal pain, but admits to having a sore throat. Past medical history is significant for a broken arm at age 10 after a skateboard accident. He denies smoking, alcohol, or other drug use. He is sexually active with one partner and uses condoms inconsistently. On physical examination the temperature is 38.5°C (101.1°F), heart rate is 100 beats per minute, respiratory rate is 18 breaths per minute, and blood pressure is 110/70 mm Hg. He is awake, alert, and in no distress. Head is without trauma. Pupils are equally reactive and round. Ears have normal pinna, canals, and tympanic membranes. The oropharynx is moist, has enlarged tonsils with white exudate, and small hemorrhages on the soft palate. Neck is supple with marked cervical adenopathy. The chest is clear. Heart has a normal S1 and S2 without murmur. The abdomen is soft and nontender. The spleen is palpable 2 cm below the left costal margin. Neurologic examination is nonfocal. GU examination is Tanner 4 without penile discharge. Testes are descended. Marked inguinal adenopathy is noted. Laboratory data show:

CBC:
    Hemoglobin: 15 g/dL
    Hematocrit: 45%
    WBC: 12,500/mm³
        Segmented neutrophils: 40%
        Band forms: 0%
        Lymphocytes: 50%
        Atypical lymphocytes: 10%
    Platelet count: 195,000/mm³

Which of the following therapies should be initiated?

a. Initiation of zidovudine
b. IV acyclovir
c. IV infusion of immunoglobulins and high-dose aspirin
d. Intramuscular penicillin
e. Avoidance of contact sports

327. A 2-year-old child is seen in the emergency center with a 10-day complaint of fever and a limp. The child has an erythrocyte sedimentation rate (ESR) of 60 mm per hour and the radiograph is shown in the photograph. Which of the following statements about this child's condition is correct?

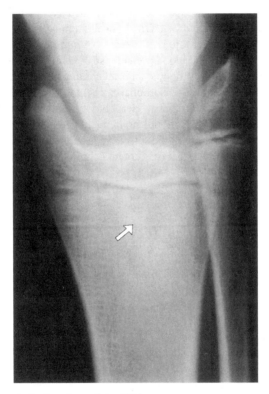

(Used with permission from Susan John, MD.)

a. It is most commonly caused by *Streptococcus pyogenes*.
b. It can arise following development of deep cellulitis.
c. It usually results in diffuse rather than localized regional tenderness.
d. It causes diagnostic radiographic changes on plain films within 48 hours of the beginning of symptoms.
e. It requires antibiotic therapy usually for 10-14 days.

328. A 16-day-old neonate is seen in the emergency center for a 6-hour history of fever, irritability, and poor feeding. The mother reports the neonate to have been in her normal state of good health until the symptoms started. The mother reports the neonate to have been born vaginally after an uncomplicated pregnancy; discharge was at 48 hours of life. She reports good breast-feeding and that the newborn had regained birth weight 2 days prior at the well-child visit. On physical examination the temperature is 38.5°C (101.1°F), heart rate is 170 beats per minute, respiratory rate is 38 breaths per minute, and blood pressure is 70/35 mm Hg. She is pale and lethargic. Head is without trauma; anterior fontanel is bulging. Pupils are equally reactive and round. The oropharynx is moist without lesions. Neck has mild rigidity. The chest is clear. Heart has a normal S1 and S2 without murmur. The abdomen is soft and nontender. The liver edge is palpable 1 cm below the costal margin; the spleen tip is barely palpable. Neurologic examination is nonfocal; lethargy is noted. Laboratory data show:

CBC:
  Hemoglobin: 15 g/dL
  Hematocrit: 45%
  WBC: 1500/mm^3
    Segmented neutrophils: 20%
    Band forms: 20%
    Lymphocytes: 60%
  Platelet count: 105,000/mm^3
Spinal fluid:
  Glucose: 25 mg/dL
  Protein: 50 mg/dL
  WBC: 200 (80% polymorphonuclear leukocytes)
  RBC: 3
  Grams stain: gram positive rods

Which of the following is the most likely diagnosis?

a. *Listeria monocytogenes*
b. Group A streptococci
c. Group B streptococci (GBS)
d. *Streptococcus pneumoniae*
e. *Staphylococcus aureus*

329. A 16-year-old boy presents to the emergency center with a 2-day history of an abscess with spreading cellulitis. While in the emergency center, he develops a high fever, hypotension, and vomiting with diarrhea. On examination, you note the erythematous rash along with injected conjunctiva and oral mucosa, and a strawberry tongue. He is not as alert as when he first arrived. This rapidly progressive symptom constellation is likely caused by which of the following disease processes?

a. Vasculitis of the medium-sized arteries, especially the coronary vessels
b. TSST-1–secreting *S aureus*
c. Shiga toxin–secreting *Escherichia coli*
d. α-Toxin–secreting *Clostridium perfringens*
e. Neurotoxin-secreting *Clostridium tetani*

330. A 14-month-old child is seen by his pediatrician for the sudden onset of fever to 40.2°C (104.4°F). His father reports that he had been in perfectly good health until about 2 hours prior when he developed the fever. He denies vomiting, diarrhea, or sick contacts. The child was born vaginally at term and has no previous serious illnesses. On physical examination on arrival temperature is 40°C (104°F), heart rate is 118 beats per minute, respiratory rate is 22 breaths per minute, and blood pressure is 100/60 mm Hg. Repeat vital signs 30 minutes after acetaminophen are: temperature 38.5°C (101.1°F), heart rate is 105 beats per minute, respiratory rate is 20 breaths per minute, and blood pressure is 100/62 mm Hg. He is now alert and in no distress. Head is without trauma. Pupils are equally reactive and round. The oropharynx is moist without lesions. Neck is supple. The chest is clear. Heart has a normal S1 and S2 without murmur. The abdomen is soft and nontender. No organomegaly is noted. Neurologic examination is nonfocal. Skin has good turgor, capillary refill, and is without lesions. Laboratory data show:

CBC:
  Hemoglobin: 12 g/dL
  Hematocrit: 36.1%
  WBC: 22,500/mm^3
    Segmented neutrophils: 70%
    Band forms: 18%
    Lymphocytes: 12%
  Platelet count; 175,000/mm^3

Which of the following is the most likely diagnosis?

a. Pneumococcal bacteremia
b. Roseola
c. Streptococcosis
d. Typhoid fever
e. Diphtheria

331. A 21-year-old woman has just delivered a term infant. She has had only one visit to her obstetrician, and that was at about 6 weeks of pregnancy. She provides her laboratory results from that visit. The delivered infant is microcephalic, and has cataracts, a heart murmur, and hepatosplenomegaly. Your further evaluation of the neonate demonstrates thrombocytopenia, mild hemolytic anemia, and, on the echocardiogram, patent ductus arteriosus and peripheral pulmonary artery stenosis. Which of the following is the most likely etiology of this neonate's condition?

a. Neonatal hepatitis B
b. Congenital syphilis
c. Congenital rubella syndrome
d. Down syndrome
e. Congenital varicella infection

332. The parents of a 7-day-old neonate bring her to your office for a swollen eye. Her temperature has been normal, but for the last 2 days she has had progressive erythema and swelling over the medial aspect of the right lower lid near the punctum. Her sclera and conjunctiva are clear. Gentle pressure extrudes a whitish material from the punctum. Which of the following ophthalmic conditions is the correct diagnosis?

a. Chalazion
b. Dacryocystitis
c. Preseptal cellulitis
d. Hyphema
e. Congenital Sjögren syndrome

333. A previously healthy 8 week-old-infant is seen for fever, cough, and rhinorrhea. He was born vaginally at term after an uneventful pregnancy. He lives at home with his 2- and 4-year old siblings; care is provided by his father. On physical examination the temperature is 38.5°C (101.1°F), heart rate is 120 beats per minutes, respiratory rate is 36 breaths per minutes, and blood pressure is 90/60 mm Hg. He is awake, alert, and in mild respiratory distress. The chest has some wheezes and a few rales; mild subcoastal and intercostal retractions. Laboratory testing shows RSV antigens to be negative. Which of the following is the most likely etiology for his condition?

a. Cystic fibrosis
b. Infection with human metapneumovirus
c. Infection with human papilloma virus
d. H-type tracheoesophageal fistula
e. Gastroesophageal reflux with silent aspiration

334. The child shown in the photograph presents with a 3-day history of malaise, fever of 41.1°C (106°F), cough, coryza, and conjunctivitis. She then develops the erythematous, maculopapular rash pictured. She is noted to have white pinpoint lesions on a bright red buccal mucosa in the area opposite her lower molars. Which of the following is most likely to be found as an associated symptom?

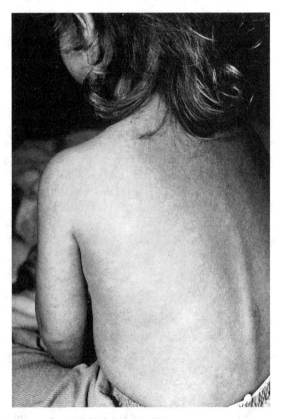

(Used with permission from Adelaide Hebert, MD.)

a. Profound anemia, if the child had sickle cell disease
b. Development of pinpoint or large petechial lesions on the soft palate (Forchheimer sign)
c. Meningitis characterized by increased CSF RBC counts
d. Increased risk for subacute sclerosing panencephalitis
e. Methicillin-resistant staphylococcal superinfection

335. A 14-year-old girl is seen by the pediatrician for tender swelling of her wrists and redness of her eyes. She reports that she awoke about 24 hours prior with a mild sore throat, low-grade fever, and a diffuse maculopapular rash. She reports no vomiting or diarrhea, exposure to sick contacts, or travel. The child reports no serious illnesses or hospitalizations. Social history is significant in that she has just been placed into foster care as her mother has recently entered the penal system. On physical examination vital signs are normal. She is alert and in no distress. Head is without trauma. Eyes have slight injection. Pupils are equally reactive and round. The oropharynx has petechiae on the soft palate. Neck is supple but with mildly tender and markedly swollen posterior cervical and occipital lymph nodes. The chest is clear. Heart has a normal S1 and S2 without murmur. The abdomen is soft and nontender. No organomegaly is noted. Neurologic examination is nonfocal. Skin has a diffuse rash (photograph). Extremities show mildly swollen and tender wrists. Four days after the onset of her illness, the social case worker calls to report the rash has vanished. Which of the following is the most likely diagnosis?

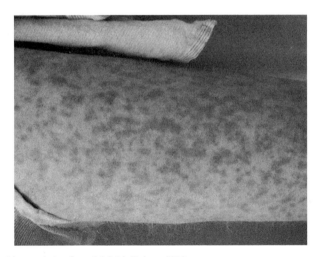

(Used with permission from Adelaide Hebert, MD.)

a. Rubella
b. Rubeola
c. Roseola
d. Erythema infectiosum
e. Erythema multiforme

336. A 2-day-old infant is seen in the normal newborn nursery with newly developing bilateral eye discharge. The 29-year-old mother lives in a nearby shelter and had scant prenatal care, but reports no complications during the pregnancy. The hospital social worker reports that the mother has five other children in CPS custody. The infant was born vaginally and Apgar scores were 9 and 9 at 1 and 5 minutes, respectively. No prenatal labs are available. He has been rooming in with mother and bottle feeding without difficulty. He has voided 6 times and stooled twice. On physical examination, the temperature is 37°C (98.5°F), heart rate is 150 beats per minutes, respiratory rate is 36 breaths per minutes, and blood pressure is 90/60 mm Hg. He is awake, alert, and in no distress. Head is with minimal molding. Neck is supple with flat fontanelles. Mucous membranes are pink, moist, and without lesions. Both eyes are swollen, red, and significant purulent material is draining from both. With some difficulty you are able to demonstrate normal extraocular eye movement and a red reflex. The oropharynx is moist without lesions. Neck is supple. The chest is clear. Heart has a normal S1 and S2 without murmur. The abdomen is soft and nontender. No organomegaly is noted. Neurologic examination is nonfocal. Skin has good turgor, capillary refill, and is without lesions. Which of the following is the most appropriate next step to manage this child's ophthalmologic condition?

a. Viral culture of the conjunctival surfaces and initiation of topical ophthalmologic acyclovir
b. Measurement of the serum rapid plasma reagin (RPR) level and daily penicillin injections for 10 days
c. Bacterial culture of the purulent material and initiation of intravenous third-generation cephalosporin
d. Measurement of maternal hepatitis titers and administration of hepatitis B immune globulin (HBIG)
e. Nucleic acid amplification testing (NAAT) of the purulent material and initiation of oral azithromycin

337. A 3-year-old boy is seen in the clinic with a 6-day history of diarrhea, low-grade fever, and poor appetite. His mother reports the diarrhea began as watery, but has now changed to a frothy appearance and is accompanied by malodorous flatulence. Past medical history is positive for occasional upper respiratory tract infections but no hospitalizations. His development appears to be normal except for some language delay which his mother states has improved since she enrolled him in day care 2 months ago. On physical examination, the temperature is 37°C (98.5°F), heart rate is 100 beats per minutes, respiratory rate is 20 breaths per minutes, and blood pressure is 90/60 mm Hg. A malodorous scent is detected upon entering the room. He is awake, alert, and in no distress; Mucous membranes are pink, moist, and without lesions. Neck is supple. The chest is clear. Heart has a normal S1 and S2 without murmur. The abdomen is bloated but without hepatosplenomegaly. Neurologic examination is nonfocal. Skin has good turgor, capillary refill, and is without lesions. Which of the following treatments is most appropriate for his condition?

a. Observation only
b. Oral trimethoprim-sulfamethoxazole for 7 days
c. Nitazoxanide orally for 3 days
d. Metronidazole orally in a single dose
e. Albendazole orally for 14 days

338. An 8-year-old boy is seen by the pediatrician for the rapid onset of fever, headache, muscle pain, and rash. His mother reports the rash began on the flexor surfaces of the wrist and has begun to extend centrally. She denies vomiting or diarrhea. Past medical history is positive only for a laceration on his leg 2 years ago that required four stitches. The mother reports no medications. He is an active participant in the Cub Scouts, returning from a camping trip 9 days prior. Family history is positive for diabetes in the maternal grandmother. On physical examination the temperature is 38.5°C (101.1°F), heart rate is 95 beats per minute, respiratory rate is 18 breaths per minute, and blood pressure is 110/69 mm Hg. He is awake, alert, and in no distress. Head is without trauma. Neck is supple with occasional shoddy cervical lymph nodes. The mucous membranes are pink, moist, and without lesions. Extraocular eye movement and fundoscopic examinations are normal. The chest is clear. Heart has a normal S1 and S2 without murmur. The abdomen is soft and nontender. No hepatosplenomegaly or adenopathy is noted. Neurologic examination is nonfocal. Extremities show a maculopapular, petechial rash on the flexor surfaces of the wrist and ankles extending toward the trunk about 3 inches at the wrist and 4-5 inches at the ankle. Which of the following is the most appropriate treatment for his likely condition?

a. Oral amoxicillin
b. Intravenous streptomycin
c. Infusion of IgG and supportive care
d. Intravenous vancomycin
e. Oral or intravenous doxycycline

339. The parents of a 7-month-old boy arrive in your office with the infant and a stack of medical records for a second opinion. The boy first started having problems after his circumcision in the nursery when he had prolonged bleeding. Studies were sent at the time for hemophilia, but factors VIII and IX activity were normal. At 2 months, he developed bloody diarrhea, which his doctor assumed was a milk protein allergy and changed him to soy; his parents note he still has occasional bloody diarrhea. He has seen a dermatologist several times for eczema, and has been admitted to the hospital twice for pneumococcal bacteremia. During both admissions, the parents were told that the infant's platelet count was low, but they have yet to attend the hematology appointment arranged for them. The infant's WBC count and differential were normal. Which of the following is the most likely diagnosis in this infant?

a. Idiopathic thrombocytopenic purpura (ITP)
b. Wiskott-Aldrich syndrome
c. Acute lymphocytic leukemia (ALL)
d. Adenosine deaminase deficiency
e. Partial thymic hypoplasia

340. A 10-year-old boy is seen by the pediatrician for pain in his right knee and a rash on his back. Since camping with his grandparents on the Connecticut coast 1 month prior the large annular rash he had on his back is improved, but the fever, headache, chills, and generalized malaise he had during that visit have since completely resolved. Past medical history is significant for mild seasonal allergies treated with loratadine. He denies other medications and sick contacts. On physical examination the vital signs are normal. He is awake, alert, and in no distress. Head is without trauma. Neck is supple with occasional shoddy cervical lymph nodes. The mucous membranes are pink, moist, and without lesions. The chest is clear. Heart has a normal S1 and S2 without murmur. The abdomen is soft and nontender. No hepatosplenomegaly or adenopathy is noted. Neurologic examination is nonfocal. Extremities show a swollen and tender right knee. Skin has a fading, 5-cm circular, slightly elevated lesion on the central back. Which of the following is the most appropriate next step in his management?

a. Aspiration of the affected knee
b. Measurement of pathogen-specific IgM antibodies
c. Administration of a course of oral doxycycline
d. Electrocardiogram (ECG)
e. Biopsy of the remaining rash

341. A previously healthy 7-year-old boy is seen by the pediatrician for a 1-day history of diarrhea. His mother reports that he has had decreased intake of food, but that he has been drinking fairly well and is urinating. She describes the stool as watery and without blood. She reports he has been having low-grade fevers, mild cramping, and intermittent vomiting. Several of his classmates have had similar symptoms. Which of the following is the most likely causative agent?

a. *Salmonella sonnei*
b. *Cryptosporidium*
c. *Sporothrix schenckii*
d. *Toxoplasma gondii*
e. *Rotavirus*

342. A 14-month-old child is seen by the pediatrician for a rash (Photograph). The mother reports that the eruption began 5 days into the course of amoxicillin initiated for an upper respiratory infection (URI) with otitis media. Which of the following would confirm the diagnosis?

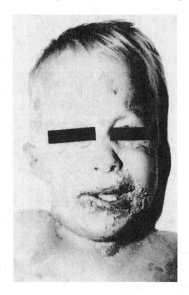

a. Results of skin prick testing
b. Viral-specific elevation of IgM
c. Subepidermal cleavage on skin biopsy of lesion
d. Thrombocytosis and coronary artery aneurysms
e. Elevation of antistreptolysin titer

343. An 8-year-old child is seen by the pediatrician with weakness, facial swelling, muscle pain, and fever. He is from Central America and is visiting his aunt in Texas for the summer. His aunt denies vomiting, headache, or change in behavior. She reports that he has been otherwise in good health, has no chronic diseases, and regularly takes no medications. On physical examination the temperature is 38.5°C (101.1°F), heart rate is 90 beats per minute, respiratory rate is 18 breaths per minute, and blood pressure is 105/68 mm Hg. He is awake, alert, in no distress, but appears tired. Head is without trauma. The face is generally swollen with edema of the eyelids. Neck is supple with occasional shoddy cervical lymph nodes. The mucous membranes are pink, moist, and without lesions. The chest is clear. Heart has a normal S1 and S2 without murmur. The abdomen is soft and non-tender. No hepatosplenomegaly or adenopathy is noted. Neurologic examination is nonfocal. Extremities show generalized myalgia. Laboratory data show:

CBC:
  Hemoglobin: 13 g/dL
  Hematocrit: 37.1%
  WBC: 8500/mm^3
    Segmented neutrophils: 40%
    Lymphocytes: 30%
    Eosinophils: 30%
  Platelet count: 175,000/mm^3

Which of the following is the most appropriate treatment?

a. Supportive care alone or a course of nitazoxanide if symptoms persist
b. Saturated solution of potassium iodine (SSKI) or itraconazole
c. Metronidazole
d. Ketoconazole
e. Mebendazole or albendazole

344. A relatively well-appearing 6-month-old infant presents with distinctive paroxysms of symptoms including machine-gun-like bursts of coughing, eyes bulging and watering, and purple face followed by post-tussive emesis. The family reports that 2 weeks prior the infant had congestion, rhinorrhea, low-grade fever, sneezing, and lacrimation, but otherwise seemed fine and had been recovering from these symptoms for a few days. They report all in the family are well except their 15-year-old daughter who has had a cough for 3 weeks. For which of the following vaccines is the 15-year old most likely delinquent explaining the younger sibling's symptoms?

a. Meningococcal bacteria (MCV)
b. HPV
c. MMR
d. Pneumococcal 13 (PCV 13)
e. Reduced diphtheria toxoid and acellular pertussis vaccine, adsorbed (Tdap)

345. A 2-month-old infant is seen by the emergency center physician for fever, rash, and seizures. The mother reports the infant to have had a fever to 40°C (104°F) at home, 2 days of nonbloody, nonbilious emesis, and increased lethargy in the previous 4 hours. She denies any sick exposures, trauma, or medications other than acetaminophen. Family history is negative for significant illnesses in young children. On physical examination his temperature is 39.2°C (102.6°F), heart rate is 150 beats per minute, respiratory rate is 40 breaths per minute, and blood pressure is 60/40 mm Hg. He is pale and lethargic. Head is without trauma. Neck is stiff with a bulging fontanelle. The mucous membranes are pale, dry, and without lesions. The chest is clear. Heart has a normal S1 and S2 without murmur. The abdomen is soft and nontender. No hepatosplenomegaly or adenopathy is noted. Neurologic examination is nonfocal. Skin has tenting and a diffuse and petechial rash, especially on the trunk and proximal extremities. Oozing of blood is noted at the insertion site of the IV and the blood draw. Laboratory data show:

CBC:
    Hemoglobin: 12 g/dL
    Hematocrit: 36.1%
    WBC: 2500/mm^3
        Segmented neutrophils: 30%
        Band forms: 28%
        Lymphocytes: 42%
    Platelet count: 33,000/mm^3
    Blood culture: Pending

As the CBC results return he has a 3-minute generalized tonic-clonic seizure that is aborted with lorazepam. Which of the infant's problems listed is a contraindication to lumbar puncture?

a. The platelet count
b. His bulging fontanel
c. Evidence of severe dehydration
d. History of recent seizure
e. Significantly elevated WBC count consistent with bacteremia

346. The mother of one of your partner's regular patients calls your office. She reports that her daughter has a 3-day history of subjective fever, hoarseness, and a "bad" barking cough. You arrange for her to be seen in your office that morning. Upon seeing this child, you would expect to find which of the following?

a. A temperature greater than 38.9°C (102°F)
b. Expiratory stridor
c. Infection with parainfluenza virus
d. Hyperinflation on chest x-ray
e. A child between 6 and 8 years of age

Questions 347 to 354

Match the disease with the associated organism. Each lettered option may be used once, more than once, or not at all.

a. *Bartonella henselae*
b. *Yersinia enterocolitica*
c. *Pseudomonas aeruginosa*
d. Rubivirus
e. *Ancylostoma braziliense*
f. Human herpes virus 6 (HHV 6)
g. *Escherichia coli*
h. *Helicobacter pylori*
i. Group B streptococci (GBS)
j. *Listeria monocytogenes*
k. Epstein-Barr virus (EBV)
l. *Toxocara cati*
m. *Campylobacter jejuni*
n. *Leishmania mexicana*
o. *Enterobius vermicularis*
p. *Francisella tularensis*

347. An 18-year-old college girl is seen by the student health physician for a diffuse, erythematous rash. She was seen about 24 hours prior at a local emergency center for a high fever and sore throat. She took one dose of the ampicillin that was prescribed for the clinically diagnosed streptococcal pharyngitis.

348. A 14-year-old boy is seen by the pediatrician for a red and swollen foot. He reports that he was exploring a construction site about 1 week prior when he stepped on a board with a protruding nail that entered his foot through his tennis shoe.

349. A 5-year-old girl is seen by the pediatrician for red and swollen axillary lymph nodes. She had been well until returning from her grandparents' farm 2 weeks prior. On physical examination she is in no distress and is happily telling you of her recent adventures on the farm where she enjoyed playing with chihuahua puppies, kittens, and ducklings. She has warm, red, and tender axillary lymph nodes. Both hands have red papules on the dorsum.

350. A 9-month-old boy has had a fever to 40°C (104°F) for the previous 2 days. Two visits to the pediatrician have shown him to be playful and active without an obvious source of infection. On the third day an evanescent, erythematous, maculopapular rash following the rapid defervescence is noted.

351. A 3-week-old uncircumcised neonate is seen in the ED for fever and irritability. His catheterized urinalysis shows 2+ protein, 20-40 WBCs/HPF, and no epithelial cells.

352. A 9-year-old boy is seen by the pediatrician for several weeks of epigastric and periumbilical pain. He reports that the pain worsens with fasting and is relieved by eating. His stool is guaiac-positive.

353. A 3-year-old girl has had for the last week an irritated and itchy vagina and is noted to be scratching her anus.

354. An 18-year-old man is seen in student health clinic having just returned from Spring Break at a Mexican beach resort. He now has several intensely pruritic, erythematous linear lesions on his left foot extending just above the heel toward the ankle.

Questions 355 to 360

Match each clinical state with the most likely cause of pneumonia. Each lettered option may be used once, more than once, or not at all.

a. *Mycoplasma pneumoniae*
b. Human metapneumovirus
c. Group B *Streptococcus*
d. *Streptococcus pneumoniae*
e. *Toxocara canis*
f. *Chlamydia trachomatis*
g. Respiratory syncytial virus
h. *Mycobacterium tuberculosis*
i. *Histoplasma capsulatum*
j. *Staphylococcus aureus*
k. *Legionella pneumophilia*
l. *Pseudomonas aeruginosa*
m. *Pneumocystis jiroveci*

355. A 12-month-old infant with failure-to-thrive since about 6 months of age has recently developed several episodes of pneumonia. He was born vaginally at term to a 22-year-old woman after an uncomplicated pregnancy. Beginning at about 3 months of age he had frequent, malodorous stools, microcytic anemia, and two episodes of rectal prolapse that required visits to the emergency room.

356. An 8-hour-old infant rooming in with his mother after a vaginal delivery is noted to have an increased respiratory rate and poor feeding. The pregnancy is thought to be term and without complications, but no prenatal records are available. On physical examination the infant has a temperature of 35.8°C (96.4°F) and respiratory rate of 80. He is pale, mottled, and has subcostal and intercostal retractions.

357. A 6-week-old infant is seen by the pediatrician for cough and rapid breathing. The mother denies fever, vomiting, or diarrhea. The infant was born vaginally at term to a 20-year-old woman whose pregnancy was complicated by gestational hypertension. The infant has had no illness other than mild eye discharge at 2 weeks of age treated with topical antibiotic drops. On physical examination she is a well-hydrated child with a respiratory rate of 50 breaths per minute, minimal subcostal retractions, and scattered rales but no wheezing throughout the lung fields.

358. A 14-year-old girl is seen by the pediatric nurse practitioner with a 3-week history of cough and intermittent temperature to 38.5°C (101.1°F). She reports that she has been tired and is unable to sleep due to the cough. On physical examination she has a few fine rales over both lung fields without focality. Chest radiograph shows an interstitial infiltrate.

359. A 2-month-old boy is admitted to the PICU after an emergent placement of a chest tube for a left-sided pneumothorax. He was admitted to the general pediatric floor 2 days prior with a several day history of URI which had suddenly worsened on the day of admission to include high fever, worsening cough, and respiratory distress. The chest radiograph upon admission showed him to have a left-sided pneumatocele. He had been receiving intravenous antibiotics, oxygen, and close observation when the sudden deterioration necessitating chest tube placement occurred.

360. An 8-year-old girl is seen by the pediatric hospitalists after having gone to the operating room for drainage of empyema and chest tube placement. She had been in good health until about 1 week prior when she developed fever, tachypnea, and a lobar infiltrate was found on chest radiograph. She had been taking amoxicillin at home, but her symptoms gradually progressed over several days when the empyema was diagnosed.

Infectious Diseases and Immunology

Answers

---

315. The answer is a. (*Hay et al, pp 1265-1266. Kliegman et al, pp 1552-1554. Rudolph et al, pp 1174-1175.*) The child in the question has classic findings of mumps. In addition to the findings described, mumps typically causes swelling of the opposite side a day or so after symptoms appear on the first side. Other findings include redness and swelling at the opening of Stensen duct, edema and swelling in the pharynx, and displacement of the uvula on the affected side. A rash would not be expected. It is important to note that while mumps has largely been eliminated with vaccination, other organisms still may cause parotitis. Measles presents in a child with a several days' history of malaise, fever, cough, coryza, and conjunctivitis followed by the typical, widespread, erythematous, maculopapular rash. Koplik spots, white pinpoint lesions on a bright red buccal mucosa often in the area opposite the lower molars, appear transiently and are pathognomonic. Symptoms of rubella, usually a mild disease, include a diffuse maculopapular rash that lasts for 3 days, marked enlargement of the posterior cervical and occipital lymph nodes, low-grade fever, mild sore throat, and, occasionally, conjunctivitis, arthralgia, or arthritis. Signs and symptoms of varicella include a prodrome of fever, anorexia, headache, and mild abdominal pain, followed 24-48 hours later by the typical clear, fluid-filled vesicles (dewdrop on a rose petal). The rash of varicella typically starts on the scalp, face, or trunk. The lesions are pruritic and appear in crops over the next several days, with old lesions crusting over as new lesions develop.

Human papilloma virus causes anogenital warts, cervical disease, anal cancer, and non-anogenital disease (such or oropharyngeal warts and respiratory papillomas). The current vaccines include protection against 9 HPV types. Meningococcal vaccine prevents meningococcemia (rapid onset multisystem organ failure with purpura fulminans) and meningococcal meningitis. Current universally recommended vaccines include coverage against serotypes A, C, Y, and W135; a separate vaccine effective against serotype B was licensed in the early 2015 and currently is recommended for high-risk groups only. Tetanus toxoid, reduced diphtheria toxoid, and acellular pertussis vaccine adsorbed is the "adolescent" booster of tetanus with pertussis protection. This vaccine is a booster dose against classic tetany associated with the bacteria *C tetani* but also provides protection against the waning immunity in pertussis seen in adolescents and young adults. In adolescents pertussis presents as prolonged and violent coughing spells classically described as having an inspiratory whoop.

316. The answer is b. (*Hay et al, pp 1271-1282. Kliegman et al, pp 1645-1666. Rudolph et al, pp 1164-1170.*) Infants born to mothers who are HIV positive require therapy as close to birth as possible, preferably within 6 to 12 hours. Infants born to mothers who were prescribed ARV therapy during the pregnancy, had sustained viral suppression near delivery, whose adherence was not questioned, and received ARV intrapartum are begun on a 4-week course of zidovudine. Infants born to mothers who do not meet these criteria require alternative therapy depending on the risk of perinatal HIV transmission. Breast-feeding in the developed world is contraindicated for the HIV positive mother. Prophylaxis against *P jirovecii* might be considered starting at 4-6 weeks and continued until the infant has been determined to be uninfected. HIV infection is not a contraindication for circumcision. Circumcision reduces the chance of heterosexually-acquired HIV infection.

317. The answer is e. (*Kliegman et al, pp 2902-2904. Rudolph et al, pp 1506-1507.*) The child in the question is at risk for Reye syndrome, an acquired mitochondrial hepatopathy that results from the interaction of an influenza (or varicella) infection and aspirin use. While the prevalence has decreased over the last few decades and it is now a rare disease, mortality remains the same at more than 40% of cases. Initial findings in the child older than about 2 years of age include abrupt onset of emesis about 3 days after the viral infection symptoms resolve. Neurologic symptoms follow including lethargy and dilated pupils. In smaller children diarrhea may be a presenting sign. Later stages of the illness result in patients with delirium, seizures, and coma. Death is usually from cerebral edema and subsequent herniation. While aspirin is no longer routinely used in children as an antipyretic or pain reliever, it is used for patients with Kawasaki disease and the increase in the use of aspirin in adults with heart disease requires specific counseling for parents of children with influenza and varicella to avoid aspirin use. In addition, the incidence of influenza and varicella is reduced with proper immunization.

318. The answer is e. (*Hay et al, pp 1322-1323. Kliegman et al, pp 1393-1396. Rudolph et al, pp 1084-1087.*) Clinical manifestations of shigellosis range from watery stools for several days to severe infection with high fever, abdominal pain, and generalized seizures. In addition, a rare and fatal "toxic encephalopathy" seen with *Shigella* infection known as Ekiri syndrome can occur. In general, about 50% of infected children have emesis, greater than two-thirds have fever, 10%-35% have seizures, and 40% have blood in their stool. Often, the seizure precedes diarrhea and is the complaint that brings the family to the physician. Fever usually lasts about 72 hours, and the diarrhea resolves within 1-2 weeks. The white count may show a dramatic left shift. Presumptive diagnosis can be made on the clinical history, and confirmation is through stool culture or PCR. Supportive care, including adequate fluid and electrolyte support, is the mainstay of therapy. Antibiotic treatment is problematic; resistance to trimethoprim-sulfamethoxazole and ampicillin is common, necessitating therapy with third-generation cephalosporins in many cases. As always, knowledge of the susceptibility patterns of the bacteria in your area is the key to using the appropriate antibiotic.

319. The answer is a. (*Hay et al, pp 1045-1046. Kliegman et al, pp 1019-1022. Rudolph et al, pp 760-761.*) Among the T-cell diseases is DiGeorge anomaly, in which defective embryologic development of the third and fourth pharyngeal pouches results in hypoplasia of both the thymus and parathyroid glands. Associated findings with DiGeorge anomaly include CATCH: C for cardiac, A for abnormal faces, T for thymic hypoplasia, C for cleft palate, and H for hypocalcemia. The pattern in option B is consistent with primary B-cell diseases that include X-linked agammaglobulinemia (XLA, or Bruton disease), a deficiency of all three major classes of immunoglobulins, as well as other selective deficiencies of the immunoglobulins or their subgroups. This condition usually presents after 3 months of age (after maternal antibodies wane) with recurrent and often simultaneous bouts of otitis media, pneumonia, diarrhea, and sinusitis, but usually without fungal and viral infections. Option C is consistent with the catastrophic combined T- and B-cell disease known as severe combined immunodeficiency disease (Swiss-type lymphopenic agammaglobulinemia or SCID) and have deficient T- and B-cells. Consequently, they have lymphopenia and agammaglobulinemia, as well as thymic hypoplasia. Chronic diarrhea; rashes; recurrent, serious bacterial, fungal, or viral infections; wasting; and early death are characteristic.

Option D is consistent with X-linked recessive Wiskott-Aldrich syndrome with mild T-cell dysfunction, diminished serum IgM, and marked elevation of IgA and IgE. These children are prone to eczema, recurrent middle-ear infections, lymphopenia, and thrombocytopenia. Option E might be seen in a patient with recurrent staphylococcal skin infections who has Job-Buckley syndrome, a disorder of phagocytic chemotaxis with increased IgE levels.

320. The answer is b. (*Hay et al, p 436. Kliegman et al, pp 3214-3215. Rudolph et al, pp 1299-1301.*) *Trichophyton tonsurans* is a major cause of tinea capitis. It produces an infection within the hair follicle that is unresponsive to topical treatment alone and requires long-term oral therapy with griseofulvin or another antifungal for eradication. Fluorescene usually is absent on examination by Wood lamp. Diagnosis is made by microscopic examination of KOH preparation of infected hairs and by culture on appropriate media. A severe manifestation of tinea capitis known as *kerion* is shown in the photograph. Enlarged occipital lymph nodes are a common finding. A diagnosis of tinea capitis, and not seborrhea, should be considered in any child between the ages of 6 months and puberty who presents with scaliness and hair loss, even if mild. Seborrhea rarely occurs in that age group. *Microsporum canis* is an occasional cause of tinea capitis, and it does fluoresce under a Wood lamp.

Traction alopecia typically is seen in children who have their hair tied tightly in bows or braids; the hair loss is linear following the area of traction, and is often associated with regional adenopathy. Alopecia areata can appear similar to fungal infections, but the hairs near the active lesion often can be extracted with gentle traction resulting in an attenuated or catagen bulb at the termination of the hair shaft (exclamation hair); it does not produce a kerion as shown in the photograph. Therapy for alopecia areata might consist of ultraviolet light therapy and topical or intradermal steroids. Children with biotinidase deficiency and those with hypothyroidism would be unlikely to have only isolated hair loss as the presenting symptom; rather, symptoms might include a variety of neurologic, dermatologic, and ocular complaints.

321. The answer is b. (*Hay et al, p 1232. Kliegman et al, pp 1568-1572. Rudolph et al, p 1559.*) The child in the question with sickle cell disease and profound anemia likely has a parvovirus B19 infection. Fifth disease (erythema infectiosum), long recognized as a benign mild exanthem of school-age children, is now known to be caused by human parvovirus B19. Replication of the virus occurs in the erythroid progenitor cells resulting in a decrease in red cell production for about a week in infected patients. While this transient drop in reticulocytes is not noticeable in normal children, patients with hemolytic conditions (such as sickle cell anemia) develop a transient aplastic crisis. A poorly functioning bone marrow (for a week or more) in a patient with a reduced red-cell life span (about 30 days) can result in profound anemia.

Other problems can result in patients infected with parvovirus B19. In patients with immunodeficiency, the B19 infection can be persistent and lead to life-threatening chronic anemia. Infection in a pregnant woman can result in severe anemia in the infected fetus, with secondary hydrops fetalis and death.

Roseola is now thought to be caused most often by the HHV 6. Coxsackie A16 virus causes hand-foot-and-mouth disease. Other causes of profound anemia might include splenic sequestration in a sickle cell patient (which would result in an enlarged spleen on examination) and leukemia, which would result in physical examination findings including bruising, petechiae, and adenopathy. Blood abnormalities might include findings in the WBC and/or platelet cell lines in addition to the anemia.

322. The answer is c. (*Hay et al, pp 877-878. Kliegman et al, p 3279. Rudolph et al, p 856.*) The child likely has transient (toxic) synovitis of the hip, a condition that is treated with rest and anti-inflammatory medications. This condition is more common in boys, occurs in children aged 3-10 years, and must be differentiated from a septic hip. Findings that are supportive of toxic synovitis is a history of a recent upper respiratory infection, low-grade fever, mild pain with movement, and normal or minimally elevated WBC, ESR, and CRP. Frog-leg views of the film are normal, and ultrasound may show a joint effusion. Children for whom concern about septic hip remains (high fever, severe pain, elevated screening labs) require further study which may include MRI or aspiration of the joint space. If septic joint is found, antibiotic therapy is appropriate. Cancer causing bone pain is always a consideration; without hepatosplenomegaly, pallor, bruising, or hematologic findings this diagnosis seems unlikely.

323. The answer is d. (*Hay et al, pp 629-630. Kliegman et al, pp 2263-2269. Rudolph et al, pp 939-941.*) The presentation of infective endocarditis can be quite variable, ranging from prolonged fever with few other symptoms to an acute and severe course with early toxicity. A high index of suspicion is necessary to make the diagnosis quickly. Identification of the causative organism (frequently *Streptococcus* sp or *Staphylococcus* sp) through multiple blood cultures is imperative for appropriate treatment. Echocardiography may identify valvular vegetations and can be predictive of impending embolic events, but a negative echocardiogram does not rule out endocarditis. Treatment usually consists of 4-6 weeks of appropriate antimicrobial therapy. Antistreptolysin antibody testing might be useful to help confirm the diagnosis of rheumatic fever; this child has none of the major criteria. Serial measurement of platelet count and initiation of aspirin would be appropriate for Kawasaki disease, but the child in the question is older than typical for Kawasaki disease (80% will present younger than the age of 5 years) and the history is not consistent with the diagnosis. Scarlet fever (rapid streptococcal test) is typically self-limited and would not be consistent with the 3-week time course. Tuberculosis can cause prolonged low-grade fever, but cardiac involvement is unusual, consisting of pericarditis; thus a friction rub would be the typical examination finding.

324. The answer is e. (*Hay et al, pp 836-837, 1304. Kliegman et al, pp 2938-2946. Rudolph et al, pp 393-394, 913-916, 2182-2184.*) The child in the question has had a change in status since his visit to his physician earlier in the day. He now has evidence of sepsis and meningitis (fever, lethargy/irritability, and petechial/purpuric rash). Bacteremia caused by *H influenzae* type B (now rare), *Neisseria meningitidis*, or *S pneumoniae* (decreasing in frequency secondary to vaccination) should be considered before prescribing treatment for otitis media in a young, febrile, toxic-appearing child. This patient now requires a lumbar puncture because of the change in his clinical status despite his supple neck (neck rigidity is a more reliable finding in children older than about 12-18 months of age).

This child needs intravenous antibiotics, but the choice would likely be a third-generation cephalosporin and vancomycin, preferably after the lumbar puncture if it can be performed quickly. Diphenhydramine and topical steroids might be considered for an allergic reaction or urticaria, but have no place in the treatment of purpura. The child now has evidence of sepsis/meningitis; a change in oral therapy for the otitis media is inappropriate. A myringotomy with culture of the fluid might help identify the causative organism, but delaying further treatment for this procedure is likely not available.

325. The answer is d. (*Hay et al, pp 1038-1042. Kliegman et al, pp 1012-1018. Rudolph et al, pp 762-765.*) Primary B-cell diseases include X-linked agammaglobulinemia (XLA, or Bruton disease), a deficiency of all three major classes of immunoglobulins, as well as other selective deficiencies of the immunoglobulins or their subgroups. This condition usually presents after 3-6 months of age (after maternal antibodies wane) with recurrent and often simultaneous bouts of otitis media, pneumonia, and sinusitis due to *S pneumonia* and *H influenzae*, and skin infections due to group A streptococci and *S aureus*. Recurrent fungal and viral infections are unusual. On physical examination the patient may be small for age owing to the frequent infections, and absence of lymphoid tissue is found.

Patients with severe combined immune deficiency present in the first few months of life with recurrent/persistent diarrhea, otitis media, sepsis, pneumonia, and skin infections. Early growth failure is noted, especially after the diarrhea ensures. Opportunistic infections including viruses, fungus, and mycobacteria are common. Patients have deficient T- and B-cells, lymphopenia and agammaglobulinemia, and thymic hypoplasia. Dysgenesis of the third and fourth pharyngeal pouches during embryogenesis with resultant hypoplasia of the thymus and parathyroid glands is at the root of DiGeorge syndrome. Associated findings might include CATCH: *C* for cardiac, *A* for abnormal faces, *T* for thymic hypoplasia, *C* for cleft palate, and *H* for hypocalcemia. The condition is suspected in a newborn with neonatal hypocalcemia, especially if associated with abnormal facies/cleft palate and conotruncal heart defects. Antibody levels are normal, parathyroid and T-cell function is decreased or absent. Wiskott-Aldrich is an X-linked recessive syndrome of mild T-cell dysfunction, diminished serum IgM, marked elevation of IgA and IgE, eczema, recurrent middle-ear infections, lymphopenia, and thrombocytopenia. Patients with X-linked lymphoproliferative syndrome have a propensity to develop hemophagocytic lymphohistiocytosis and fulminant infectious mononucleosis. Mean age of onset is 3-5 years with fever, pharyngitis, hepatosplenomegaly, lymphadenopathy, and jaundice. Fatal mononucleosis infection occurs in about 60% of patients; about 30% of patients develop high-grade (Burkitt) lymphoma.

326. The answer is e. (*Hay et al, pp 1253-1254. Kliegman et al, pp 1586-1590. Rudolph et al, pp 1154-1158.*) To prove a diagnosis of infectious mononucleosis caused by EBV, a triad of findings should be present. First, physical findings can include diffuse adenopathy, tonsillar enlargement, an enlarged spleen, small hemorrhages on the soft palate, and periorbital swelling. Second, the hematologic changes should reveal a predominance of lymphocytes with at least 10% of these cells being atypical. Third, the characteristic antibody response should be present. Traditionally, heterophil antibodies can be detected when confirming a diagnosis of infectious mononucleosis. These antibodies may not be present, however, particularly in young children. Alternatively, specific antibodies against viral antigens on the EBV can be measured. Antibodies to viral capsid antigen (VCA) and to anti-D early antigen are elevated prior to the appearance of Epstein-Barr nuclear antigen (EBNA) and are, therefore, markers for acute infection. IgG VCA and EBNA persist for life, whereas anti-D disappears after 6 months. Adolescents with this condition, because of the enlarged spleen and risk of splenic rupture, should avoid contact sports until the splenomegaly has resolved.

While some features of the other conditions can overlap with EBV infection, the totality of the presentation in the case strongly suggests EBV as the causative agent. Initiation of zidovudine would be indicated if the child were proven to have HIV disease. IV acyclovir might be indicated for varicella infection. IV infusion of immunoglobulins and high-dose aspirin suggest a diagnosis of Kawasaki disease, which is unusual at this age. Intramuscular penicillin might be helpful in streptococcal pharyngitis, but atypical lymphocytes are not usually seen with this condition.

327. The answer is b. (*Hay et al, pp 874-877. Kliegman et al, pp 3322-3327. Rudolph et al, pp 934-939.*) The radiograph shown demonstrates lytic lesions in the proximal tibia; when combined with the history, the scenario is consistent with osteomyelitis. Acute osteomyelitis tends to begin abruptly, with fever and marked, localized bone tenderness that usually occurs at the metaphysis. Redness and swelling frequently follow. Although usually the result of hematogenous bacterial spread, particularly of *S aureus*, acute osteomyelitis can follow an episode of deep cellulitis or septic joint. Diagnosis often must be based on clinical grounds because early soft tissue changes on plain radiograph will take several days to develop, and diagnostic bone changes may not be visible on plain films for up to 12 days after onset of the disease. Bone scans with radionuclides, however, can be useful in the diagnosis of osteomyelitis within 24-48 hours of symptoms and in its differentiation from cellulitis and septic arthritis. Magnetic resonance imagining (MRI) has become more widely used for the diagnosis of osteomyelitis, as it is very sensitive and specific.

Caution must be exercised, however, when interpreting a normal bone scan in a patient suspected of having osteomyelitis; falsely normal bone scans do occur in patients with active bone infection. Antibiotic treatment must be initiated immediately to avoid further extension of infection into bone, where adequate drug levels are difficult to achieve. Treatment is usually continued for at least 3 weeks.

328. The answer is a. (*Hay et al, pp 59, 836-837, 1316. Kliegman et al, pp 920-922, 2086-2095. Rudolph et al, pp 1045-1046, 1097-1099.*) The presentation is that of a newborn with fever, leukopenia with significant left shift, mild thrombocytopenia, and abnormal spinal fluid (low glucose, high protein, elevated WBCs that are polymorphonuclear leukocytes, and Gram stain positive for gram-positive rods). Many organisms can cause meningitis in the neonate, including *E coli*, *L monocytogenes*, *H influenzae*, gram-negative rods, groups B and D streptococci, and coagulase-positive and coagulase-negative staphylococci. Statistically, the most likely cause in this case would be late-onset GBS. However, in this case the neonate has gram-positive rods, an indication of *L monocytogenes*. Early-onset listeriosis usually presents in the first day and always by day 3; fetal distress is common. These neonates have rashes and hepatosplenomegaly on presentation and a history of maternal fever is common. Late-onset *Listeria* typically presents with purulent meningitis. Early-onset GBS is seen in the first 7 days of life and is associated with maternal complications such as prolonged rupture and chorioamnionitis; late-onset GBS occurs after 7 days of life and is not related to maternal issues but rather environmental exposures. As expected, the incidence of early-onset GBS has been steadily dropping with maternal prophylaxis; the incidence of late-onset GBS and listeriosis has remained unchanged during the same time period. Clinical manifestations of meningitis in neonates include lethargy, bulging fontanel, seizures, and nuchal rigidity. The diagnosis is made with examination and culture of the CSF. Treatment is begun while awaiting the results of the spinal fluid analysis. Appropriate initial antibiotic coverage must include activity against gram-positive and gram-negative organisms (ampicillin and gentamicin or ampicillin and cefotaxime are common choices).

329. The answer is b. (*Hay et al, p 1232. Kliegman et al, pp 1320-1321. Rudolph et al, pp 1090-1094.*) Toxic shock syndrome (TSS) is usually caused by *S aureus*, but a similar syndrome (sometimes called toxic shock-like syndrome [TSLS]) may be caused by *Streptococcus* sp. The strains of *S aureus* secrete toxic shock syndrome toxin 1 (TSST-1), and can cause "menstrual" TSS (associated with intravaginal devices like tampons, diaphragms, and contraceptive sponges) or "non-menstrual" TSS (associated with pneumonia, skin infection [as in this patient], bacteremia, or osteomyelitis). The diagnosis is made clinically, and the case description is typical. Treatment includes blood cultures followed by aggressive fluid resuscitation and antibiotics targeting *S aureus*. Kawasaki (vasculitis of medium-sized arteries throughout the body with a predilection to causing coronary artery aneurysms) is not typically seen in adolescents and is not so rapidly progressive. Shiga toxin–producing strains of *E coli* and *Shigella* are usually associated with hemolytic-uremic syndrome. *Clostridium perfringens* can secrete several toxins; one is an α-toxin that causes hemolysis, platelet lysis, increased vascular permeability, and hepatotoxicity. The neurotoxin secreted by *C tetani* causes tetanus.

330. The answer is a. (*Hay et al, pp 1294-1298. Kliegman et al, pp 1323-1327. Rudolph et al, pp 398, 893-895, 1078-1080.*) In a child who appears otherwise normal, the sudden onset of high fever, together with a marked elevation and shift to the left of the WBC count, suggests pneumococcal bacteremia. The incidence of pneumococcal disease producing this picture has decreased with the widespread use of the pneumococcal vaccine. Viral infections such as roseola occasionally can present in a similar fashion but without such profound shifts in the blood leukocyte count. Streptococcosis refers to prolonged, low-grade, insidious nasopharyngitis that sometimes occurs in children infected with group A β-hemolytic streptococci. Neither typhoid fever nor diphtheria produces markedly high WBC counts; both are characterized by headache, malaise, and other systemic signs. Other bacteria that should be considered in a child with this presentation include *H influenzae* type B (rare in the vaccinated child) and meningococcus.

331. The answer is c. (*Hay et al, p 291. Kliegman et al, pp 1548-1552. Rudolph et al, pp 1177-1180.*) When German measles (rubella) occurs during the first 2 months of pregnancy, it has a severe effect on the fetus, including cardiac defects, cataracts, and glaucoma. The most common cardiac defects are patent ductus arteriosus, which can be accompanied by peripheral pulmonary artery stenosis, and atrial and ventricular septal defects. Myriad other complications vary in incidence with the timing of the infection during pregnancy, including thrombocytopenia, hepatosplenomegaly, hepatitis, hemolytic anemia, microcephaly, and a higher risk of developing insulin-dependent diabetes mellitus. The mother's negative rubella titer early in the pregnancy indicates she is susceptible to the infection and its sequelae; her titer undoubtedly now is positive.

Hepatitis B can spread from mother to infant, but is not a teratogen. A positive hepatitis B surface antibody in the mother indicates successful vaccination or old, resolved infection. A positive maternal hepatitis B surface antigen suggests ongoing maternal infection and the need to treat the neonate with hepatitis B immune globulin in addition to routine immunization at birth. Congenital syphilis is asymptomatic in most cases although testing (RPR) will demonstrate elevation in the newborn and the need for treatment. Alternatively, affected infants may be stillborn, born prematurely, or have findings of hepatosplenomegaly, pneumonia, a bullous skin rash (pemphigus syphiliticus), and skeletal abnormalities. Down syndrome presents with a wide variety of features including hypotonia, epicanthal folds, single palmer crease, cardiac lesions (VSD or atrioventricular [AV] canal), intellectual disability, and a propensity for leukemia. Congenital varicella infection can present with low-birth weight, skin findings including hypertrophic scars, hypoplasia of the arms, legs, fingers and/or toes, cortical atrophy, and ventriculomegaly. Cardiac defects are not a common finding.

332. The answer is b. (*Hay et al, pp 463-465. Kliegman et al, pp 3035-3036, 3062-3064. Rudolph et al, pp 2307-2308.*) Dacryocystitis is an infection of the nasolacrimal sac. In newborns it is associated with congenital nasolacrimal duct obstruction, which is seen in about 6% of normal infants. Nasolacrimal duct obstruction is thought to be caused by the failure of epithelial cells forming the duct to canalize. Treatment of this benign, usually self-limited condition involves nasolacrimal massage and cleaning the area with warm washcloths; failure to open the duct by 6 months usually results in a referral to ophthalmology for surgical opening. When the lacrimal sac is infected, as in dacryocystitis, the patient requires a course of antibiotics to clear the infection.

Chalazion is a firm, nontender nodule that results from a chronic granulomatous inflammation of the meibomian gland. Preseptal (periorbital) and orbital cellulitis may be distinguished by clinical examination. Blood in the anterior chamber of the eye is called a hyphema. Congenital Sjögren syndrome is not recognized as an entity; however, mothers with Sjögren syndrome may have infants with congenital lupus.

333. The answer is b. (*Hay et al, pp 1238-1239. Kliegman et al, pp 2044-2048. Rudolph et al, p 965.*) The child in the question likely has bronchiolitis, and of the choices the most likely causative agent is human metapneumovirus since the respiratory syncytial virus testing is negative. The clinical picture of bronchiolitis caused by human metapneumovirus is similar to that caused by RSV and includes cough, congestion, rhinorrhea, wheezing, and respiratory distress. Other viral causes on bronchiolitis include para-influenza, adenovirus, influenza, rhinovirus, coronavirus, and enterovirus. A variety of laboratory tests are available to confirm the pathogen, but in actual practice the diagnosis is suspected if the RSV testing is negative. Like RSV infection, the treatment is supportive.

Cystic fibrosis classically presents with delayed passage of meconium, and then later with large, foul-smelling stools, failure to thrive, and recurrent pneumonias. Maternal HPV may present in a child with a hoarse cry as a result of lesions growing in the upper airway and on the vocal cords. An H-type tracheoesophageal fistula might present with recurrent coughing or cyanotic episodes associated with feedings, or unexplained aspiration-like pneumonias. The typical child with gastroesophageal reflux has repeated episodes of visible emesis of ingested foods that may be worse immediately after meals. In severe cases failure to thrive may result and aspiration of this material may result in repeated pneumonia.

334. The answer is d. (*Hay et al, pp 1261-1262. Kliegman et al, pp 1542-1548. Rudolph et al, pp 1170-1173.*) The picture and clinical history presented are most common for the diagnosis of measles (rubeola). This is an uncommon disease in areas where immunization rates are high, but sporadic outbreaks do occur. The rash typically lasts 6 days. Complications are common, including pneumonia, laryngitis, myocarditis, and encephalitis. Subacute sclerosing panencephalitis, a chronic but progressive form of encephalitis, is associated with a prior measles infection.

Parvovirus B19 causes erythema infectiosum (fifth disease), which presents with low-grade fever, headache, and mild URI symptoms; the rash is "slapped cheek" in appearance. In the child with sickle cell disease, parvovirus infection also results in bone marrow suppression and profound anemia. Rubella in this age of child would present with mild URI symptoms, retroauricular, posterior cervical and post-occipital lymphadenopathy, and then a diffuse erythematous maculopapular rash that clears in about 72 hours. Pinpoint or larger petechial lesions on the soft palate (Forchheimer sign) may also be seen in rubella disease. Herpes, when localized to the skin only presents as thin-walled vesicles on an erythematous base. When its spread includes meningitis, results in the spinal fluid include an increased number of RBCs and WBCs. Varicella presents with fever, malaise, headache, moderate fever 37.8°C-38.9°C (100°F-102°F), and then crops of intensely pruritic red macules that evolve into fluid-filled vesicles. These lesions have a higher chance of developing a methicillin-resistant staphylococcal superinfection.

335. The answer is a. (*Hay et al, pp 1262-1264. Kliegman et al, pp 1548-1552. Rudolph et al, pp 1177-1180.*) Symptoms of rubella (German measles), usually a mild disease, include a diffuse maculopapular rash that lasts for 3 days, marked enlargement of the posterior cervical and occipital lymph nodes, low-grade fever, mild sore throat, and, occasionally, conjunctivitis, arthralgia, or arthritis; it has become a rare disease in the United States. Persons with rubeola (measles) develop a severe cough, coryza, photo-phobia, conjunctivitis, and a high fever that reaches its peak at the height of the generalized macular rash, which typically lasts for 5 days. Koplik spots on the buccal mucosa are diagnostic; it, too, is a rare disease in the United States in areas of high vaccination. Roseola is a viral exanthem of infants in which the high fever abruptly abates as a rash appears. Erythema infectiosum (fifth disease) begins with bright erythema on the cheeks ("slapped cheek" sign), followed by a red maculopapular rash on the trunk and extremities, which fades centrally at first. Erythema multiforme is a poorly understood syndrome consisting of skin lesions and involvement of mucous membranes. A number of infectious agents and drugs have been associated with this syndrome.

336. The answer is c. (*Hay et al, p 1306. Kliegman et al, p 3038. Rudolph et al, pp 177, 1069-1070.*) The most likely diagnosis is ophthalmia neonato-rum caused by *Neisseria gonorrhoeae*; culture for this organism and treat-ment with ceftriaxone or cefotaxime is warranted. While overlap is seen, conjunctivitis in the first day of life classically is caused by topical prophy-lactic silver nitrate or erythromycin administered shortly after birth. In the next 24-96 hours bilateral purulent discharge is likely gonococcal. Beyond 5 days conjunctivitis is classically caused by *C trachomatis* (treated with oral macrolides) or herpes (treated with topical and intravenous acyclovir). Syphilis and hepatitis B typically do not cause conjunctivitis. Of note, early administration of oral macrolides is associated with an increased incidence in the development of hypertrophic pyloric stenosis at a later date.

337. The answer is c. (*Hay et al, pp 1371-1372. Kliegman et al, pp 1692-1694. Rudolph et al, pp 1219-1220.*) Infection with Giardia may be asymptomatic (especially in adults) but more commonly in children it causes diarrhea associated with malodorous flatulence, occasional low-grade fever, nausea, and anorexia; vomiting is not a prominent feature. Abdominal cramps and bloating, abdominal distension, and weight loss is seen. This condition is commonly spread in day care centers, but is endemic in some parts of the world. Peaks in incidence occur in summer months, probably owing to spreading of the cysts in community pools. Recommended treatment is nitazoxanide orally for 3 days or tinidazole orally once. Metronidazole orally for 5-7 days and albendazole orally for 5 days are alternatives. Trimethoprim-sulfamethoxazole might be considered for bacterial enteritis such as salmonella, although resistance to this drug is common.

338. The answer is e. (*Hay et al, pp 1268-1269. Kliegman et al, pp 1500-1504. Rudolph et al, pp 1110-1111.*) The child in the question likely has Rocky Mountain spotted fever (RMSF); the incubation period for RMSF has a range of 1-14 days. A brief prodromal period consisting of headache and malaise is typically followed by the abrupt onset of fever and chills. A maculopapular rash starts on the second to fourth day of illness on the flexor surfaces of the wrists and ankles before moving in a central direction. Typically, the palms and soles are involved. The rash can become hemorrhagic within 1 or 2 days. Hyponatremia and thrombocytopenia may be seen. Doxycycline is the appropriate treatment, and it must be started early in the course to be effective, but should not be used in children younger than 8 years of age.

In the differential diagnosis of RMSF are a number of other diseases. A morbilliform eruption can precede a petechial rash caused by *N meningitidis*. Viral infections, particularly by the enteroviruses, can cause a severe illness that resembles RMSF. Atypical measles is seen primarily in persons who received the killed measles vaccine before 1968. After exposure to wild-type measles, such a person can develop a prodrome consisting of fever, cough, headache, and myalgia. This is usually followed by the development of pneumonia and an urticarial rash beginning on the extremities. TSS is a disease characterized by sudden onset of fever, diarrhea, shock, inflammation of mucous membranes, and a diffuse macular rash resulting in desquamation of the hands and feet; vancomycin would be part of the treatment.

Lyme disease is seen with an early period of localized disease including erythema migrans, possibly with flu-like symptoms, followed by a distinctive period of erythema migrans, arthralgia, arthritis, meningitis, neuritis, and carditis.

339. The answer is b. (*Hay et al, pp 1044-1045. Kliegman et al, p 1026. Rudolph et al, pp 761-762.*) The patient described has Wiskott-Aldrich syndrome, an X-linked recessive combined immunodeficiency characterized by thrombocytopenia, eczema, and increased susceptibility to infection. Problems occur early, and prolonged bleeding from the circumcision site may be the first clue. The thrombocytopenia also manifests as bloody diarrhea and easy bruising. Patients have impaired humoral immunity with a low serum IgM and a normal or slightly low IgG; they also have cellular immunity problems, with decreased T cells and depressed lymphocyte response. Few live past their teens, frequently succumbing to malignancy caused by EBV infection.

ITP is an isolated and usually transient thrombocytopenia thought to be secondary to a viral infection. These children do not have increased susceptibility to infection. ALL usually presents with abnormalities in all three cell lines, and does not have a prolonged course as in the described patient. Adenosine deaminase deficiency is a type of severe combined immunodeficiency (SCID) but patients always have lymphopenia from birth; platelets are not affected. Partial thymic hypoplasia (partial DiGeorge) patients usually do not have problems early on and can grow up normally, and they do not have thrombocytopenia.

340. The answer is c. (*Hay et al, pp 1350-1352. Kliegman et al, pp 1483-1487. Rudolph et al, pp 1046-1048.*) Lyme disease, caused by the spirochete *Borrelia burgdorferi* and transmitted mostly by ticks of the Ixodes family, is a clinical diagnosis. It is characterized by a unique skin lesion, recurrent attacks of arthritis, and occasional involvement of the heart and CNS. Illness usually appears in late summer or early fall, 2-30 days after a bite by an infecting tick. Erythema chronicum migrans begins as a red macule, usually on the trunk at the site of tick attachment, which enlarges in a circular fashion with central clearing. In the right epidemiologic setting this rash is virtually pathognomonic for Lyme disease. Nonspecific systemic signs include headache, fever, and malaise. Joint involvement generally occurs days to years after onset of the rash. Cardiac disease consists primarily of disturbances of rhythm. Involvement of the CNS is evidenced by headache and stiff neck. The diagnosis should be suspected when any of the signs and symptoms occurs, because the disease can present in an atypical manner and the laboratory data often are normal when only the rash is present. The characteristic lesion of erythema chronicum migrans, as well as the history of tick bite, is frequently not noted by the patient. It is not until later that joint, heart, or neurologic manifestations occur, and Lyme disease is suspected, that serologic evidence confirms the etiology. Serologic evidence is sought when the patient has spent time in summer months in endemic areas or there is a risk of tick bite. Treatment with amoxicillin in the patient younger than 8 years or doxycycline in the older patient results in a faster resolution of symptoms and prevention of later complications, especially if given early in the course of the disease.

341. The answer is e. (*Hay et al, pp 678-679. Kliegman et al, pp 1616-1618. Rudolph et al, pp 945-946.*) The most common cause of diarrhea in the United States is rotavirus. Within about 48 hours of exposure vomiting (80-90%), low-grade fever, and watery diarrhea lasting 4-8 days is typically seen. Testing is usually not done since the therapy for all common viral agents is supportive. Use of the rotavirus vaccine has reduced dramatically the rate of hospitalization for this virus. *Salmonella sonnei* causes shigellosis which includes fever, cramping, rectal pain, nausea and vomiting, and typically bloody or mucous-containing diarrhea. *Cryptosporidium* has become an important cause of diarrhea in immunocompromised patients. It causes vomiting in about 80% of children; this feature is less common in adults. Fever occurs in about 30%-50% of cases. Chronic cases result in failure to thrive and weight loss. Sporotrichosis is a fungal infection of the cutaneous and subcutaneous tissue that typically does not cause diarrhea. Acquired *T gondii* can infest any body tissue. Infection can result in fever, myalgia, lymphadenopathy, maculopapular rash, hepatomegaly, pneumonia, encephalitis, chorioretinitis, or myocarditis. This intracellular parasite does not ordinarily cause diarrhea.

342. The answer is c. (*Hay et al, p 1232. Kliegman et al, pp 3142-3144. Rudolph et al, pp 1277-1279.*) The combination of erythema multiforme and vesicular, ulcerated lesions of the mucous membranes of the eyes, mouth, anus, and urethra defines the Stevens-Johnson syndrome (erythema multiforme major). Fever is common, and even pulmonary involvement occasionally is noted; the mortality rate can approach 10%. Common complications include corneal ulceration; dehydration due to severe stomatitis with poor fluid intake; and urinary retention caused by dysuria. Among the known causes of the Stevens-Johnson syndrome are allergy to various drugs (including phenytoin, barbiturates, sulfonamides, and penicillin) and infection with a variety of organisms including *M pneumoniae* or herpes type 1. Erythema multiforme is sometimes confused with urticaria early in the course because both can have a target-like lesion. The former has a target center that contains a papule or vesicle, which progresses to blister and necrosis. In contrast, urticaria can have a bluish center, but the lesions are transient (often lasting < 24 hours) and are pruritic. If the clinical presentation is not diagnostic for Stevens-Johnson, a biopsy of a lesion will demonstrate subepidermal cleavage. Skin prick testing may help identify the offending agent in urticaria but rarely is required. Kawasaki disease is an acute febrile illness of unknown etiology, sharing many of its clinical manifestations with scarlet fever. Scarlatiniform rash, desquamation, erythema of the mucous membranes that produces an injected pharynx and strawberry tongue (but not sloughing, as in the case presentation), and cervical lymphadenopathy are prominent findings in both. Kawasaki disease is associated with thrombocytosis and coronary aneurysms. Streptococcal pharyngitis causes elevated ASO titers. Persons with rubeola develop a severe cough, coryza, photophobia, conjunctivitis, and a high fever that reaches its peak at the height of the generalized macular rash, which typically lasts for 5 days. The oral changes include Koplik spots (transient white pinpoint lesions on a bright red buccal mucosa often in the area opposite the lower molars) but not sloughing. Elevation of viral specific (rubeola) IgM levels would be diagnostic if the clinical and epidemiologic picture were not clear.

Drug rash, eosinophilia, and systemic symptoms (DRESS) is another consideration in this patient. The condition is usually associated with anticonvulsants, but has been associated with other medications such as antibiotics. The skin findings are the same as erythema multiforme but patients may also have lymphadenopathy; eosinophilia; leukocytosis; fever; and liver, kidney, and lung involvement.

343. The answer is e. (*Hay et al, p 1379. Kliegman et al, pp 1744-1745. Rudolph et al, pp 1197-1199.*) One to seven days following the ingestion of pork or other improperly cooked meat infected with *T spiralis*, symptoms develop, including abdominal pain, nausea, vomiting, and malaise. These symptoms occurred prior to his arrival to Texas. During the second week, muscle invasion occurs, which causes edema of eyelids, myalgia, weakness, fever, and eosinophilia. The muscle organisms can become encysted and remain viable for years. Therapy is with mebendazole or albendazole.

344. The answer is e. (*Hay et al, pp 1331-1333. Kliegman et al, pp 1377-1382. Rudolph et al, pp 1075-1077.*) The patient in the question has a classic case of pertussis, likely contracted from her adolescent sister. Humans are the only know reservoir for pertussis; infants who have not yet completed the primary immunization series are at risk of infection from unimmunized adults. Recommendations now include vaccination with reduced diphtheria toxoid and acellular pertussis vaccine, adsorbed (Tdap) for all adolescents, parents and grandparents, and for healthcare workers and adults routinely exposed to the children.

345. The answer is a. (*Hay et al, pp 798-799. Rudolph et al, p 2183.*) The importance and urgency of the lumbar puncture in cases of suspected meningitis outweigh the usual niceties in the performance of procedures. Infants and children require adequate restraints, preferably local anesthesia, and sometimes sedation. Contraindications are few and include increased intracranial pressure in the patient without an open fontanelle that can result in herniation; severe cardiorespiratory distress; skin infection at the puncture site; and severe thrombocytopenia or other coagulation disorder, suggested by the oozing IV and venipuncture sites and thrombocytopenia on the CBC.

346. The answer is c. (*Hay et al, pp 545-546. Kliegman et al, pp 2031-2036. Rudolph et al, pp 1950-1952.*) The description is that of croup. This infection involves the larynx and trachea; it usually is caused by parainfluenza or respiratory syncytial viruses. The usual age range for presentation is 6 months-6 years. Symptoms include low-grade fever, barking cough, and hoarse, inspiratory stridor without wheezing. The pharynx can be normal or slightly red and the lungs are usually clear. In children with severe respiratory distress, prolonged dyspnea can progress to physical exhaustion and fatal respiratory failure. Expiratory stridor is usually associated with a fixed obstruction, such as a tumor or vascular ring. Because agitation can be a sign of hypoxia, sedation should not be ordered. Hyperinflation on chest x-ray is seen in asthma, not croup. One condition in the differential in this child is epiglottitis, a now rare disease owing to widespread use of the *H influenzae* type B vaccine. Its presentation is more abrupt, with higher fever in rather toxic-appearing patients.

347-354. The answers are 347-k, 348-c, 349-a, 350-f, 351-g 352-h, 353-o, 354-e. (*Hay et al, pp 659-661, 752-775, 1249, 1287-1293, 1317-1318, 1325-1327, 1333-1334, 1343-1344, 1374-1378. Kliegman et al, pp 1337-1341, 1349-1352, 1403-1408, 1413-1419, 1423-1426, 1586-1590, 1594-1597, 1698-1701, 1736-1738, 1743-1744, 1816-1819, 2556-2562. Rudolph et al, pp 950-956, 1026-1030, 1106, 1109-1110, 1149-1152, 1154-1158, 1183, 1194-1195, 1221-1226, 1456-1457.*) EBV can produce a number of clinically important syndromes, one of which is mononucleosis as described in the college-age patient with fever and sore throat. Other symptoms might include headache, profound fatigue, abdominal pain, and myalgia. Splenic enlargement is common, and contact sports are to be avoided. The rash (ampicillin rash) is poorly understood but occurs so commonly as to be diagnostic when seen; it is self-resolving.

Pseudomonas is a ubiquitous organism. Most infections with the organism are opportunistic, involving several organs. Skin infections related to burns, trauma (such as in a puncture wound through a tennis shoe), and use of swimming pools are not uncommon. Injuries through a tennis shoe are prone to pseudomonal infections because of the warm, moist nature of the shoe's environment. In contrast, a wound through a bare foot would be associated with cutaneous flora such as *Staphylococcus.*

Bartonella henselae is the major etiologic agent for cat-scratch disease (the 5-year old with a feline scratch). History of a scratch or a bite from a kitten is often positive, and fleas are often a factor in transmission. Diagnosis is usually by history and presenting signs and symptoms, as described in the question. Another form of the disease, Parinaud oculoglandular syndrome, occurs when the primary site of inoculation occurs in or near the conjunctivae, resulting in a moderately severe conjunctivitis and preauricular lymph adenopathy.

Roseola (exanthema subitum) is a common acute illness of young children (such as the 9-month-old infant with fever and transient rash), characterized by several days of high fever followed by a rapid defervescence and the appearance of an evanescent, erythematous, maculopapular rash. HHV 6 has been identified as its primary cause.

Urinary tract infections are the most common cause of bacterial infections in the young neonate. The incidence is slightly higher in the uncircumcised as compared to the circumcised male. *E coli* is a leading cause.

Infection with *H pylori* is associated with antral gastritis and primary duodenal ulcer disease, with the symptoms described in the question of the 9-year old with abdominal pain and blood in the stool. Culture for *H pylori* requires endoscopy and gastric biopsy. The biopsied tissue can be tested for urease activity and examined histologically after special staining. Alternatively, noninvasive tests involving detection of metabolic products of *H pylori* (urease activity) or antibodies against *H pylori* can be demonstrated.

Enterobius vermicularis is the causative agent of pinworm, an intensely pruritic perianal (and sometime vaginal) infestation.

Ancylostoma braziliense is the causative agent for cutaneous larva migrans, classically described as a pruritic, creeping eruption of the lower extremities. A common source of acquiring this infestation includes walking barefoot on a beach where animal feces may have been deposited.

Listeria monocytogenes in a pregnant woman presents as flu-like symptoms in the second and third trimesters, frequently resulting in stillbirth or premature delivery. Early-onset neonatal listeriosis presents in listeria-exposed women as sepsis with meningitis and widespread microabscesses and granulomas (granulomatous infantiseptica) in the first days of life; the infant typically is premature and small for gestational age. In contrast, women with GBS lack the flu-like presentation and typically have an uncomplicated pregnancy. Early-onset GBS disease (first 7 days of life) is characterized by rapidly progressive sepsis without the microabscess formation. The incidence of this GBS disease has diminished owing to peripartum treatment of GBS colonized women.

Yersinia enterocolitica causes diarrhea, fever, and abdominal pain along with mesenteric lymphadenitis that may mimic symptoms of appendicitis. Rubivirus (rubella) in the neonate can cause neonatal rubella syndrome (hearing loss, persistent ductus arteriosus, microcephaly with developmental delay, cataracts, hepatosplenomegaly, and "blue berry muffin" baby). In older children it causes "3-day" or "German measles" which is usually a mild disease, including a diffuse maculopapular rash that lasts for 3 days, marked enlargement of the posterior cervical and occipital lymph nodes, low-grade fever, mild sore throat and, occasionally, conjunctivitis, arthralgia, or arthritis. *Toxocara cati* (and *canis* which is more common) are the causes of visceral and ocular larva migrans. The classic presentation is eosinophilia, fever, and hepatomegaly in a toddler with a history of pica and exposure to puppies. *Campylobacter jejuni* is a common cause of diarrhea which begins with a prodrome of fever, headache, and myalgias followed by crampy abdominal pain, and loose, watery stools (occasionally bloody). *Leishmania mexicana* causes a form of leishmaniasis characterized by nonulcerating macules, papules, or plaques commonly involving the face and extremities that resemble leprosy. *Francisella tularensis* causes tularemia.

It occurs after the bite of an infected tick or other insect, or after exposure to an infected animal carcass. Signs and symptoms include sudden onset of fever, lymphadenopathy, hepatosplenomegaly, and skin lesions.

355 to 360. The answers are 355-l, 356-c, 357-f, 358-a, 359-j, 360-d. (*Hay et al, pp 60-61, 551-552, 561-574, 1287-1293, 1317-1318, 1339-1340, 1378. Kliegman et al, pp 1315-1327, 1337-1341, 1412-1416, 1421-1423, 1445-1461, 1489-1490, 1492-1493, 1525-1527, 1606-1611, 1743-1744, 2088-2094. Rudolph et al, pp 962-965, 1031-1034, 1043-1044, 1066-1068, 1078-1080, 1090-1094, 1097-1099, 1197, 1977-1986.*) *Pseudomonas aeruginosa* is an unusual cause of pneumonia in the immunocompetent patient, but is a common finding in a patient with cystic fibrosis. The patient in the question has classic findings of cystic fibrosis including failure to thrive, evidence of fat-malabsorption resulting in malodorous stools, poor caloric intake, and fat-soluble vitamin deficiency (anemia due to vitamin E deficiency). Rectal prolapse in children is distinctly unusual and would strongly suggest CF.

Pneumonia due to group B *Streptococcus* presents in the newborn typically in the first 24 hours of life as part of early-onset neonatal GBS disease. This condition is characterized as a rapidly progressive sepsis with findings such as poor feeding, hypothermia, apnea, lethargy, tachypnea, grunting, nasal flaring, and retractions. Prenatal diagnosis of GBS carriage by the mother allows prophylactic antibiotics to be provided to her just prior to delivery, thus reducing the chance of infection by the baby.

Approximately 10%-20% of infants born to mothers with *C trachomatis* infection develop pneumonia. The presentation of this pneumonia usually occurs between 1 and 3 months of age, with cough, tachypnea, and lack of fever. Examination reveals rales but not wheezing. Laboratory data suggestive of *C trachomatis* infection include an increase in eosinophils in the peripheral blood. The chest radiograph shows hyperinflation with interstitial infiltrates.

Mycoplasma pneumoniae is a common cause of pneumonia in the school-age child or young adult. Usual presentation includes the gradual onset of headache, malaise, fever, and lower respiratory symptoms. Typically, the cough (often nonproductive) worsens for the first 2 weeks of the illness, and then slowly resolves over the ensuing 3-4 weeks. Early in the disease, the physical examination is remarkable for a paucity of signs; the patient usually has a few fine rales. Later, the dyspnea and fever become worse. Radiographic findings include an interstitial or bronchial pattern, especially in the lower lobes, and commonly on only one side. The diagnosis usually is made on clinical grounds.

Staphylococcal pneumonia is caused by *S aureus*. It is a rapidly progressive and life-threatening form of pneumonia most commonly seen in infants younger than 1 year of age. Commonly, the infant has a URI for several days, with the abrupt onset of fever and respiratory distress. Pleural effusion, empyema, and pyopneumothorax are common complications. Laboratory evidence of this disease can include a markedly elevated WBC count with left shift. Radiographic findings include nonspecific bronchopneumonia early in the disease, which later becomes more dense and homogeneous and involves an entire lobe or hemithorax.

Pneumococcal pneumonia often presents with sudden onset of fever, cough, and chest pain. This child may have failed outpatient therapy because of increased incidence of resistant organisms. Pleural effusions or empyema are commonly seen; chest tube evacuation of the fluid is often required. Depending on sensitivity patterns in a particular community, therapy with high-dose penicillin, cefuroxime, amoxicillin/clavulanate, or even vancomycin may be required.

A high index of suspicion is needed to diagnose tuberculosis. An exposure history is helpful but not always present. Many children who are infected have a positive PPD as the only evidence. Children at higher risk of active disease include those who are very young, malnourished, immunodeficient or immunosuppressed, or diabetic. Most active disease is pulmonary, but can also be disseminated and involve the CNS, bone, skin, and abdomen. Pulmonary disease includes a parenchymal focus and regional lymphadenopathy. The pleura is frequently involved.

Fungal infections can resemble TB, and can be difficult to diagnose. In the United States, *Histoplasma* is found in the Ohio and Mississippi River valleys. Human-to-human transmission does not occur, so exposure to an endemic area is required. About half of histoplasmosis infection is asymptomatic and diagnosed based on scattered calcifications in the lungs. In immunocompetent individuals, the disease usually resolves in 2 weeks. Other clinically significant fungi that cause lung disease include *Coccidioides*, *Cryptococcus*, *Blastomyces*, and *Aspergillus*. *Pneumocystis jiroveci* (formerly *P carinii*) is technically a fungus but responds to antiparasitic medications.

Respiratory syncytial virus and human metapneumovirus classically present in the fall and winter months in infants less than about a year of age as bronchiolitis. Upper respiratory tract signs and symptoms progress to coughing, wheezing, tachypnea, respiratory distress, poor feeding and hypoxia. Chest radiographs show hyperexpansion, peribronchial thickening, and interstitial infiltrates. *Toxocara canis* can cause visceral larva migrans, the classic presentation including eosinophilia, fever, and hepatomegaly in a toddler with a history of pica and exposure to puppies. The lung findings include wheezing and bronchopneumonia. *Legionella pneumophilia* in the pediatric population is most commonly reported in children aged 15-19 or in children less than 1 year. The true incidence of this condition in the pediatric population is unknown, but the reported incidence is low. Presentation is similar to other pneumonias such as *S pneumonia* with cough (productive or nonproductive), fever, congestion, and chest pain. Chest radiographs are classically described as rapidly progressive alveolar-filling infiltrates, in actual practice they are variable; pleural effusion is less common with legionella disease. *Pneumocystis jiroveci* is an interstitial pneumonia commonly associated with immunocompromised conditions, especially HIV. Presentation of HIV in newborns is variable, but classically includes common conditions (otitis media, sinusitis, thrush) that are prolonged or more severe than expected. Failure to thrive and opportunistic infections are found as the disease progresses.

Hematologic and Neoplastic Diseases

Questions

361. A 2-year-old child is seen in the emergency center with the complaint of bruising. His parents report that for the previous 2 days he has developed bruising on his legs, back, and arms. He has been in good health his entire life with occasional upper respiratory infections, the last about 2 weeks ago, and one episode of otitis media at age 8 months. He lives with his parents and 4-year-old sibling. On physical examination the temperature is 37°C (98.6°F), heart rate is 100 beats per minute, respiratory rate is 20 breaths per minute, and blood pressure is 100/70 mm Hg. He is awake, alert, and in no distress. Neck is supple. The mucous membranes are pink, moist, and without lesions; a tiny bit of blood oozing from the gums is noted. Pupils are equally round and reactive. The chest is clear. Heart has a normal S1 and S2 without murmur. The abdomen is soft and nontender without hepatosplenomegaly. No adenopathy is noted. Neurologic examination is nonfocal. Numerous fresh-appearing bruises are noted over the shins and scattered over the arms and back; generalized petechiae is found. Laboratory data show:

White count: 8000/μL
Hemoglobin: 12.3 g/dL
Hematocrit: 36%
Platelet count: 15,000/μL

Which of the following therapies is most appropriate?

a. Desmopressin 0.3 μg/kg IV
b. Vincristine weekly for 4 weeks
c. Observation alone
d. Platelet transfusion
e. Plasmapheresis

362. An 11-month-old African American boy is seen at the local Women, Infants, and Children (WIC) clinic. Screening laboratory testing at that site showed a hematocrit of 24%. He is referred to your clinic for further testing. On physical examination the temperature is 37°C (98.6°F), heart rate is 110 beats per minute, respiratory rate is 18 breaths per minute, and blood pressure is 105/72 mm Hg. Length, weight, and head circumference are at the 50th percentile. He is awake, alert, and in no distress. Neck is supple. The mucous membranes are pink, moist, and without lesions. Pupils are equally round and reactive. The chest is clear. Heart has a normal S1 and S2 without murmur. The abdomen is soft and nontender without hepatosplenomegaly. Neurologic examination is nonfocal. Laboratory testing shows:

White blood count: 12,200/µL
   Neutrophils: 39%
   Bands: 6%
   Lymphocytes: 55%
Hemoglobin: 7.8 g/dL
Hematocrit: 22.9%
Mean corpuscular volume (MCV): 64 fL
Smear: Hypochromia
Platelet count: 175,000/µL
Reticulocyte count: 0.2%
Free erythrocyte protoporphyrin (FEP): 114 µg/dL (normal 0-34 µg/dL)
Lead level: 4 µg/dL (normal 0-5 µg/dL)
Sickle cell preparation negative
Stool guaiac negative

Which of the following is the most appropriate recommendation?

a. Blood transfusion
b. Oral ferrous sulfate
c. Intramuscular iron dextran
d. Daily penicillin and folate
e. Calcium EDTA

363. A previously healthy 2-year-old child is known to have sickle cell disease; she now has a 1-hour history of left-sided weakness and ataxia. Which of the following therapies is the most appropriate first step in the management of her likely diagnosis?

a. Iron chelation with deferoxamine
b. Initiation of broad-spectrum antibiotics after obtaining appropriate cultures
c. Cranial ultrasound
d. Arrange for an outpatient MRI of the brain
e. Initiation of a stat blood transfusion

364. A 1-year-old child is seen for a well-child visit. On physical examination the temperature is 37°C (98.6°F), heart rate is 114 beats per minute, respiratory rate is 20 breaths per minute, and blood pressure is 110/72 mm Hg. Length, weight, and head circumference are at the 25th-50th percentile. He is awake, alert, crying, and in no distress. Neck is supple. The mucous membranes are pink, moist, and without lesions. Pupils are equally round and reactive. The chest is clear. Heart has a normal S1 and S2 without murmur. The abdomen is soft and nontender without hepatosplenomegaly. Neurologic examination is nonfocal. No adenopathy is appreciated. Office testing shows his hematocrit to be 30%. Additional testing shows:

White blood count: 12,500/µL
  Neutrophils: 40%
  Bands: 5%
  Lymphocytes: 50%
Hemoglobin: 9.8 g/dL
Hematocrit: 31%
Mean corpuscular volume (MCV): 59 fL
Smear: Microcytosis
Platelet count: 175,000/µL
Reticulocyte count: 0.2%
Free erythrocyte protoporphyrin (FEP): 20 µg/dL (normal 0-34 µg/dL)
Lead level: 2 µg/dL
Hemoglobin electrophoresis:
  HbA1: 85% (normal 95%-98%)
  HbA2: 10% (normal 1.5%-3.5%)
  HbF: 5% (<2%)

The most appropriate next step in the management of this child's condition is which of the following?

a. Initiate oral iron therapy.
b. Provide family counseling alone.
c. Begin oral, daily folate, and penicillin therapy.
d. Arrange for a bone marrow aspiration.
e. Initiate therapy with dimercaptosuccinic acid (succimer).

365. After being delivered following a benign gestation, a newborn is noted to have a 3-cm red, raised, rubbery vascular plaque on the abdomen. Over the next several weeks the lesion is noted to enlarge. The physical examination is otherwise normal. Which of the following therapies is most appropriate?

a. Oral propranolol
b. Oral prednisolone
c. Surgical excision
d. Observation and reassurance
e. Subcutaneous administration of interferon alfa

366. A 4-year-old boy is seen in the office with the complaint of "dark urine" and pallor. His mother reports that he has been in good health until about 1 week ago when he developed an ear infection for which he was started on trimethoprim-sulfamethoxazole at an urgent care center. She denies recent travel or exposure to any illnesses. A review of his chart shows his birth to have been normal, his development as expected, no serious illness, and his immunizations up to date. On physical examination the temperature is 37°C (98.6°F), heart rate is 120 beats per minute, respiratory rate is 18 breaths per minute, and blood pressure is 105/70 mm Hg. Height and weight are 25th percentile and 50th percentile, respectively. He is awake, alert, and in no distress. Neck is supple. The mucous membranes are pale, moist, and without lesions. Pupils are equally round and reactive; conjunctivae are icteric. The chest is clear. Heart has a normal S1 and S2 without murmur. The abdomen is soft and nontender without hepatosplenomegaly. Neurologic examination is nonfocal. Testing shows:

White blood count: 10,500/μL
  Neutrophils: 40%
  Bands: 2%
  Lymphocytes: 48%
Hemoglobin: 9.9 g/dL
Hematocrit: 33%
Platelet count: 175,000/μL
Serum electrolytes:
  Sodium: 139 mEq/L
  Potassium: 4.5 mEq/L
  Chloride: 110 mEq/L
  Bicarbonate: 22 mEq/L
  Glucose: 100 mg/dL
  Creatinine: 0.4 mEq/L
  Blood urea nitrogen (BUN): 10 mEq/L
Bilirubin total: 14.1 mg/dL

Which of the following is the most likely cause of this patient's symptoms?

a. Infection with hepatitis B virus
b. Infection with hepatitis A virus
c. Infection with *E coli* O157:H7
d. Reduced bilirubin uridine diphosphate glucuronosyltransferase (bilirubin-UGT)
e. Deficiency in glucose-6-phosphate dehydrogenase activity

367. A 4-year-old girl is noted to have an orange-yellow, hairless patch on her scalp (photo). Her mother reports the lesion to have been present since birth when it was more "velvety" in nature. Which of the following is the most appropriate therapy for this condition?

a. Topical 1% hydrocortisone cream
b. Surgical removal by puberty
c. Referral to pediatric neurologist
d. Topical application of 50% salicylic acid
e. Referral for carbon dioxide laser therapy

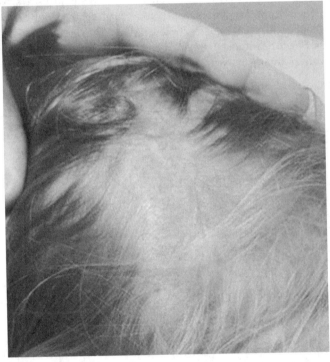

(Used with permission from Adelaide Hebert, MD.)

368. A 2950-g (6.5 lb) African American baby boy is born in the ambulance en route to the hospital. The mother is a 27-year-old gravida 5 woman who had good prenatal care and reports no complications during the pregnancy. Emergency responders report no delivery complications and gave the infant Apgar scores of 9 and 9 at 1 and 5 minutes, respectively. On physical examination the temperature is 36.1°C (97.9°F), heart rate is 150 beats per minute, respiratory rate is 36 breaths per minute, and blood pressure is 100/70 mm Hg. He is awake, alert, pale, but in no distress. Neck is supple. The mucous membranes are pale, moist, and without lesions. Pupils are equally round and reactive; conjunctivae are clear; red reflex is present. The chest is clear. Heart has a normal S1 and S2 without murmur. The abdomen is soft and nontender; spleen tip and liver edges are barely palpable. Neurologic examination is nonfocal. Skin is pale but without lesions. Laboratory studies reveal the following:

    Mother's blood type A, Rh-positive
    Baby's blood type O, Rh-positive
    Hemoglobin: 11 g/dL
    Hematocrit: 34%
    Reticulocyte count: 5%

Which of the following is the most likely cause of this infant's condition?

a. Fetomaternal transfusion
b. ABO incompatibility
c. Physiologic anemia of the newborn
d. Sickle cell anemia
e. Maternal iron deficiency

369. A father brings his 3-year-old daughter to the emergency center after noting her to be pale and tired and with a subjective fever for several days. Her past history is significant for an upper respiratory infection 4 weeks prior, but she had been otherwise healthy. The father denies emesis or diarrhea, but does report his daughter has had leg pain over the previous week, waking her from sleep. Testing shows:

White blood count: 8000/μL
  Neutrophils: 20%
  Bands: 2%
  Lymphocytes: 48%
  Atypical lymphocytes: 30%
Hemoglobin: 4 g/dL
Hematocrit: 12.5%
Platelet count: 7000/μL

Which of the following diagnostic studies is the most appropriate next step in the management of this child?

a. Epstein-Barr virus titers
b. Serum haptoglobin
c. Antiplatelet antibody assay
d. Reticulocyte count
e. Bone marrow biopsy

370. A couple brings their newly-adopted 2-year-old son for a routine office visit. The family has few details of this international adoption, but report the child to have been born at term, to have had few or no illness, and to be current on immunizations. The family reports they received the child 3 days previously and that he seems to be adapting well to his new home. On physical examination the temperature is 37°C (98.6°F), heart rate is 90 beats per minute, respiratory rate is 18 breaths per minute, and blood pressure is 120/80 mm Hg. Height and weight are 25th percentile, and head circumference is at the 50th percentile. He is awake, alert, and in no distress; he is notably enlarged on the left side of his body. Neck is supple. The mucous membranes are pink, moist, and with poor dentition. Pupils are equally round with absence of iris; conjunctivae are pink. The chest is clear. Heart has normal S1 and S2 without murmur. The abdomen is soft, non-tender, and without hepatosplenomegaly. A baseball-sized, firm mass is felt over the left lower abdomen. Neurologic examination is nonfocal. Skin is dry and without lesions. Testes are descended, hypospadias is noted. Which of the following is the most likely diagnosis for this child?

a. Neuroblastoma
b. Wilms tumor
c. Hepatoblastoma
d. Rhabdomyosarcoma
e. Testicular cancer

371. A 16-year-old boy has a several week history of pain in his left leg not associated with an episode of trauma. Over the last 10 days he has had low-grade fever and his mother reports that he has lost about 8 lb. On physical examination he has pain and swelling over the mid-shaft of his femur. Plain radiographs of the leg demonstrate an "onion skin" periosteal reaction and a "moth eaten" cortical irregularity in the area of the swelling. Which of the following is the most likely diagnosis?

a. Osteomyelitis
b. Osteosarcoma
c. Rhabdomyosarcoma
d. Ewing sarcoma
e. Non-Hodgkin lymphoma

372. A previously healthy 16-year-old boy is seen in the emergency center for a laceration to his knee. On physical examination the temperature is 37°C (98.6°F), heart rate is 90 beats per minute, respiratory rate is 18 breaths per minute, blood pressure is 115/70 mm Hg, and oxygen saturation is 94%. His physical examination is normal other than the deep, 2 cm laceration to his right knee. The area is anesthetized with lidocaine, irrigated thoroughly to remove debris, and repaired successfully with sutures. He was given a booster dose of Tdap (Adacel). As the family is preparing to leave the emergency room the patient develops central cyanosis but no other symptoms. Oxygen is placed via face mask, and repeat vital signs include: temperature 37°C (98.6°F), heart rate 100 beats per minute, respiratory rate 22 breaths per minute, blood pressure 112/75 mm Hg, and oxygen saturation 91%. Which of the following is the most appropriate next step in his management?

a. Arrange for hyperbaric oxygen therapy
b. Partial exchange transfusion
c. Administration of ascorbic acid
d. Administration of methylene blue
e. Intravenous hydration and acidification of urine

373. A 3200-g (7 lb) African American boy is born to a 21-year-old woman at term. She had good prenatal care and reports no pregnancy complications except first trimester hyperemesis. Delivery was vaginal and with infant Apgar scores of 9 and 9 at 1 and 5 minutes, respectively. On physical examination at 18 hours of age the temperature is 36.1°C (97.9°F), heart rate is 150 beats per minute, respiratory rate is 35 breaths per minute, and blood pressure is 90/70 mm Hg. He is awake, alert, jaundiced, but in no distress. Head is normocephalic with mild molding. Neck is supple. The mucous membranes are moist and without lesions. Pupils are equally round and reactive; conjunctivae are clear; red reflex is present. The chest is clear. Heart has a normal S1 and S2 without murmur. The abdomen is soft and nontender; spleen tip and liver edges are barely palpable. Neurologic examination is nonfocal. Skin is jaundiced but without lesions. Laboratory studies reveal the following:

> Mother's blood type A, Rh-positive, antibody screen negative
> Baby's blood type B, Rh-positive, Coombs negative
> White blood count: 18,000/μL
>> Neutrophils: 60%
>> Bands: 2%
>> Lymphocytes: 35%
> Hemoglobin: 12.5 g/dL
> Hematocrit: 36%
> Platelet count: 157,000/μL
> Smear: Many nucleated RBCs and some spherocytes
> Reticulocyte count: 11%
> Bilirubin total: 18 mg/dL

Which of the following is the most likely diagnosis?

a. Pyruvate kinase deficiency
b. Hereditary spherocytosis
c. Sickle cell anemia
d. Rh incompatibility
e. Polycythemia

374. A 10-year-old boy is admitted to the hospital because of bleeding. Pertinent laboratory findings include a platelet count of 50,000/μL, prothrombin time (PT) of 15 seconds (control 11.5 seconds), activated partial thromboplastin time (aPTT) of 51 seconds (control 36 seconds), thrombin time (TT) of 13.7 seconds (control 10.5 seconds), and factor VIII level of 14% (normal 38%-178%). Which of the following is the most likely cause of his bleeding?

a. Immune thrombocytopenic purpura (ITP)
b. Vitamin K deficiency
c. Disseminated intravascular coagulation (DIC)
d. Hemophilia A
e. Hemophilia B

375. A 17-year-old adolescent comes to your office seeking help for "heavy" menses. Your review of systems also reveals weekly epistaxis. Her only significant past history includes a tonsillectomy at age 6 after which she required blood transfusion for excessive bleeding. Her family history includes several people who seem to bleed and bruise more easily than others. The patient's mother required a hysterectomy after child birth for excessive hemorrhage. You order a variety of laboratory tests. The patient has hemoglobin of 6.5 g/dL with an MCV of 60 fL; her platelet count is 350,000/μL. Her von Willebrand antigen and her von Willebrand factor (vWF) activity (ristocetin cofactor activity) are decreased. Her vWF is reported as normal but in decreased amounts. You have been unable to reach her to report the findings, but when she calls about 1 week later, she reports she is having a mild to moderate nosebleed. You initiate therapy with which of the following?

a. Aminocaproic acid (Amicar)
b. vWF concentrate alone
c. vWF with factor VIII
d. Desmopressin (DDAVP)
e. Intravenous immunoglobulin (IVIG)

376. A 13-year-old white boy is seen for a well-child visit. His family reports that he has been in good health, has been getting good grades in school, and has had no significant injuries. When questioned alone he reports over the previous 2-3 weeks deep pains in his leg that awaken him from sleep. He states he has had swelling in his leg to which he attributes to his being kicked while playing soccer about 1 week ago; he has not told his family since the state tournament is starting in 3 days. He has had no fever, headaches, weakness, bruising, or other symptoms. He denies smoking, tobacco, and other drug use. He has a girlfriend, but denies sexual activity beyond "petting." On physical examination the temperature is 37°C (98.6°F), heart rate is 90 beats per minute, respiratory rate is 18 breaths per minute, and blood pressure is 105/70 mm Hg. Height and weight are 25th percentile and 50th percentile, respectively. He is awake, alert, and in no distress. Neck is supple. The mucous membranes are pink, moist, and without lesions. Pupils are equally round and reactive; conjunctivae are pink. The chest is clear. Heart has a normal S1 and S2 without murmur. The abdomen is soft, nontender, and without hepatosplenomegaly. Neurologic examination is nonfocal. Extremities and joints are normal except for left lower leg which has a distal firm, palpable mass with slightly decreased range of motion in the joint.

A radiograph of the leg is shown in the photograph. Which of the following is the most appropriate next step?

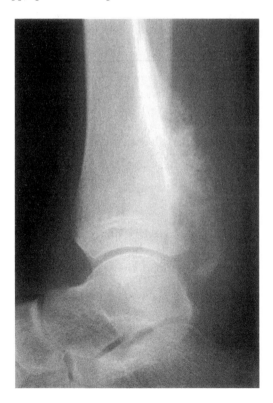

a. Reassurance to the family of the benign nature of the condition
b. Bone marrow aspiration
c. Serial blood cultures and initiation of intravenous vancomycin
d. Splinting of leg and reduction in activity
e. Bone biopsy

377. A 17-year old is seen with a 6-month complaint of cough, possible weight loss, and nocturnal fevers. He reports no nausea, vomiting, diarrhea, bleeding, or other problems. He is a senior in high school, makes "fair" grades, and works at a local supermarket. He currently has a girlfriend with whom he is sexually active; he reports condom use "most of the time." He lives at home with his parents and younger sister. Household pets include one dog and two cats. He denies drug or tobacco use; he occasionally uses alcohol. On physical examination the temperature is 37.2°C (99°F), heart rate is 90 beats per minute, respiratory rate is 18 breaths per minute, and blood pressure is 105/70 mm Hg. Weight is 25th percentile (down from previous visit at the 50th percentile) and height is 75th percentile for age. He is awake, alert, healthy-appearing, and in no distress. Neck is supple with prominent adenopathy. The mucous membranes are moist, and without lesions. Pupils are equally round and reactive; conjunctivae are pink. The chest is clear. Heart has a normal S1 and S2 without murmur. The abdomen is soft, nontender, and without hepatosplenomegaly. Neurologic examination is nonfocal. Inguinal, axillary, and supraclavicular nodes are palpable. He is Tanner V with descended testes, and no urethral discharge is noted. Extremities and joints are normal. Which of the following would be the appropriate next step?

a. Biopsy of a node
b. CBC and differential
c. Trial of antituberculosis drugs
d. Chest radiograph
e. Cat-scratch titers

378. A 6-month-old girl presents with an abdominal mass, fever, and irritability. The parents also report periorbital "shiners" of unknown etiology, and deny physical abuse or fall. An MRI of her abdomen shows a mass is arising from her left adrenal gland. Homovanillic acid (HVA) and vanillyl-mandelic acid (VMA) are elevated. The tumor is most likely:

a. Wilms tumor
b. Pheochromocytoma
c. Neuroblastoma
d. Rhabdomyosarcoma
e. Ovarian tumor

Questions 379 to 382

For each disorder listed later, select the peripheral blood smear with which it is most likely to be associated. Each lettered option may be used once, more than once, or not at all.

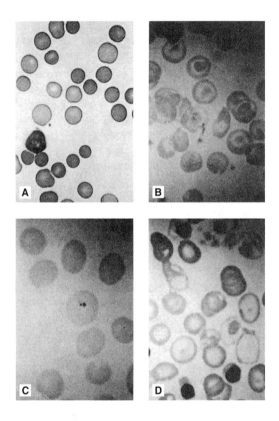

379. A 14-year-old patient has hemoglobin of 8 g/dL and repeated hospital admissions for hand pain and swelling, and one episode of priapism.

380. A 9-month-old boy recently moves into your area having been adopted by a family member when his biologic family was unable to care for him. His adoptive family states that they know that he developed progressive anemia over the first months of his life resulting in an admission at about 6 months of age for heart failure and generalized weakness. He has had "a swollen spleen forever" and has had blood transfusions each of the last 3 months.

381. A 2-day-old newborn in the neonatal ICU is receiving phototherapy and has a hemoglobin of 10 g/dL and a bilirubin of 22 mg/dL.

382. A completely asymptomatic, healthy 1-year-old boy has hemoglobin of 12 g/dL. His 35-year-old father states that he has had "mild anemia" his whole life and had a cholecystectomy 2 years ago.

Hematologic and Neoplastic Diseases

Answers

361. The answer is c. (*Hay et al, pp 859-861. Kliegman et al, pp 2390-2392, 2402-2404, 2437-2445. Rudolph et al, pp 1582-1583.*) In children, ITP is the most common form of thrombocytopenic purpura. In most cases, a preceding viral infection can be noted. Autoantibodies to platelet membrane antigens cause increased platelet destruction by macrophages, particularly those in the spleen. No diagnostic test identifies this disease; exclusion of the other diseases listed in the question is necessary. In this condition, the platelet count is frequently less than 20,000/μL, but other laboratory tests yield essentially normal results, including the bone marrow aspiration (if done). Complications are uncommon; significant bleeding occurs in only 5% of cases and intracranial hemorrhage is even rarer. The treatment of childhood ITP is controversial. Patients with mild symptoms such as bruising and self-limited epistaxis may be observed, while patients with significant bleeding should be treated. IVIG and corticosteroids are effective in causing a rapid increase in platelet count, but controversy exists surrounding the use of prednisone before ruling out leukemia with a bone marrow aspirate. For Rh-positive patients with a working spleen, the use of anti-D immunoglobulin also results in an increase in platelet count. Platelet transfusion usually is not indicated, as antiplatelet autoantibodies will target the transfused platelets as well. Only in cases of life-threatening hemorrhage (such as an intracranial hemorrhage) is transfusion appropriate. For patients with chronic (> 1 year) ITP, a splenectomy may be necessary.

vWD might be expected to present with bleeding and not just bruising; treatment options would include desmopressin. It is unlikely that acute leukemia would present with thrombocytopenia only; the induction phase includes vincristine weekly followed by the consolidation and the maintenance phases of therapy. TTP is rare in children; treatment is with plasmapheresis.

362. The answer is b. (*Hay et al, pp 838-839. Kliegman et al, pp 2323-2326. Rudolph et al, pp 1546-1548.*) Response to a therapeutic trial of iron is an appropriate and cost-effective method of diagnosing iron-deficiency anemia. A prompt reticulocytosis and rise in hemoglobin and hematocrit follow the administration of an oral preparation of ferrous sulfate. Intramuscular iron dextran should be reserved for situations in which compliance cannot be achieved since this treatment is expensive, painful, and no more effective than oral iron. The gradual onset of iron-deficiency anemia enables a child to adapt to surprisingly low hemoglobin concentrations. Transfusion is rarely indicated unless a child becomes symptomatic or is further compromised by a superimposed infection.

When the iron available for production of hemoglobin is limited, free protoporphyrins accumulates in the blood. Levels of erythrocyte protoporphyrin (EP) are also elevated in lead poisoning. Iron-deficiency anemia can be differentiated from lead intoxication by measuring blood lead, which should be less than 5 μg/dL. Calcium EDTA is one of the treatments of lead poisoning. Daily folate and penicillin are not warranted since the negative sickle cell prep has excluded that diagnostic possibility.

363. The answer is e. (*Hay et al, pp 846-848. Kliegman et al, pp 2336-2344. Rudolph et al, pp 1556-1560.*) This child has evidence of a stroke. Emergency imaging of the brain (preferably MRI but CT with contrast, if necessary), urgent transfusion of blood to reduce the number of circulating sickled cells, and hospitalization (likely in the intensive care unit) to observe for further neurologic deterioration are indicated. As recovery begins, physical therapy is instituted and the patient is enrolled in a chronic blood transfusion program to reduce the risk of recurrence.

Iron chelation with deferoxamine might be indicated long term with the chronic transfusion program, but iron overload is not currently this child's problem. The cranial ultrasound might have been part of the "well-child" care of this patient prior to the stroke, and if it showed high flow, the chronic transfusion program might previously have been started in an effort to prevent a stroke, but it has no use at this point. Antibiotics and cultures would be indicated in this child if she also has the signs and symptoms of sepsis.

364. The answer is b. (*Hay et al, pp 844-846. Kliegman et al, pp 2352-2353. Rudolph et al, pp 1563-1566.*) The concentration of hemoglobin A2 is increased in β-thalassemia trait (also called β-thalassemia minor). Patients have a single abnormal gene for the β-globin component of hemoglobin; they do not typically have problems aside from a mild microcytic anemia. It is important to distinguish between β-thalassemia trait and the more common iron-deficiency anemia, as iron is not useful to patients with β-thalassemia trait. In severe iron deficiency, hemoglobin A2 may be decreased. In mild to moderate iron deficiency, the level of hemoglobin A2 is normal. Hemoglobin A2 is also normal in patients with sickle cell anemia (for whom appropriate treatment might be daily folate and penicillin), chronic systemic illness (for whom a bone marrow aspiration might be indicated), and lead poisoning (treated with dimercaptosuccinic acid).

365. The answer is a. (*Hay et al, p 431. Kliegman et al, pp 2226-2228. Rudolph et al, pp 1283-1285.*) The child in the question likely has a hemangioma, a benign tumor of the capillary bed. The classic course is rapid growth over the first year of life with slow involution over the next several years. Observation alone and corticosteroids have been replaced by administration of oral propranolol, especially when the lesion is located in a vital area such as an airway or near the eye, or if it is located in a potentially disfiguring or trauma-prone area. Surgical intervention and α-interferon (also used for Kaposi sarcoma) are options to consider only if the lesion failed to respond to more conservative therapies and was encroaching on a vital structure such as an airway.

366. The answer is e. (*Hay et al, pp 849-850. Kliegman et al, pp 2355-2357. Rudolph et al, p 1554.*) Synthesis of the RBC enzyme glucose-6-phosphate dehydrogenase (G6PD) is determined by genes on the X chromosome, and the pattern of inheritance is X-linked recessive. The enzyme found in most populations is termed G6PDB1. There are more than 380 deficient variants of the enzyme, affecting over 100 million people worldwide. Among them is variant G6PDA1, a mutant enzyme affecting about 13% of African American men and 2% of African American women. The disease occurs, though less commonly, in other ethnic groups, including Middle Eastern, African, and Asian groups. Deficiency of G6PD compromises the generation of reduced glutathione and upon exposure to oxidant agents such as sulfa drugs, antimalarials, nitrofurans, naphthalene mothballs, or infection, a hemolytic episode can occur. The degree of hemolysis depends on the nature of the oxidant and severity of the enzyme deficiency. In African Americans, the older, more G6PD-deficient cells are destroyed, but since young cells have sufficient enzyme to prevent further RBC destruction even if the inciting factor is still present, the hemolytic crisis is usually self-limited. Blood transfusion may be unnecessary. In African Americans, premature testing for the enzyme immediately after a hemolytic episode can lead to a false-negative result, since the newly produced RBCs in the circulation have a higher G6PD enzyme activity. The older RBCs containing Heinz bodies (insoluble precipitates resulting from oxidation), the "bite cells" (RBCs after the removal of the Heinz bodies), and cell fragments are removed from the circulation within 3-4 days. In the severe Mediterranean type, young as well as old RBCs are enzyme deficient. Recovery is signaled by the appearance of reticulocytes and a rise in hemoglobin.

Hepatitis A or B will often occur after exposure to an infected individual, and typically does not cause anemia as a presenting sign. Immunization against both in the first 2 years of life is standard practice in the United States. Gilbert syndrome (bilirubin uridine diphosphate glucuronosyltransferase [bilirubin-UGT]) presents with episodes of jaundice, but not anemia. Hemolytic-uremic syndrome (infection with *E coli* O157:H7) must be considered in a clinical situation similar to that presented, but the absence of uremia makes the diagnosis less likely.

367. The answer is b. (*Hay et al, pp 854-855. Kliegman et al, p 1051. Rudolph et al, pp 1590-1591.*) The child in the question has nevus sebaceous (aka nevus sebaceous of Jadassohn), a potentially premalignant condition found at birth or in early childhood. The treatment of choice is excision before adolescence. These lesions typically present as yellowish, hairless plaque on the scalp and less commonly on the face; some sources suggest about a 14% chance of tumor development, including basal cell carcinoma. If they are widespread, they may represent epidermal nevus syndrome which may have associated neurologic and orthopedic abnormalities; in such cases pediatric neurology or orthopedics consultation would be appropriate. Topical 1% hydrocortisone cream is commonly used for a variety of conditions including refractory seborrheic dermatitis on the scalp of a newborn (a greasy, flaky lesion); nevus sebaceous would not respond to such therapy. Topical application of 50% salicylic acid is one of the appropriate therapy for warts. Carbon dioxide laser therapy has been used to alter the surface appearance of nevus sebaceous, but the malignant potential of the deeper dermal tissue remains.

368. The answer is a. (*Hay et al, pp 58-59. Kliegman et al, pp 880-883. Rudolph et al, pp 226-227.*) The absence of a major blood-group incompatibility and the finding of a normal reticulocyte count argue strongly in favor of a recent fetomaternal transfusion, probably at the time of delivery. A Kleihauer-Betke stain for fetal hemoglobin-containing RBCs in the mother's blood would confirm the diagnosis. After birth, erythropoiesis ceases, and the progressive decline in hemoglobin values, reaching a nadir at 6-8 weeks of age, has been termed physiologic anemia of infancy. Iron-deficiency anemia can be seen in a formerly term infant between 9 and 24 months of age when the iron stores derived from circulating hemoglobin have been exhausted and an exogenous dietary source of iron has not been provided. Maternal iron deficiency, unless profound, does not result in fetal anemia. The manifestations of sickle cell disease typically do not appear until 4-6 months of life, coincident with the replacement of fetal hemoglobin with sickle hemoglobin.

369. The answer is e. (*Hay et al, pp 882-885. Kliegman et al, pp 2437-2443. Rudolph et al, pp 1620-1630.*) Children who present with symptoms that suggest leukemia with bone marrow failure require a bone marrow biopsy as soon as possible to clarify the diagnosis. Leukemias are the most common childhood malignancy, accounting for about 40% of all malignancies in children younger than 15 years of age. Two thousand children a year are diagnosed with acute lymphoblastic leukemia (ALL) in the United States. Most are between the ages of 2 and 6 years; a male predominance is noted. All of the symptoms in the vignette are typically found with leukemia: clinical and laboratory evidence of marrow failure with anemia and thrombocytopenia. The WBC count can be normal, high, or low. Automated systems initially may report blast forms as atypical lymphocytes. A reticulocyte count would reflect lack of marrow response, but is nonspecific. EBV can cause fever and listlessness with lymphadenopathy, but is usually not associated with significant anemia and thrombocytopenia as described here. Haptoglobin may help distinguish hemolytic from nonhemolytic anemia, and an antiplatelet antibody would not explain the anemia.

370. The answer is b. (*Hay et al, pp 899-901. Kliegman et al, pp 2464-2467, 3023-3026. Rudolph et al, pp 1644-1647.*) An abdominal mass is palpated in 85% of patients with Wilms tumor; abdominal pain is present in 40%, hypertension in about 60% (as in this case), and hematuria in 12%-24%. Because of the association of hemihypertrophy and aniridia with Wilms tumor, children with these findings should be followed with periodic physical examinations and abdominal sonograms, especially during their first 5 years. Wilms tumor and aniridia are associated with abnormalities on chromosome 11 as part of the WAGR syndrome (Wilms tumor, aniridia, genitourinary abnormalities, and mental retardation).

Neuroblastoma should also be considered in the differential diagnosis of abdominal mass, especially if fever, irritability, bone pain, limp, and diarrhea are present. In the case presented, however, the other features such as aniridia (and horseshoe kidney which was ultimately found on ultrasound) make this diagnosis less likely than Wilms tumor.

371. The answer is d. (*Hay et al, p 1011. Kliegman et al, pp 2473-2474. Rudolph et al, pp 1639-1641.*) Ewing sarcoma can occur in any bone of the body, especially in flat bones such as the pelvis, vertebrae, ribs, and skull. When they present in long bones (as in this case) they typically arise midshaft or in the diaphysis (in contrast to osteosarcoma which arises from metaphysis). Presenting signs are pain, swelling, and limitation of motion. The diagnosis is strongly suggested by radiographic findings of lytic bone lesions and the characteristic periosteal onion skinning. Confirmation is biopsy.

Osteomyelitis classically presents as a localized pain and systemic signs such as fever. Initially routine radiographs are normal, but eventually demonstrate a more lytic lesion; serial blood cultures and IV antibiotics are also indicated. Osteosarcoma presents similarly to Ewing sarcoma, but on radiograph the expected "sunburst" pattern of bone formation is seen. Rhabdomyosarcoma are soft tissues tumors with common sites of presentation including the head and neck, orbit, GU tract, and extremities. The radiographic findings described above would be unusual. Non-Hodgkin lymphoma classically presents in children more acutely than in adults with signs and symptoms depending on the location of the tumor. Commonly seen are pain; lymphadenopathy; cough, chest pain, and superior vena cava obstruction (supradiaphragmatic disease); and abdominal pain, constipation, and masses (subdiaphragmatic disease).

372. The answer is d. (*Hay et al, p 958. Kliegman et al, pp 2347-2349. Rudolph et al, pp 1562-1564.*) The patient has a classic presentation for methemoglobinemia. The most appropriate next step in his management is administration of intravenous methylene blue. Administration of methylene blue is contraindicated in patients with G6PD deficiency, so his negative family history is reassuring although close observation for improvement in cyanosis and lack of hemolysis is warranted. Of the other choices, ascorbic acid is an option for the patient with known G6PD deficiency or in areas where methylene blue is unavailable; its onset of action is considerably slower. Hyperbaric oxygen therapy and transfusion may be considered as adjunctive therapy in a patient with severe symptoms incompletely responsive to methylene blue. Intravenous hydration and alkalization of the urine are additional supportive measures, especially for a patient with severe symptoms.

373. The answer is b. (*Hay et al, pp 841-842. Kliegman et al, pp 2330-2333. Rudolph et al, pp 1553-1554.*) The patient in the question has a hemolytic anemia and spherocytes on the smear. An increased number of spherocytes on peripheral smear can be seen in such conditions as hyperthermia, hereditary spherocytosis, G6PD deficiency, or ABO incompatibility (but usually not Rh incompatibility). Neonatal hyperbilirubinemia can be seen in patients with hereditary spherocytosis. The hemolytic manifestations of ABO incompatibility and hereditary spherocytosis are very similar. The blood types of the mother and of the infant should be determined along with the results of a direct Coombs test on the infant and the presence or absence of a family history of hemolytic disease (spherocytosis). The negative maternal antibody screen and negative Coombs test points away from blood type incompatibility as the diagnosis.

Sickle cell disease would not be expected to cause problems in newborns because of protection by fetal hemoglobin. Hyperbilirubinemia can be caused by polycythemia, but the spherocytes would be unusual, and the patient in the question had anemia for a newborn. Pyruvate kinase deficiency can cause neonatal hemolytic anemia, but spherocytes are not commonly seen.

374. The answer is c. (*Hay et al, pp 867-868. Kliegman et al, pp 2384-2389. Rudolph et al, p 1576.*) In DIC, there is consumption of fibrinogen; factors II, V, and VIII; and platelets. Therefore, there is prolongation of PT, aPTT, and TT and a decrease in factor VIII level and platelet count. In addition, the titer of fibrin split production is usually increased. D-dimer is a fibrin breakdown product and may also be elevated in DIC.

The prolongation of PT, aPTT, and TT excludes the diagnosis of ITP. PT tests principally for factors I, II, V, VII, and X and is not prolonged in hemophilia A (factor VIII deficiency) or hemophilia B (factor IX deficiency). In vitamin K deficiency, there is a decrease in the production of factors II, VII, IX, and X, and PT and aPTT are prolonged. The TT, which tests for conversion of fibrinogen to fibrin, however, should be normal, and the platelet count should also be normal.

375. The answer is d. (*Hay et al, pp 866-867. Kliegman et al, pp 2390-2392. Rudolph et al, pp 1571-1573.*) Von Willebrand disease (vWD) is the most common heritable bleeding disorder, with some studies suggesting prevalence of 1%-2% in the general population. vWF participates in clot formation by adhering to areas of vascular damage and causing platelets to attach and activate. About 85% of cases of vWD are type I, resulting from decreased production of normal vWF. Several variants of type II vWD are described, with abnormal or dysfunctional vWF the etiology. Patients with type III, the most rare, have undetectable levels of vWF. In type I, DDAVP alone can transiently increase the levels of vWF three- to fivefold, so it is frequently used for acute bleeding episodes.

Aminocaproic acid interferes with fibrinolysis and stabilizes a clot (once it is already formed) by inhibiting plasmin, but does not replace DDAVP in treating patients with vWD. vWF concentrate and vWF with factor VIII are used in other types of vWD, but are not usually used first in type I for mild to moderate bleeding. IVIG is not used in vWD.

376. The answer is e. (*Hay et al, pp 788-790, 882-885, 901-903. Kliegman et al, pp 2471-2474. Rudolph et al, pp 1637-1639.*) The patient in the question likely has osteosarcoma, and the radiograph shows the expected "sunburst" pattern of bone formation. Osteosarcoma occurs most commonly in the second decade of life, and a bit more commonly in boys than in girls. It occurs in all ethnic groups (in contrast, Ewing sarcoma, another bone malignancy, rarely occurs in African Americans). The lesion of osteosarcoma is found in the metaphyses of long bones, and usually presents with local pain and swelling. Predisposing factors include a history of retinoblastoma, Li-Fraumeni syndrome, Paget disease, or radiotherapy. Any bone or joint "injury" not responding with conservative therapy within a short period of time should be evaluated.

"Growing pains" are commonly seen in the school-age child. They present with deep, aching pain, usually in the muscles of the leg. They are most common in the evening, gone by the morning, and do not cause joint swelling, redness, heat, or systemic signs or symptoms. The etiology is unknown, but, despite the name, it is not related to growing; family reassurance is indicated. Leukemia can present with deep bone pain, but often other signs and symptoms, such as bruising, adenopathy, hepatosplenomegaly, fever, and pallor, will also be seen; a bone marrow aspiration is indicated to diagnose this condition. Osteomyelitis can present as a localized pain, but systemic signs (such as fever) would also be expected.

The radiograph of osteomyelitis would eventually demonstrate a more lytic lesion; serial blood cultures and IV antibiotics are also indicated. Bone fractures can occur in the active child, but the presentation might include a better history of trauma, and the radiograph would demonstrate a fracture or callus formation rather than a sunburst pattern of bone growth.

377. The answer is d. (*Hay et al, pp 893-894. Kliegman et al, pp 2445-2452. Rudolph et al, pp 1632-1636.*) The patient in this question, especially with the pulmonary findings, may have Hodgkin disease. In underdeveloped countries, the peak incidence of Hodgkin disease is in children younger than 10 years of age; however, in developed countries, the peak incidence occurs in late adolescence and young adulthood. Systemic symptoms of Hodgkin disease include fever, night sweats, malaise, weight loss, and pruritus. The first step would involve a radiograph, which may show mediastinal mass suspicious for Hodgkin disease. Depending on the results of the radiograph, a biopsy of a node may be indicated, especially if the question of Hodgkin (or other malignancy) remained high.

A tuberculosis skin test may be indicated, but a trial of antituberculosis drugs without a chest radiograph, a positive purified protein derivative (PPD), or other diagnostic evaluation indicating tuberculosis would be unwise. In Hodgkin disease, the CBC is not diagnostic, but may show nonspecific findings of anemia, neutropenia, or thrombocytopenia; they are useful in the staging process after the diagnosis has been confirmed by biopsy. The presenting complaint with multiple groups of swollen nodes is unlikely to be related to cat-scratch disease (CSD); lymphadenopathy in CSD is typically unilateral and even singular.

378. The answer is c. (*Kliegman et al, pp 2461-2464. Rudolph et al, pp 1647-1651.*) Neuroblastoma, a tumor of the sympathetic nervous system, is the most common solid tumor outside the central nervous system. The tumor accounts for about 10% of all childhood malignancies, and about 15% of childhood malignancy deaths. Peak incidence is around 2 years of age, and most cases are diagnosed before the age of 5. Half of all tumors originate in the adrenal medulla, and another third originate in other abdominal sites such as paravertebral ganglia. Metastasis is common on presentation; sites include lymph nodes, bone cortex, bone marrow, orbits (resulting in periorbital ecchymoses), and liver.

Neuroblastoma has several paraneoplastic syndromes with which it is occasionally associated; because the presenting symptoms can be vague, diagnosis can be difficult and delayed. Neuroblastomas can secrete vaso-active intestinal peptide (VIP), causing persistent secretory diarrhea with dehydration and electrolyte disturbances. Another group of related symptoms includes opsoclonus and myoclonus (dancing eyes and dancing feet) in which the child has uncontrolled uncoordinated eye movement, myoclonic jerks, and cerebellar ataxia. Finally, because most neuroblastomas usually excrete catecholamines, they sometimes present with tachycardia, hypertension, flushing, sweating, and palpitations. Most children with extensive metastasis have a poor prognosis; for unknown reasons, children with metastasis limited to the liver, skin, and bone marrow (and not cortical bone), staged as 4S, tend to have a good long-term prognosis. Some infants with small adrenal masses will actually see spontaneous tumor reduction without therapy.

Pheochromocytoma is rare in pediatrics. Presenting signs and symptoms include headache, "racing heart," abdominal pain, dizziness, sustained hypertension (in contrast to adults where it is episodic), and instances of pallor and sweating. Rhabdomyosarcomas are the most common soft tissue sarcomas in children. The most common sites of presentation are the head and neck, orbit, GU tract, and extremities. The presentation is a mass. HVA and VMA are not elevated; diagnosis is made on typical biopsy features. Ovarian masses are unusual in children and ovarian malignancies are rare. Cysts may be an incidental finding on physical examination, or may be accompanied by nausea, vomiting, or urinary frequency or retention. HVA and VMA are not expected to be elevated with ovarian lesions; rather, α-fetoprotein, carcinoembryonic antigen (CEA), and antigen CA-125 are used to diagnose and follow therapy results. Wilms tumor classically presents as an abdominal mass with abdominal pain, hypertension, and frequently hematuria. It can be isolated, but often is associated with hemihypertrophy and aniridia.

379 to 382. The answers are 379-c, 380-d, 381-a, 382-b. (*Hay et al, pp 841-842, 848, 874. Kliegman et al, pp 2330-2333, 2336-2353. Rudolph et al, pp 1544, 1553-1554, 1558, 1563-1566.*) Howell-Jolly bodies (Photograph C) are small, spherical, nuclear remnants seen in the reticulocytes and, rarely, erythrocytes of persons who have no spleen (because of congenital asplenia or splenectomy) or who have a poorly functioning spleen (eg, in hyposplenism associated with sickle cell disease).

A target cell is an erythrocyte with a membrane that is too large for its hemoglobin content; a thin rim of hemoglobin at the cell's periphery and a small disk in the center give the cell a target-like appearance. Target cells, which are more resistant to osmotic fragility than are other erythrocytes, are seen in children who have α- or β-thalassemia, hemoglobin C disease, or liver disease (eg, obstructive jaundice or cirrhosis). Thalassemia major (Photograph D) presents in the second 6 months of life with severe anemia requiring transfusion, heart failure, hepatosplenomegaly, and weakness. Later, the typical facial deformities (maxillary hyperplasia and malocclusion) can be seen in a patient inadequately transfused. The diagnosis can be made on peripheral blood smear by the presence of poorly hemoglobinized normoblasts in addition to target cells in the peripheral blood.

Although hemoglobin C disease (Photograph B) is frequently a mild disorder, target cells constitute a far greater percentage of total RBCs than in thalassemia major. In the heterozygous state, no anemia or disease is noted, but target cells are seen. In the homozygous state, a moderately severe hemolytic anemia, reticulocytosis, and splenomegaly are seen, along with a smear containing a large number of target cells.

Uniformly small microspherocytes (< 6 μm in diameter) are typical of hereditary spherocytosis (Photograph A). Because of a decreased surface to volume ratio, these osmotically fragile RBCs have an increased density of hemoglobin. Although spherical RBCs also can appear in other hemolytic states (eg, immune hemolytic anemia, microangiography, ABO incompatibility, and hypersplenism), their cellular volume is only irregularly augmented. Patients with hereditary spherocytosis can present in the newborn period with anemia, hyperbilirubinemia, and reticulocytosis. They may remain asymptomatic until adulthood, when they develop symptoms. After infancy, hepatosplenomegaly and gallstones are common.

Endocrine, Metabolic, and Genetic Disorders

Questions

383. A 6-month old presents to the emergency center with seizures. The family denies fever and trauma, but does note the infant has had intermittent emesis for the last several weeks and has become progressively irritable and lethargic. They report no sick contacts or travel. The only recent change in the infant's routine has been the introduction of baby foods and fruit juice after the 6-month checkup 1 week ago. On physical examination the temperature is 37°C (98.6°F), heart rate is 120 beats per minute, respiratory rate is 25 breaths per minute, and blood pressure is 90/55 mm Hg. She is irritable, but consolable and mildly jaundiced. Head is without trauma. Neck is supple. The mucous membranes are pink, moist, and without lesions. Pupils are equally round and reactive; sclera are icteric. The chest is clear. Heart has a normal S1 and S2 without murmur. The abdomen is soft and nontender. The liver edge is palpable 3 cm below the costal margin. Neurologic examination is nonfocal. Laboratory studies show:

Sodium: 140 mEq/L
Potassium: 4.5 mEq/L
Chloride: 102 mEq/L
Bicarbonate: 22 mEq/L
Glucose: 50 mg/dL
Creatinine: 0.5 mEq/L
Blood urea nitrogen (BUN): 10 mEq/L
Aspartate aminotransferase (AST): 95 IU/L
Alanine aminotransferase (ALT): 110 IU/L
Albumin 2.5 g/dL
Urinalysis: specific gravity 1.010, glucose, protein, white cells negative; reducing substances positive

Which of the following is likely to explain this infant's condition?

a. Tyrosinemia
b. Galactosemia
c. Hereditary fructose intolerance
d. α_1-Antitrypsin deficiency
e. Glucose-6-phosphatase deficiency

384. A 12-year-old healthy girl has some dizziness while at synagogue. At the community ED where she is seen laboratory testing shows her to have a hemoglobin of 8 mg/dL, a white blood cell (WBC) count of 4000/μL, and a platelet count of 98,000/μL. Physical examination reveals an enlarged spleen. Her urine pregnancy test is negative, as are her chest radiographs and ECG. As she was no longer dizzy, she was discharged home to follow-up with you. She arrives 3 days later having sustained an injury to her thigh. You obtain a radiograph of her femur; the radiologist report is negative for fracture, but does note relative constriction of the diaphysis and flaring of the metaphysis of the distal femur. Putting together the clinical picture, you order a bone marrow biopsy and measure which of the following?

a. Sphingomyelinase activity
b. Hexosaminidase A
c. Sulfatase A
d. Glucocerebrosidase
e. Ceramide trihexosidase

385. A neonate is born to a woman who has received very little prenatal care. The mother is anxious, complains of heat intolerance and fatigue, and reports that she has not gained much weight despite having an increased appetite. On examination, the mother is tachycardic, has a tremor, and has fullness in her neck and in her eyes. The newborn is most likely at risk for development of which of the following?

a. Constipation
b. Heart failure
c. Macrocephaly
d. Third-degree heart block
e. Thrombocytosis

386. An otherwise healthy 8-year-old girl is brought to your office by her father because she has some acne, breast development, and fine pubic hair. Which of the following is the most appropriate next action in the care of this child?

a. Computerized tomographic (CT) scan of the ovaries
b. Administration of gonadotropin-releasing hormone (GnRH) analogues
c. Magnetic resonance imaging (MRI) of the brain
d. Evaluation of the home for missing birth control pills
e. Reassurance for the father

387. The parents of a 14-year-old boy are concerned about his short stature and lack of sexual development. By history, you learn that his birth weight and length were at the 50th percentile. His early childhood development was on par with his two siblings, and his school performance has been good. His past medical history is significant only for occasional upper respiratory tract infections and a broken finger when he was 6 years old. He takes no medicines and denies alcohol, tobacco, and other drugs. On physical examination vital signs are normal; blood pressure is 110/65 mm Hg. He is alert and in no distress. HEENT examination is normal; fundoscopic examination is normal. Neck is supple. The mucous membranes are pink, moist, and without lesions; dentition is good. The chest is clear; fine axillary hair is seen. Heart has a normal S1 and S2 without murmur. The abdomen is soft and nontender; he has no hepatosplenomegaly nor masses. Neurologic examination is nonfocal. GU examination shows a small amount of fine pubic hair and no scrotal pigmentation. Testes measure 4.0 cm^3 and his penis is 6 cm in length. His growth curve is shown in the photograph. In this situation, which of the following is the most appropriate course of action?

a. Measure pituitary gonadotropin.
b. Obtain an MRI of the pituitary area.
c. Order chromosome analysis.
d. Measure serum testosterone levels.
e. Reassure the parents that the boy is normal.

2–20 years: Boys
Stature-for-age and Weight-for-age percentiles

NAME _____

RECORD # _____

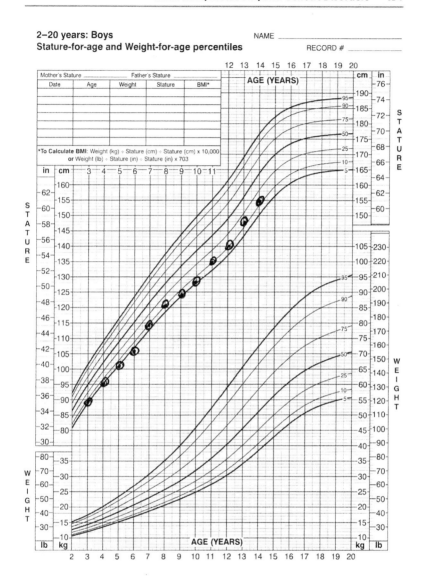

388. A neonatologist is called to the delivery room to evaluate a newborn that has cleft lip and palate, microphthalmia, and a 2-cm area on the scalp that appears to be void of skin and hair. The pregnancy was at term to a 23-year-old woman whose pregnancy was complicated by no prenatal care. Further examination in the neonatal intensive care unit demonstrates rocker-bottom feet, postaxial polydactyly, and a loud heart murmur. Chromosome analysis is likely to demonstrate which of the following?

a. 47XXY karyotype
b. Trisomy 13 karyotype
c. Trisomy 8 mosaicism karyotype
d. Trisomy 21 karyotype
e. XO karyotype

389. A 13-year-old asymptomatic girl is shown in the photograph. She states that the findings demonstrated began more than a year ago. Antithyroglobulin antibodies are positive; thyroid-stimulating hormone (TSH) is 3.1 mIU/L. Which of the following is the most likely diagnosis?

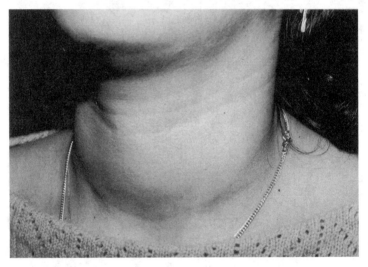

(Used with permission from Adelaide Hebert, MD.)

a. Iodine deficiency
b. Congenital hypothyroidism
c. Graves disease
d. Exogenous ingestion of Synthroid
e. Lymphocytic (Hashimoto) thyroiditis

390. A 14-year-old boy is seen in the weight management clinic as a referral from a pediatric pulmonologist who has diagnosed him with sleep apnea. His foster family knows little of his history other than he has relatively poor school performance. On physical examination his weight is well over the 99th percentile and his height is at the 10th percentile. He has almond-shaped eyes and strabismus. His abdomen is obese with a well-healed scar on the left side. He has small hands and feet, and is tanner stage 1 with overall hypogenitalism. His condition is most likely related to which of the following?

a. Microdeletion on chromosome 22q11.2
b. Submicroscopic deletion on chromosome 16p13.3
c. Microdeletion on chromosome 13q14
d. Loss of the paternally inherited allele of chromosome 15q11
e. Loss of the maternally inherited allele of chromosome 15q11

391. A 6-year-old boy is seen for the complaint of head banging, as well as biting of his hands, arms, and lips. He has a history of being normal at birth, but by about 3 months of age he was diagnosed with cerebral palsy after findings of hypotonia and failure to reach expected milestones were noted. His mother reports no problems with her pregnancy, but does report that he often had what appeared to be "orange sand" in his diapers which was attributed to concentrated urine reacting with baby powder. In the ensuing years he has continued to have poor development, cannot walk, and also has dystonia, chorea, and ballismus. Which of the following is the most likely mechanism of his disease?

a. Purine metabolism defect
b. Abnormal accumulation of glycogen
c. Fatty acid oxidation disorder
d. Lysosomal acid lipase deficiency
e. Defect in copper metabolism

392. A large-for-gestation age newborn is noted in the delivery room to have a large omphalocele. Further findings in the nursery include an enlarged tongue, hypertelorism, and unusual creases on his ears. His jitteriness prompts glucose checks, which require infusion of dextrose containing fluids to prevent recurring hypoglycemia. His mother had limited prenatal care, but states the pregnancy seemed to be uncomplicated. His constellation of findings is consistent with which of the following conditions?

a. Beckwith-Wiedemann syndrome
b. Sotos syndrome
c. Infant of a diabetic mother
d. Trisomy 13
e. Trisomy 18

393. A 2-week-old neonate is seen in the emergency center with the complaint of emesis and listlessness. His parents report a normal pregnancy without complications with care provided by a midwife. Delivery was at home, and he has had no medical visits since birth. The parents do not feel that he has gained much weight. On examination, you find a dehydrated, listless, and irritable neonate. He has significant jaundice. His abdominal examination is significant for both hepatomegaly and splenomegaly. Laboratory values include a total bilirubin of 15.8 mg/dL and a direct bilirubin of 5.5 mg/dL. His liver function tests are elevated and his serum glucose is 38 mg/dL. His admit urinalysis is negative for glucose but positive for gram-negative rods; his urine and his blood ultimately grow *Escherichia coli*. Which of the following nutritional considerations should be considered in this neonate?

a. Administration of high doses of vitamin B_6
b. Initial diet free of branched-chain amino acids
c. Lactose-free formula
d. Protein restriction and supplementation with citrulline
e. Initiation of a diet low or free of phenylalanine

394. You see in consultation a 2-year-old child from a local home for chronically ill children. He was born term and without reported complications, but significant developmental delay was noted in the first months of life. Early in his life he had significant vomiting and was once evaluated for pyloric stenosis although the testing for this was negative. He is now hyperactive, and has purposeless movements with rhythmic rocking and athetosis. The family notes that his only other illnesses have been mild seborrhea and eczema, which have got better over time. As you compare him to his two older siblings in the room, you note that his skin is of lighter color. You note a distinctive, unpleasant "mousy" smell in the room. Which of the following testing results is likely to explain this child's condition?

a. Elevated quantitative fecal fat levels
b. Elevated levels of blood or urine succinylacetone
c. Finding of high blood levels of methionine and homocystine
d. Elevated serum phenylalanine levels
e. Finding on plasma amino acid analysis elevations of leucine, isoleucine, valine, and alloisoleucine and depression of alanine

395. A 7-year-old boy is seen for a well-child checkup. His family, who has recently moved into the area, reports that he is doing well in school but they are concerned he is the shortest child in his class. He was born vaginally at term after an uneventful pregnancy to a 28-year-old gravida 3 woman. He met developmental milestones at the same rate as his brother who is 2 years older than him. On physical examination the temperature is 37°C (98.6°F), heart rate is 88 beats per minute, respiratory rate is 19 breaths per minute, and blood pressure is 90/72 mm Hg. Height is less than the 5th percentile and weight at the 5th percentile for age. He is a small but normal appearing child who is alert and in no distress. HEENT examination is normal. The chest is clear. Heart has a normal S1 and S2 without murmur. The abdomen is soft and nontender; no hepatosplenomegaly nor masses are noted. Neurologic examination is nonfocal. GU examination shows normal tanner 1 external. Which of the following findings is most likely related to his growth disorder?

a. Mutation in the fibroblast growth factor receptor 3 (FGFR3) gene
b. Deficiency of N-acetylgalactosamine-6-sulfatase (MPS-IVA) or β-galactosidase (MPS-IVB)
c. Low serum levels of triiodothyronine (T_3), thyroxine (T_4), and elevated serum TSH level
d. Reduced levels of insulin-like growth factor and insulin-like growth factor-binding protein
e. Mutation in the fibrillin-1 (FBN1) genes on chromosome 15

396. An 11-year-old boy comes to your office for a second opinion. His parents report progressive difficulty walking and weakness that started at about the age of 4 with a staggering gait, and since the last year he has been using a wheelchair. He has had multiple admissions to the local hospital for pneumonia. During the admission the treating physician ordered a serum IgM level, which was high, and serum IgE and IgA levels, which were very low. CD4+ T cells were reduced. HIV was negative. Expected examination findings in this child would include which of the following?

a. Dilated small blood vessels in the bulbar conjunctiva and on both his ears
b. Eczema with easy bruising
c. Retention of deciduous teeth, evidence of recurrent fractures, and oral candidiasis
d. Hypopigmented elliptical macules and angiofibromas on the malar region of the face
e. Multiple hyperpigmented macules with axillary freckling

397. A 1-year-old boy presents with the complaint from his parents of "not developing normally." He was the product of an uneventful term pregnancy and delivery, and reportedly was normal at birth. His previous health-care provider noted his developmental delay, and also noted that the child seemed to have an enlarged spleen and liver. On your examination, you confirm the developmental delay and the hepatosplenomegaly, and also notice that the child has short stature, macrocephaly, hirsutism, a coarse facies, and decreased joint mobility. Which of the following is the most likely etiology of his condition?

a. Beckwith-Wiedemann syndrome
b. Crouzon syndrome
c. Trisomy 18 (Edwards syndrome)
d. Jeune syndrome
e. Hurler syndrome

398. A 13-year-old boy comes to your office expressing concern about his height. He had first seen you a year prior for his routine checkup and a preparticipation sports physical for soccer (Growth curve photograph). Now in the eighth grade, all of his friends are taller than him, and he is at a disadvantage on the soccer field playing against much larger boys. After obtaining height information from his parents, you order a skeletal bone age radiograph. Which of the following results would allow you to assure him of an excellent prognosis for near-normal adult height?

a. A bone age of 9 years
b. A bone age of 13 years
c. A bone age of 15 years
d. Insulin-like growth factor levels elevated for chronologic age
e. Being at the 3rd percentile for weight

2–20 years: Boys
Stature-for-age and Weight-for-age percentiles

NAME _____

RECORD # _____

Mother's Stature _____		Father's Stature _____		
Date	Age	Weight	Stature	BMI*

*To Calculate BMI: Weight (kg) ÷ Stature (cm) ÷ Stature (cm) x 10,000
or Weight (lb) ÷ Stature (in) ÷ Stature (in) x 703

AGE (YEARS)

STATURE

WEIGHT

399. In counseling the parents of the child photographed, which of the following statements is true?

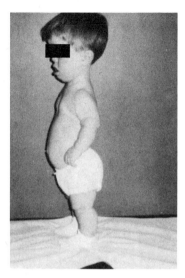

a. Delayed motor milestones is likely.
b. Normal intelligence is expected.
c. Infertility is a likely outcome.
d. Ventriculoperitoneal shunting for hydrocephalus will likely be required.
e. Ultimate normal height and weight is expected.

400. An otherwise healthy and developmentally normal 7-year-old child is brought to you to be evaluated because he is the shortest child in his class. Careful measurements of his upper and lower body segments demonstrate normal body proportions for his age. Which of the following disorders of growth should remain in your differential?

a. Achondroplasia
b. Morquio disease
c. Hypothyroidism
d. Growth hormone deficiency
e. Marfan syndrome

401. The 16-month-old male child was recently brought from a developing country to the United States (Photograph). The family history reveals that his father had an eye and a leg removed. Which of the following is the most likely diagnosis?

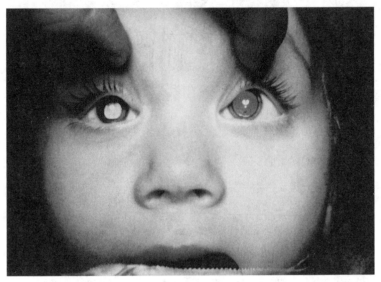

(Used with permission from Kathryn Musgrove, MD.)

a. Coloboma of the choroid
b. Retinal detachment
c. Nematode endophthalmitis
d. Retinoblastoma
e. Persistent hyperplastic primary vitreous

402. A 4-year-old child has intellectual disability, shortness of stature, brachydactyly (especially of the fourth and fifth digits), and obesity with round facies and short neck. The child is followed by an ophthalmologist for subcapsular cataracts, and has previously been noted to have cutaneous and subcutaneous calcifications, as well as perivascular calcifications of the basal ganglia. This patient is most likely to have which of the following features?

a. Hypercalcemia
b. Hypophosphatemia
c. Elevated concentrations of parathyroid hormone
d. Advanced height age
e. Decreased bone density, particularly in the skull

403. A 15-year-old boy has been immobilized in a double hip spica cast for 6 weeks after having fractured his femur in a skiing accident. He has become depressed and listless during the past few days and has complained of nausea and constipation. He is found to have microscopic hematuria and a blood pressure of 150/100 mm Hg. Which of the following is the most appropriate course of action?

a. Begin fluoxetine (Prozac) 10 mg daily and increase as needed to 20 mg after several weeks.
b. Apply a 24-hour ambulatory blood pressure monitor.
c. Collect urine for measurement of the calcium to creatinine ratio.
d. Order a renal sonogram and intravenous pyelogram (IVP).
e. Begin lisinopril 0.1 mg/kg/d.

404. A 7-year-old boy is seen in the metabolic clinic. He has bitemporal narrowing, an upturned nares, ptosis, a small chin, cryptorchidism, and syndactyly of the second and third toes. He has had poor growth and has severe developmental delay. Serum cholesterol level is < 20 mg/dL. Which of the following is the most likely diagnosis?

a. Wolman disease
b. Niemann-Pick disease
c. Familial dysbetalipoproteinemia
d. Smith-Lemli-Opitz syndrome
e. Gaucher disease

405. A 7-day-old boy is admitted to a hospital for vomiting. His parents report that he was born vaginally at term after an uneventful pregnancy; he was discharged after about 24 hours of age having passed stool and urine. Birth weight was 3200 g (7 lb), and discharge weight was 3000 g (6.6 lb). He was taking 20 to 30 cc of infant formula in the hospital and for the first days at home, but over the previous 24 hours his intake has decreased to about 15 cc/feeding. On physical examination the temperature is 37°C (98.6°F), heart rate is 180 beats per minute, respiratory rate is 45 breaths per minute, and blood pressure is 80/58 mm Hg. Weight is 2720 g (6 lb). He is sleepy and somewhat difficult to arouse. Head is normocephalic with a sunken fontanelle. Mucous membranes are dry. The chest is clear with hyper-pigmentation of the nipples. Heart has tachycardia with a normal S1 and S2 without murmur. The abdomen is soft and nontender; no hepatospleno-megaly or masses are noted. Neurologic examination is nonfocal. Skin is without lesions; capillary refill is 5 seconds. Laboratory data show:

Sodium: 119 mEq/L
Potassium: 9.1 mEq/L
Chloride: 90 mEq/L
Bicarbonate: 15 mEq/L
Glucose: 35 mg/dL

Which of the following testing is most likely to result in this neonate's diagnosis?

a. Ultrasound of the pylorus
b. Measurement of his 17-hydroxyprogrosterone level
c. Measurement of his T_3, T_4, and TSH levels
d. MRI of the pituitary
e. Chemical analysis of the commercial formula being fed to the newborn

406. A 14-year-old boy presents with the complaint of "breast swelling." The boy reports that he has been in good health and without other problems, but has noticed over the past month or so that his left breast has been "achy" and that he has now noticed some mild swelling under the nipple. He has never seen discharge; the other breast has not been swelling; and he denies trauma. Your examination demonstrates a quarter-sized area of breast tissue under the left nipple that is not tender and has no discharge. The right breast has no such tissue. He has a normal genitourinary examination, and is Tanner stage 3. Which of the following is the best next course of action?

a. CT scan of the pituitary gland
b. Measurement of serum luteinizing hormone (LH) and follicle-stimulating hormone (FSH)
c. Measurement of serum testosterone
d. Reassurance of the normalcy of the condition
e. Chromosomes

407. An infant is brought to a hospital because her wet diapers turn black when they are exposed to air. Physical examination is normal. Urine is positive both for reducing substance and when tested with ferric chloride. This disorder is caused by a deficiency of which of the following?

a. Homogentisic acid oxidase
b. Phenylalanine hydroxylase
c. L-histidine ammonia lyase
d. Ketoacid decarboxylase
e. Isovaleryl-CoA dehydrogenase

408. An 18-year-old girl has hepatosplenomegaly, an intention tremor, dysarthria, dystonia, and deterioration in her school performance. She also developed abnormal urine with excess glucose, protein, and uric acid. She has a several-year history of elevated liver enzymes of unknown etiology. Which of the following best explains her condition?

a. Indian childhood cirrhosis
b. α_1-Antitrypsin deficiency
c. Menkes syndrome
d. Dubin-Johnson syndrome
e. Wilson disease

409. A 3-month-old infant without significant past history was brought to the emergency center by her mother with a generalized tonic-clonic seizure. She is found to have glucose of 5 mg/dL. After correction of her hypoglycemia, she is admitted to your service for further evaluation. Several hours later, her nurse calls to tell you that her bedside glucose check was now 10 mg/dL. You order laboratory work suggested by the pediatric endocrinology team and again correct the infant's hypoglycemia. The results of the laboratory tests you drew include an elevated serum insulin level of 50 μU/mL, and a low IGFBP-1 (plasma insulin-like growth factor binding protein-1). C-peptide levels are not detectable. Which of the following is the likely cause of this infant's recurrent hypoglycemia?

a. Nesidioblastosis (persistent hyperinsulinemic hypoglycemia of infancy)
b. Pancreatitis
c. Beckwith-Wiedemann syndrome
d. Galactosemia
e. Factitious hypoglycemia

410. An 11-year-old boy is seen in the local high school gym during a mass sports physical event. He reports that he has been in good health, takes no medications, has had no previous sports injuries but was hospitalized 1 year ago for a spontaneous pneumothorax. On physical examination vital signs are normal, height is 99th percentile, and weight is 65th percentile. Hearing is normal and his corrected vision is 20/20. He has a high-arched palate with dental crowding, pectus excavatum, and somewhat hypermobile joints. Heart has a midsystolic click. His echocardiogram is likely to show which of the following?

a. Atrial septal defect
b. Ventricular septal defect
c. Hypertrophic cardiomyopathy
d. Aortic root dilation
e. Coarctation of the aorta

411. A very upset mother brings her 8-month-old infant to the emergency room because he will not move his leg. She reports that when she was carrying him to the car about half an hour ago, she slipped on some ice and fell on top of him. The mother, an 18-year-old African American woman, has been exclusively breast-feeding her infant. She has only recently started him on cereals, and has not supplemented his diet with vitamins. A radiograph of the infant's leg is shown in the photograph. Which of the following laboratory findings would be expected?

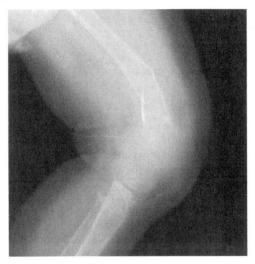

a. Hypocalcemia
b. Hypophosphaturia
c. Reduced serum alkaline phosphatase
d. Hypocalciuria
e. Hyperphosphatemia

412. A healthy 18-year-old girl is seen for routine checkup. She reports that over the previous several months she has been having hoarseness and difficulty swallowing. On physical examination you note that she has a lump at the base of her neck just above her larynx, which is especially notable when she swallows. She has had no fever, weight loss, or other findings. Family history is positive for her mother and two aunts that died at a young age of some type of "throat cancer". With further evaluation of this young lady, which of the following is most likely to be an associated finding?

a. Hypertension
b. Reduced serum calcitonin level
c. Hypocalcemia
d. Hypercalciuria
e. Reduced serum carcinoembryonic antigen (CEA) levels

413. A 1-day-old normal-appearing neonate develops tetany and convulsions. He was born at 34 weeks' gestation with Apgar scores of 2 and 4 (at 1 and 5 minutes, respectively) to a woman whose pregnancy was complicated by diabetes mellitus and pregnancy-induced hypertension. Which of the following serum chemistry values is likely to be the explanation for his condition?

a. Serum bicarbonate level of 22 mEq/dL
b. Serum calcium of 6.2 mg/dL
c. Serum glucose of 45 mg/dL
d. Serum magnesium level of 5.0 mg/dL
e. Intracranial hemorrhage

414. A small-for-gestation-age neonate is born at 30 weeks' gestation. At 1 hour of age, his serum glucose is noted to be 20 mg/dL (normally more than 40 mg/dL). Which of the following is the most likely explanation for hypoglycemia in this neonate?

a. Inadequate stores of nutrients
b. Adrenal immaturity
c. Pituitary immaturity
d. Insulin excess
e. Glucagon deficiency

415. A 13-year-old boy is seen for a well-child visit. He is accompanied by his father, whom you have not seen for several years, as his mother usually brings him to the office. You note the father to be moving slowly and rigidly, is unstable when he walks, and has some challenges in speaking fluently. Upon questioning the father reports he is followed by a neurologist for this condition which first began with uncontrolled movements of his arms that have progressed to his current state. You are concerned that your adolescent patient is at risk for a genetically inherited condition caused by which of the following?

a. Defect of paternal chromosome 15
b. Defect of maternal chromosome 15
c. Triplet repeat expansion disorder
d. Sex chromosome imbalance
e. Karyotype mosaicism

416. A 4-year-old child is seen for a well-child examination. He was delivered vaginally after a term, uneventful pregnancy. The mother reports that his development continues to be normal and on par with her other two children from a previous marriage. His past medical history is positive for peanut allergy for which he has been prescribed an EpiPen, three bouts of otitis media, and three broken bones. Mom reports the first fracture was on his left arm at 1 year of age when he tripped over one of his toys, the second when he was about 2 years of age when mom noted after returning from the playground with his father that his leg was deformed, and the most recent was his arm about 6 weeks ago after falling from his bicycle. She reports all healed well. On physical examination vital signs are normal. Weight is at the 45th percentile, length and head circumference is at the 50th percentile. He is awake, alert, and active. Head is normocephalic. Mucous membranes are moist; teeth are without caries. Ear canals are clean and tympanic membranes are clear. Pupils are equally round and reactive, sclera are azure, red reflex normal, conjunctiva without lesions. Nose is patent without discharge. Neck is supple with adenopathy. The chest is clear. Heart has regular rate and rhythm without murmur. The abdomen is soft and nontender; no hepatosplenomegaly or masses are noted. Neurologic examination is normal. Skin is without lesions. No boney or joint abnormalities are noted. Which of the following is the most likely explanation for his condition?

a. Physical abuse
b. Defect in COL1A1 allele
c. Normal childhood development
d. Dietary deficiency of vitamin D
e. Impaired renal production of 1,25-dihydroxycholecalciferol

417. A 3-month-old girl is seen with her family for failure to thrive. The family reports the child to be a challenge to feed since birth, seemingly uninterested in eating, and to have frequent non-projectile vomiting. They bring birth records that show her to have been a term, vaginal delivery after an uneventful pregnancy. Birth weight was 1900 g (4 lb). Her 8-year-old sister is in the room. She is small in size, had similar feeding challenges, and currently is noted to have erythematous plaques and telangiectasia in a butterfly pattern over her face, which her family says occurs when she gets into the sun. Which of the following is the most likely explanation for these findings?

a. Systemic lupus erythematosus
b. Bloom syndrome
c. Ataxia telangiectasia
d. Erythropoietic protoporphyria
e. Cockayne syndrome

418. Since about 3 months of age a 1-year-old girl has had repeated episodes of hypoglycemic seizures and bouts of lactic acidosis. She has a protuberant abdomen due to her massive hepatomegaly, a doll-like facies, thin extremities, and is short for her age. Upon drawing her blood, you are struck by the "milky" appearance. Which of the following is the most likely diagnosis?

a. von Gierke disease
b. Infantile Pompe disease
c. McArdle disease
d. Hers disease
e. Tarui disease

Questions 419 to 424

All the conditions below are associated with an overweight state or abnormal fat distribution. For each of the clinical findings that follow, select the condition with which it is most likely to be associated. Each lettered option may be used once, more than once, or not at all.

a. Kallmann syndrome
b. Prader-Willi syndrome
c. Down syndrome
d. Laurence-Moon-Biedl syndrome
e. Cushing syndrome
f. Hypothyroidism
g. Leptin deficiency
h. Pseudohypoparathyroidism
i. Polycystic ovary syndrome
j. Nephrotic syndrome
k. Cohen syndrome
l. Maternal uniparental disomy of chromosome 14
m. Type 2 diabetes
n. Williams syndrome

419. A 15-year-old defensive lineman for his high school football team whose mother reports that his shoulder pads have permanently stained his neck.

420. A 6-day-old boy with severe hypotonia, cryptorchidism, scrotal hypoplasia, and a disinterest in feeding since birth.

421. A 5-year-old boy with intellectual disability has a very gregarious and affectionate personality. At birth he was noted to have an elfin-like facies, hypercalcemia, and supravalvular aortic stenosis.

422. A 5-day-old girl with brachydactyly, round facies, and short neck.

423. A 15-year-old girl with menstrual irregularities and hirsutism.

424. A 14-year-old boy with hypogonadism and night blindness with retinitis pigmentosa.

Questions 425 to 428

For each of the following disorders, select the serum concentrations (mEq/L) of sodium (Na^+) and potassium (K^+) with which it is most likely to be associated in a dehydrated patient. Each lettered option may be used once, more than once, or not at all.

a. Na^+ 118, K^+ 7.5
b. Na^+ 125, K^+ 3.0
c. Na^+ 134, K^+ 6.0
d. Na^+ 144, K^+ 2.9
e. Na^+ 155, K^+ 5.5
f. Na^+ 140, K^+ 4.0

425. An 11-year-old boy has been involved in an automobile accident. During his recovery in the intensive care unit he is noted to have large amounts of what appears to be dilute urine output.

426. A 1-year-old girl has recently moved into your area. The family members who bring her to see you have no paperwork and they seem to be developmentally delayed. You can glean from them that the girl, like several other family members, urinates a great deal, has had multiple hospitalizations for dehydration, and her previous doctors have told the family to "make sure she gets plenty to drink."

427. A 4-year-old boy is noted to have blood pressure measurements about 30 mm Hg higher than normal but appears to be otherwise fine. On close evaluation of the family history, you find that many in his family have had the early onset hypertension and several have had strokes. In addition to abnormal electrolytes, this child also has elevated serum levels of aldosterone but low plasma renin activity.

428. An 8-year-old boy has a diagnosis of Addison disease. However, he is on vacation at his grandmother's house when he is involved in an automobile crash and sustains a fractured femur; his grandmother is intubated in the surgical intensive care unit. While his family is arriving from out of state, he develops a number of electrolyte abnormalities.

Questions 429 to 435

Patients with genetic disorders or those affected by specific teratogens *in utero* typically have certain characteristic dysmorphic features. Match the physical description with the genetic or teratogenic abnormality. Each lettered option may be used once, more than once, or not at all.

a. Isotretinoin
b. Trisomy 21 (Down syndrome)
c. Fragile X syndrome
d. Trisomy 18 (Edwards syndrome)
e. Phenytoin
f. Marfan syndrome
g. Ehlers-Danlos
h. Valproic acid
i. Holt-Oram syndrome
j. Diabetic embryopathy
k. Tetracycline
l. Fetal alcohol syndrome
m. Turner syndrome (45,XO)
n. Klinefelter syndrome (47,XXY)
o. Lithium
p. Angiotensin-converting enzyme inhibitors (ACE)

429. A 10-year-old boy with hypermobile joints and poor wound healing.

430. A 6-year-old girl with cognitive delay, a blowing holosystolic heart murmur, short stature, round face, bilateral trans-palmar crease, upslanting palpebral fissures, small ears, and epicanthal folds.

431. A newborn has low sloping shoulders, right hand attached at elbow with agenesis of the forearm, cardiac abnormalities, missing chest wall musculature, and a bifid thumb.

432. A 2-year-old boy, less than the 5th percentile for weight and height, is in early childhood intervention for developmental delay. He has a short nose, thin upper lip with thin vermillion border, a ventricular septal defect (VSD), and short palpebral fissures.

433. A 14-year-old girl with short stature, thick neck, minimal pubertal development, repaired coarctation of the aorta, and normal intelligence.

434. A small for gestation age newborn with a large VSD, clenched hands, cleft palate, rounded heels, and a horseshoe kidney.

435. A newborn with hypoglycemia, hypocalcemia, and hypoplastic lower extremities.

Endocrine, Metabolic, and Genetic Disorders

Answers

383. The answer is c. (*Hay et al, p 999. Kliegman et al, pp 727-728. Rudolph et al, pp 608-609.*) The patient in the question has new symptoms of emesis, irritability, and lethargy along with low serum glucose and albumin, elevated serum liver function studies, and reducing substances in the urine. These changes are likely due to hereditary fructose intolerance, manifest only when fructose in fruit juice is provided in the diet. Galactosemia, fructosemia, tyrosinosis, and glucose-6-phosphatase deficiency represent diseases in which a congenital deficiency of enzyme causes an interruption of a normal metabolic pathway and an accumulation of metabolic precursors that damage vital organs. Galactose (found in milk) and fructose (found in fruit juices) produce urinary reducing substances in their respective disorders. The mode of inheritance of galactosemia, fructosemia, and most forms of glucose-6-phosphatase deficiency is autosomal recessive. In galactosemia and fructosemia, errors in carbohydrate metabolism cause the accumulation of toxic metabolites when specific dietary sugars are introduced (lactose in galactosemia; fructose and sucrose in fructosemia). Exclusion of the offending carbohydrate from the diet will prevent liver damage. In tyrosinemia type I, or tyrosinosis, the accumulation of tyrosine and its metabolites is associated with severe dysfunction of the liver, kidney, and CNS. Manifestations of acute liver failure can appear in infancy. A chronic form of the disorder presents as progressive cirrhosis and leads to liver failure or hepatoma. Dietary management does not prevent liver disease. Glucose-6-phosphatase deficiency (also known as glycogen storage disease type 1, or von Gierke disease) often presents at 3-4 months of age with failure to thrive, hypoglycemia, hepatomegaly, and acidosis. α_1-Antitrypsin deficiency causes liver disease through accumulation of an abnormal protein, caused by a single amino acid substitution in the SERPINA1 gene on the long arm of chromosome 14. It has a variable and bimodal presentation, but the following are common in infancy: cholestasis; bleeding into the CNS, gastrointestinal (GI) tract, or at the umbilical stump; and elevation of transaminase concentrations. Affected children may have chronic hepatitis with cirrhosis and portal hypertension; pulmonary symptoms such as emphysema tend to dominate in adults.

384. The answer is d. (*Hay et al, pp 746-747, 1013. Kliegman et al, pp 708-710. Rudolph et al, pp 634-635, 2252-2253.*) The most common lysosomal storage disease, Gaucher disease is characterized by β-glucocerebrosidase deficiency, which causes an abnormal accumulation of glucocerebroside in the reticuloendothelial system. Bone marrow aspirate shows the typical Gaucher cells engorged with glucocerebroside. Replacement of marrow with these cells leads to anemia, leukopenia, and thrombocytopenia. The liver and spleen can also be involved. Serum acid phosphatase activity is elevated. X-ray evaluation demonstrates an Erlenmeyer-flask appearance of the long bones. The diagnosis of Gaucher disease is confirmed by reduced glucocerebrosidase activity in peripheral leukocytes, in cultured skin fibroblasts, and in liver cells. While a bone marrow may be performed as part of the evaluation of pancytopenia, the diagnosis can be made on enzyme analysis alone. Prenatal diagnosis by enzyme analysis is now possible. In the most common form of Gaucher disease, type I, there is no involvement of the CNS. Therefore, MRI of the brain is not indicated. Enzyme replacement therapy is available.

Sphingomyelinase deficiency causes type A Niemann-Pick disease; hexosaminidase A deficiency causes Sandhoff disease; sulfatase A deficiency causes juvenile metachromatic leukodystrophy; and serum trihexosidase deficiency causes Fabry disease.

385. The answer is b. (*Hay et al, pp 957-958. Kliegman et al, pp 2684-2685. Rudolph et al, p 2040.*) The neonate is likely at risk for neonatal thyrotoxicosis caused by transplacental passage of thyroid stimulating hormone receptor antibodies (TSHR-Ab) from the mother to the fetus. Neonatal thyrotoxicosis usually disappears within 2-4 months as the concentration of maternally acquired TSHR-Ab falls. Unlike TSHR-Ab, TSH does not cross the placenta. All forms of thyrotoxicosis are more common in girls, with the exception of neonatal thyrotoxicosis, which has an equal sex distribution. Symptoms include tachycardia and tachypnea, irritability and hyperactivity, low-birth weight with microcephaly, severe vomiting and diarrhea, thrombocytopenia, jaundice, hepatosplenomegaly, and heart failure. In severely affected infants, the disease can be fatal if not treated vigorously and promptly. Third-degree heart block is not a feature of this disease, but is sometimes seen in infants born to mothers with systemic lupus erythematosus.

386. The answer is e. (*Hay et al, pp 112-113, 969-971. Kliegman et al, pp 2614-2615. Rudolph et al, pp 2077-2082.*) The patient in the question appears to have "true sexual precocity," implying that the gonads have matured in response to the secretion of pituitary gonadotropins and have begun secreting sex steroids, causing the development of secondary sexual characteristics. Ovarian tumors and exogenous estrogens, which suppress the function of the pituitary gland, do not cause true precocious puberty; rather, they cause isolated premature thelarche and/or vaginal bleeding without pubic hair, body odor, and acne. In girls, the most common form of true precocious puberty is idiopathic and is thought to be caused by early maturation of an otherwise normal hypothalamic-pituitary-gonadal feedback system. In boys, true precocious puberty is relatively rare and is more likely to be caused by lesions of the CNS and would require imaging of the brain. Hypothalamic hamartomas are a possible cause of precocious puberty in both genders and produce GnRH; surgery for these hamartomas usually is not indicated, since GnRH analogs usually are effective therapy. In general the onset of puberty in girls is between the ages of 10 and 14 with African American girls being earlier than Caucasians, while in boys it is between 12 and 16. The onset of puberty in Caucasian girls before age 7, African American girls before age 6, and in boys before age 9 is considered precocious and requires evaluation.

387. The answer is e. (*Hay et al, pp 946, 973. Kliegman et al, p 1643. Rudolph et al, pp 2082-2083.*) A child with constitutionally short stature and delayed puberty will have a consistent rate of growth below, but parallel to, the average for his or her age, whereas patients with organic disease do not follow a given percentile but progressively deviate from their prior growth percentile. Knowledge of the patterns of growth and sexual maturation of family members is helpful, because such patterns are often familial. Reassurance that normal sexual development will occur and that a normal adult height (usually a midparental height) will be attained is frequently the only therapy indicated.

Puberty is said to be delayed in boys if physical changes are not apparent by 14 years of age. Identification of the earliest signs of sexual maturation by means of careful physical examination avoids unnecessary workup. In this case, measurement of pituitary gonadotropins is unnecessary because the child already shows evidence of pubertal development (a penile length of more than 2.5 cm and a testicular volume more than 3.0 cm^3). The single most useful laboratory test is the radiographic determination of bone age. In those of constitutionally short stature with delayed pubertal maturation, the bone age is equal to the height age, both of which are behind chronologic age. In familial short stature, bone age is greater than the height age and equal to chronologic age. In a child at any age, the administration of human chorionic gonadotropin (hCG) will stimulate interstitial cells of testes to produce testosterone, thereby serving as a method of assessing testicular function. The finding of testicular enlargement is evidence of pituitary secretion of gonadotropins and of testicular responsiveness and obviates the need for administration of hCG. Elevated serum gonadotropins are found in children 12 years of age or older who have primary hypogonadism due to Klinefelter syndrome (for whom chromosomes would be diagnostic), or bilateral gonadal failure from trauma or infection. Because the secretion of gonadotropins is not constant but occurs in spurts, children with constitutional delay of puberty may have normal or low levels of gonadotropins.

388. The answer is b. (*Hay et al, pp* 1151-1154. *Kliegman et al, pp 610-616. Rudolph et al, pp 691-697.*) Trisomy 13 occurs in about 1:5000-12,000 live births. In most cases, all or a majority of the extra chromosome 13 is present. Findings at birth may include cleft lip and palate (60%-80%), cutis aplasia, microphthalmia, microcephaly, congenital heart disease (80% of cases), clinodactyly, and polydactyly. Failure to thrive, seizures, severe developmental delay, and death in the first 6 months of life are common.

Findings at birth in trisomy 18 might include measuring small for gestational age, microcephaly, narrow head, micrognathia, low-set ears, short sternum, rocker bottom feet, clinodactyly, and a variety of cardiac defects. Cleft lip/palate is less common; cutis aplasia is not a common feature. Klinefelter syndrome boys (47XXY) at birth typically appear normal. Later they are tall with long arms and legs and a eunuchoid body habitus. They have delayed and/or incomplete puberty with firm and fibrotic testes. Learning disabilities (esp. language) is common. Infants with Trisomy 8 mosaicism karyotype have long faces with high forehead, an upturned nose, everted lower lip, micrognathia, low-set ears, and deep plantar and palmar creases.

Down syndrome has many diagnostic features at birth, including short length, microcephaly, centrally placed hair whorl, small ears, redundant skin on the nape of the neck, upslanting palpebral fissures, epicanthal folds, flat nasal bridge, Brushfield spots, protruding tongue, short and broad hands, simian creases, widely spaced first and second toe, and hypotonia. Cardiac lesions are found in 30%-50% of children with Down syndrome, including endocardial cushion defect (30%), VSD (30%), and tetralogy of Fallot (about 30%). At birth, duodenal atresia is a common finding. It causes bilious emesis and a characteristic plain abdominal radiographic finding of a double bubble (dilatation of the stomach and the proximal duodenum).

Common features of Turner syndrome (XO karyotype) at birth include female phenotype, webbed neck, lymphedema of the hands and the feet, and coarctation of the aorta. Later they develop short stature, have sexual infantilism, streak gonads, and a broad chest, and the low hairline becomes more apparent.

389. The answer is e. (*Hay et al, pp 956-957. Kliegman et al, pp 2675-2680. Rudolph et al, pp 2037-2038.*) The photograph shows thyromegaly. Lymphocytic thyroiditis is an organ-specific autoimmune disease characterized by lymphocytic infiltration of the thyroid gland, with or without goiter. It is the most common cause of juvenile hypothyroidism in developed countries, peaking in adolescence, and affecting as many as 1% of school children. The condition is four to seven times more prevalent in girls than in boys and may persist for many years without symptoms. Patients are initially euthyroid (with the occasional child having elevated TSH levels) but, with the eventual atrophy of the gland, they become hypothyroid (decreased triiodothyronine [T_3] and T_4, elevated TSH). Spontaneous remission can occur in one-third of the affected adolescents. Hashimoto thyroiditis is not related to endemic goiter caused by iodine deficiency. Autoimmune thyroiditis is associated with many other autoimmune disorders; its association with Addison disease and/or insulin-dependent diabetes mellitus is called polyglandular autoimmune syndrome type II. Family clusters of autoimmune thyroiditis are common; nearly 50% of the patients have siblings with antithyroid antibodies.

Children with Graves disease will be symptomatic, with increasing nervousness, tachycardia, palpitations, weight loss despite an increased appetite, and exophthalmos. In Graves disease TSH is suppressed. Congenital hypothyroidism would have been manifested before the age of 13. Iodine deficiency can cause goiter and hypothyroidism, but this condition has been almost eliminated in developed countries with iodine supplementation.

390. The answer is d. (*Hay et al, p 1161. Kliegman et al, pp 602-603. Rudolph et al, pp 681-682.*) The child in the question likely has Prader-Willi syndrome, a disorder consisting of profound hypotonia and poor feeding in the newborn period (often requiring a feeding tube as hinted at by the scar on the abdomen). After the newborn period hypogonadism, hyperphagia, hypomentia, and obesity become apparent. The short stature is likely related to growth hormone deficiency, another common finding with this condition. The etiology is most commonly a paternally-acquired deletion of a portion of chromosome 15; the maternally acquired loss in this region is associated with Angelman syndrome. Microdeletion on chromosome 22q11.2 results in a variety of signs and symptoms historically known as DiGeorge syndrome, velocardiofacial syndrome, or Shprintzen syndrome. Submicroscopic deletion on chromosome 16p13.3 is associated with Rubinstein-Taybi syndrome. A 13q14 microdeletion is associated with retinoblastoma.

391. The answer is a. (*Hay et al, p 1125. Kliegman et al, pp 747-748. Rudolph et al, p 671.*) The child in the question demonstrates a classic presentation of Lesch-Nyhan disease, a purine recycling defect linked to a mutation in the HPRT1 gene. Such children usually are born normal, developing hypotonia and developmental delay by 3 months or so. Affected children typically are wheel-chair bound, have chorea and ballismus, and in classic cases have self-injury behavior including head banging and biting of extremities, lips, and tongue. The "orange sand" in the diaper was probably uric acid accumulation. Abnormal accumulation of glycogen (for instance, von Gierke disease) would present at about 3 months of age with poor feeding (especially at night), seizures due to hypoglycemia, lactic acidosis, and hyperuricemia. Older children develop deposition in the liver leading to a protuberant abdomen. The most common fatty acid oxidation disorder is medium-chain-acyl-CoA dehydrogenase deficiency, a condition that is similar in frequency to PKU which, unfortunately, often presented as a sudden infant death with the findings of fatty liver at autopsy. This condition is included in most newborn screening programs. Lysosomal acid lipase deficiency includes a variety of conditions in which excess amounts of lipid accumulate throughout the body. The most severe forms begin in infancy, while other forms develop in childhood or later. Hepatosplenomegaly, malabsorption, diarrhea, vomiting, and cirrhosis of the liver are common presenting findings. The prototypical defect in copper metabolism is Menke syndrome which is characterized by sparse, kinky hair in the failure to thrive child who fails to meet expected milestones. Hypotonia, seizures, and early death are typically seen.

392. The answer is a. (*Hay et al, p 1161. Kliegman et al, pp 2747-2748. Rudolph et al, p 270.*)

The constellation of signs described suggest Beckwith-Wiedemann syndrome, a condition linked to abnormal gene expression on chromosome 11p15. In addition to the omphalocele, macroglossia, hypertelorism, unusual ear creases and large-for-gestational status, affected children frequently have hemihypertrophy. Hypoglycemia is common. Affected children have a significantly increased incidence of cancer, especially Wilms tumor, and require abdominal ultrasounds every 3 months until about age 8 years. In addition to overgrowth in childhood, Sotos syndrome patients have characteristic facies including long, narrow face; high forehead; small, pointed chin; and flushed cheeks. Infants born to mother with uncontrolled diabetes frequently are large and are at risk for hypoglycemia due to excess infant insulin production owing to maternal hyperglycemia. Other classic findings include birth trauma, cardiomyopathy, microcolon, polycythemia, jaundice, and limb reduction syndromes. Trisomy 13, 18, and 21 infants can have omphalocele, but all generally are small for gestation age. Trisomy 13 children also have cleft lip and palate (60%-80%), cutis aplasia, microphthalmia, microcephaly, congenital heart disease (80% of cases), clinodactyly, and polydactyly. Failure to thrive, seizures, severe intellectual disability, and death in the first 6 months of life are common. Trisomy 18 (Edwards syndrome) babies have low-set ears, a prominent occiput, a short sternum, a closed hand with overlapping fingers, cardiac defects, rocker-bottom (rounded) feet, cleft lip and/or palate, and renal and genital abnormalities. Mortality is 50% in the first week and 90% in the first year. Trisomy 21 features include the typical facies (flat face, upwardly slanting palpebral fissures, epicanthal folds, brachycephaly, microcephaly, small ears), protuberant tongue, poor tone, short neck with redundant skin, short fifth digit, single transverse palmar crease, and high risk of heart defect.

393. The answer is c. (*Hay et al, pp 998-999. Kliegman et al, pp 726-727. Rudolph et al, pp 607-608.*) The patient has classic findings of galactosemia. Galactose is a component of lactose, found in breast milk and most infant formulas. Symptoms of galactosemia occur in the first weeks of life. While screening for classic galactosemia typically is part of the newborn metabolic panel, patients fitting the clinical presentation as outlined in the question must be evaluated promptly. Signs and symptoms in addition to those presented in the vignette include cataracts and ascites. While three different errors in galactose metabolism are known, most cases result from the deficiency in galactose-1-phosphate uridyl transferase. Urine-reducing substances can be positive, but a routine urinalysis will be negative, as the urine strips do not react with galactose. Patients are at increased risk for *E coli* sepsis, and this infection may precede the diagnosis of galactosemia. Prompt removal of galactose from the diet usually reverses the symptoms, including cataracts.

The use of a phenylalanine-free diet would be appropriate for a patient with phenylketonuria (PKU), protein restriction and supplementation with citrulline might be used for treating ornithine transcarbamylase deficiency, a diet free from branched-chain amino acids would be appropriate for maple syrup urine disease, and part of the treatment for a patient with homocystinuria is high doses of vitamin B_6.

394. The answer is d. (*Hay et al, pp 1002-1003. Kliegman et al, pp 636-640. Rudolph et al, pp 561-563.*) The child in the question likely has PKU; the clinical picture described was entirely preventable with universal newborn metabolic screening, presymptomatic dietary intervention, and therapy with a newly-approved medication (pegvaliase-pqpz [Palynziq]). PKU is a disease that affects about 1 in 15,000 people in the United States, being more common in Caucasians and Native Americans than in African Americans, Hispanics, and Asians. It is inherited in an autosomal recessive manner. In addition to the features in the question, children born to women with PKU and who do not follow a low-PKU prenatal diet are at risk for a syndrome similar to fetal-alcohol exposure including microcephaly, developmental delay, and malformations of the heart and great vessels. Infants that are not diagnosed as part of the newborn screening program or for whom postnatal dietary manipulation is not achieved have additional signs and symptoms that can include seizures.

Elevated levels of fecal fat might be associated with cystic fibrosis or some other malabsorption syndrome; this would not be expected to cause developmental delay or any of the other symptoms listed. Elevated blood or urine succinylacetone is associated with tyrosinemia, a condition that results in liver and renal tubular dysfunction, growth failure, rickets, and a variety of neurologic symptoms such as peripheral neuropathy. Elevated methionine and homocystine levels are associated with methioninemia, a condition that can be asymptomatic or can result in a "cabbage smell" and potentially manifest with delays in walking, developmental delay, and muscle weakness. Elevated levels of leucine, isoleucine, valine, and alloisoleucine with depression of alanine suggest maple syrup urine disease that, in its classic form, results in poor feeding, vomiting, lethargy, developmental delay, seizures, coma, and death.

395. The answer is d. (*Hay et al, pp 945-951. Kliegman et al, pp 1878-1881. Rudolph et al, pp 2012-2017.*) Of the choices, only growth hormone deficiency (reduced levels of insulin-like growth factor and insulin-like growth factor-binding protein) would be expected to have a child who is normal appearing, that is, the upper to lower segment ratio is normal, often without other signs or symptoms. In achondroplasia (mutation in the fibroblast growth factor receptor 3 [FGFR3] gene) a disproportion in growth between the limbs and the trunk (the limbs are relatively short) is noted. The head in achondroplasia is also disproportionately large. Marfan syndrome (mutation in the fibrillin-1 [FBN1] genes on chromosome 15) is an autosomal dominant inherited condition with predominant findings of bilateral subluxation of the lens, dilatation of the aortic root, and disproportionately long limbs in comparison with the trunk. Morquio syndrome (deficiency of N-acetylgalactosamine-6-sulfatase [MPS-IVA] or β-galactosidase [MPS-IVB]) is one of the mucopolysaccharidoses (MPS IV) in which abnormal amounts of keratan sulfate accumulate with widespread storage of this material in the body resulting in problems in morphogenesis and function. Skeletal malformations are similar to those seen in osteochondrodysplasias, namely, short trunk with short stature, marked slowing of growth, severe scoliosis, pectus carinatum, and short neck. Thyroid hormone is necessary for physical growth and development and, along with sex hormones, has an essential role in development of bone and linear growth. Thyroid deficiency results in delayed puberty in most cases and in stunting of growth with persistence of immature body proportions; signs and symptoms of hypothyroidism are also frequently seen.

396. The answer is a. (*Kliegman et al, p 1027. Rudolph et al, pp 761-763.*) The constellation of immunodeficiency and progressive cerebellar ataxia with dilated small vessels on the bulbar conjunctiva, ears, neck, and popliteal and antecubital fossae is seen in the autosomal recessive immunodeficiency ataxia-telangiectasia. Underlying the disorder is the defective repair of damaged DNA. These children have increased sensitivity to ionizing radiation. Other associated findings may include gonadal dysgenesis and insulin-resistant diabetes. These patients are at significantly increased risk for developing malignancies.

Eczema with easy bruising or bleeding (thrombocytopenia) in conjunction with eosinophilia, elevated IgE, and skin infection with *Staphylococcus aureus* is known as Wiskott Aldrich syndrome, an X-linked immunodeficiency. These patients have defects in both cellular and humoral immunity, and are also at high risk of developing malignancy. Serum IgA and IgE levels are elevated, while the serum IgM level is decreased and the serum IgG level is normal.

Hyper IgE syndrome, also known as Job syndrome, is transmitted in both an autosomal dominant and autosomal recessive pattern, with different phenotypes. The findings of autosomal dominant version include recurrent fractures, retained "baby" teeth, and impaired inflammatory response with altered neutrophil chemotaxis leading to frequent bacterial infections. The recessive version does not have skeletal manifestations but is associated with recurrent viral infections such as varicella, HSV, and molluscum.

Hypopigmented "ash-leaf" spots and angiofibromas on the face are characteristics of tuberous sclerosis complex (TSC), an autosomal dominant mutation in either the TSC1 or the TSC2 gene. The condition is characterized by benign tumor formation in the brain, heart, skin, eyes, lungs, and kidneys. The characteristic skin findings of neurofibromatosis are hyperpigmented macules called "café-au-lait" spots. Staggering gait and immunodeficiency are not part of either TSC or NF.

397. The answer is e. (*Hay et al, pp 1015-1016. Kliegman et al, pp 737-743. Rudolph et al, pp 624-626.*) Patients born normal who then have progressive developmental delay (and in particular developmental regression, or loss of milestones) and hepatosplenomegaly with coarse facial features are likely to have a storage disease. Hurler syndrome, mucopolysaccharidosis type I, is an autosomal recessive condition caused by a deficiency of α-l-iduronidase, which results in deposition of dermatan sulfate and heparan sulfate in the body, and excessive excretion in the urine. Other features of this condition include umbilical hernia, kyphoscoliosis, deafness, cloudy corneas, and claw hand deformity. Death is common in childhood, a result of respiratory or cardiac compromise.

In none of the other choices would one expect to see the development of hepatosplenomegaly or a loss of normal childhood developmental milestones. Jeune syndrome (asphyxiating thoracic dystrophy) is notable for short stature, long and narrow thorax, hypoplastic lungs, fibrotic liver, and short limbs. Death is common, a result of pneumonia or asphyxia because of the abnormally shaped thorax. Crouzon syndrome is an autosomal dominant condition that results in craniosynostosis (usually coronal), proptosis, brachycephaly, hypertelorism and strabismus, "beak" nose, midface hypoplasia, and high and narrow palate. Trisomy 18 (Edwards syndrome) is a condition marked by low birth weight, low-set and malformed ears, micrognathia, clenched hands with overlapping digits, a variety of cardiac defects, and poor subcutaneous fat deposition. About 50% of children with the condition die in the first weeks of life, and less than 10% survive beyond the first year; severe intellectual disability is uniform. At birth, patients with Beckwith-Wiedemann syndrome are macrosomic with macroglossia, abdominal wall defects, linear ear creases, and organomegaly; they often have hypoglycemia in the newborn period. They have an increased incidence of developing malignancy, especially Wilms tumor, hepatoblastoma, and gonadoblastoma. Intellect is usually normal.

398. The answer is a. (*Hay et al, p 946. Kliegman et al, p 2643. Rudolph et al, pp 2013-2016.*) The determination of bone age by the radiographic examination of ossification centers provides a measure of a child's level of growth that is independent of his or her chronologic age. Since the pattern of ossification is predictable, radiologists compare the patient's wrist and hand ossification with images in one of several standard atlases. The report will contain the patients "bone age" as compared to his "chronologic age." Height age is the age that corresponds to the 50th percentile for a child's height. When bone age and height age are equally retarded several years behind chronologic age, a child is described as having constitutional short stature. Such a child is usually shorter than peers in adolescence because of the delayed growth spurt, but the prognosis for normal adult height is relatively good because potential for growth remains. Detailed questioning will usually identify other family members with a history of delayed growth and sexual maturation but with ultimately normal stature. Children with genetic or familial short stature grow at an adequate rate, but remain small throughout life; their ultimate height is consistent with predictions based on parental heights. Bone age is within the limits of normal for chronologic age, and puberty occurs at the normal time. In all cases, a thorough history and physical examination are necessary to identify any other cause of growth delay. Laboratory findings would include IGF-1 levels low for chronologic age but normal for bone age.

399. The answer is b. (*Hay et al, pp 782, 1041-1042. Kliegman et al, pp 3370-3373. Rudolph et al, pp 718-720.*) Achondroplasia, occurring with an incidence of approximately 1 in every 26,000 live births, is the most common genetic form of skeletal dysplasia. Affected persons bear a striking resemblance to one another and are identified by their extremely short extremities; prominent foreheads; short, stubby fingers; and marked lumbar lordosis. Although they go through normal puberty, affected females must have children by cesarean section because of the pelvic deformity. Other complications include hydrocephalus, muscle weakness, apnea, and sudden death secondary to bony overgrowth at the foramen magnum. Achondroplasia is inherited in an autosomal dominant manner, but most cases represent spontaneous mutations in unaffected parents. Intelligence is normal.

400. The answer is d. (*Hay et al, pp 1056-1063. Kliegman et al, p 88. Rudolph et al, pp 2027-2028.*) Alteration of body proportion results from selective regional rates of growth at different stages during the developmental period. At birth, the head is large for the body size, the limbs are short, and the average upper to lower segment ratio (crown to pubis/pubis to heel) of 1.7 is high. As the growth of the limbs exceeds that of the trunk from infancy to adolescence, there is a change in body proportions reflected in the upper to lower segment ratios: 1.3 at 3 years, 1.1 at 6 years, and 1.0 at 10 years of age. In growth hormone deficiency, the upper to lower segment ratio is normal, often without other signs or symptoms. In achondroplasia, there is a disproportion between the limbs and the trunk; that is, the limbs are relatively short. The head in this condition is also disproportionately large. Achondroplasia is the most common genetic skeletal dysplasia. This disorder has an autosomal dominant mode of inheritance. Marfan syndrome is a serious disease of connective tissue that is inherited in the autosomal dominant mode. The predominant findings in this condition are bilateral subluxation of the lens, dilatation of the aortic root, and disproportionately long limbs in comparison with the trunk. The decreased upper to lower segment ratio in Marfan syndrome reflects this relative increase in the length of the legs compared with the trunk. Morquio syndrome is one of the mucopolysaccharidoses (MPS IV). Abnormal amounts of keratan sulfate accumulate as a result of an enzyme deficiency, and widespread storage of this material in the body results in problems in morphogenesis and function. Skeletal malformations are similar to those seen in osteochondrodysplasias, namely, short trunk with short stature, marked slowing of growth, severe scoliosis, pectus carinatum, and short neck. Thyroid hormone is necessary for physical growth and development and, along with sex hormones, has an essential role in development of bone and linear growth. Thyroid deficiency results in delayed puberty in most cases and in stunting of growth with persistence of immature body proportions; signs and symptoms of hypothyroidism are also frequently seen.

401. The answer is d. (*Hay et al, pp 904-905. Kliegman et al, pp 2476-2477. Rudolph et al, pp 1661-1662.*) The child pictured has an asymmetric "red" reflex (one eye is lighter than the other). Although all the listed options can produce the symptoms described, the family history supports the diagnosis of retinoblastoma, the most common intraocular tumor in children. Early detection can result in a survival rate of over 90%. The pattern of inheritance of retinoblastoma is complicated: the hereditary form of the disease can be transmitted by means of autosomal dominant inheritance from an affected parent, from an unaffected parent carrying the gene, or from a new germinal mutation. Familial occurrences are usually bilateral. A second primary tumor develops in 15%-90% of survivors of bilateral retinoblastoma, the most common of which is osteosarcoma, increasing in incidence with time. Retinoblastoma is associated with a mutation or deletion of the long arm of chromosome 13. In addition to specialized ophthalmologic care, management of retinoblastoma includes molecular genetic investigation of the family to identify those who have inherited the tumor-predisposing retinoblastoma gene.

402. The answer is c. (*Hay et al, pp 963-964. Kliegman et al, pp 2693-2694. Rudolph et al, p 2090.*) The patient with the features listed likely has pseudohypoparathyroidism (Albright hereditary osteodystrophy). Such patients have chemical findings of hypoparathyroidism (low calcium, high phosphorus), but parathyroid hormone levels are high, indicating resistance to the action of this hormone. Parathyroid hormone infusion does not produce a phosphaturic response. Phenotypically, these patients demonstrate shortness of stature with delayed bone age, developmental delay, increased bone density throughout the body (especially evident in the skull), brachydactyly (especially of the fourth and fifth digits), obesity with round facies and short neck, subcapsular cataracts, cutaneous and subcutaneous calcifications, and perivascular calcifications of the basal ganglia.

403. The answer is c. (*Hay et al, p 965. Kliegman et al, p 2697. Rudolph et al, pp 2093-2096.*) Hypercalcemia can develop in children who are immobilized following the fracture of a weight-bearing bone. Serious complications of immobilization hypercalcemia, and the hypercalciuria that occurs as a result, include nephropathy, nephrocalcinosis, hypertensive encephalopathy, and convulsions. The early symptoms of hypercalcemia—namely, constipation, anorexia, occasional vomiting, polyuria, and lethargy—are nonspecific and may be ascribed to the effects of the injury and hospitalization. Therefore, careful monitoring of these patients with serial measurements of the serum ionized calcium and the urinary calcium to creatinine clearance ratio is critical during their immobilization. A ratio of more than 0.2 suggests a diagnosis of metabolic or nephrogenic hypercalciuria. Although complete mobilization is curative, additional measures, such as vigorous intravenous hydration with a balanced salt solution, dietary restrictions of dairy products, and administration of diuretics, can be instituted. For patients who are at risk for symptomatic hypercalcemia, short-term therapy with calcitonin is highly effective in reducing the concentration of serum calcium by inhibiting bone resorption. Treatment of this child for depression (fluoxetine) and hypertension (Lisinopril) without addressing the cause of the symptoms is imprudent. Ambulatory blood pressure monitors are helpful to determine "real" from "white coat" elevations of blood pressure; this hospitalized patient has symptoms beyond hypertension suggesting "real" hypertension. Neither a renal sonogram nor an IVP would add information for his management.

404. The answer is d. (*Hay et al, p 1159. Kliegman et al, pp 700, 2759. Rudolph et al, p 645.*) The child has classic features of Smith-Lemli-Opitz syndrome, a condition caused by a metabolic defect in the final states of cholesterol production. The result is a low serum cholesterol and an elevated 7-dehydrocholesterol (7-DHC) level. Clinical features are as described; treatment to prevent progression of the disease is supplemental cholesterol (egg yolk). Wolman disease is a lysosomal acid lipase deficiency resulting in large amounts of lipids accumulate throughout the body. Severe forms begin in infancy, while other forms develop in childhood or later. Hepatosplenomegaly, malabsorption, diarrhea, vomiting, and cirrhosis of the liver are common presenting findings. Niemann-Pick disease is caused by a deficiency of acid sphingomyelinase resulting in an accumulation of sphingomyelin and other lipids throughout the monocyte-macrophage system. In this condition normal children develop hepatosplenomegaly by about 3 months of age, then feeding problems, failure to thrive, and progressive motor delays. Familial dysbetalipoproteinemia is an inherited form of hypercholesterolemia resulting in elevated cholesterol and less-elevated lipids. Gaucher disease is the most common lysosomal storage disease caused by β-glucocerebrosidase deficiency which results in abnormal accumulation of glucocerebroside in the reticuloendothelial system, including the bone marrow. Presentation includes anemia, leukopenia, and thrombocytopenia.

405. The answer is b. (*Hay et al, pp 1089-1091. Kliegman et al, pp 2714-2722. Rudolph et al, pp 2048-2052.*) Salt-losing congenital adrenal hyperplasia (adrenogenital syndrome, 21-hydroxylase deficiency) usually manifests during the first 5-15 days of life as anorexia, vomiting, diarrhea, and dehydration (the history in the vignette suggests poor intake; vital signs and physical examination suggest dehydration). Hypoglycemia can also occur. Affected neonates can have increased pigmentation, and female newborns show evidence of virilization with ambiguous external genitalia. Hyponatremia, hyperkalemia, and urinary sodium wasting are the usual laboratory findings and result from a deficiency of aldosterone. Death can occur if the diagnosis is missed and appropriate treatment is not instituted.

Although adrenal hypoplasia, an extremely rare disorder, presents a similar clinical picture, it has an earlier onset than adrenal hyperplasia, and virilization does not occur. In classic 21-hydroxylase deficiency, serum levels of 17-hydroxyprogesterone are markedly elevated beyond 3 days of life (in the first 3 days of life they can be high in normal newborns). Blood cortisol levels are usually low in salt-losing forms of the disease.

Pyloric stenosis (diagnosed with an ultrasound) seems unlikely in this infant in that the vomiting with this disease usually begins after the third week of life. Hypothyroidism would present as a lethargic, poor-feeding infant with delayed reflexes, persistent jaundice, and hypotonia. Panhypopituitarism usually presents with apnea, cyanosis, or severe hypoglycemia. Analysis of the infant's formula for incorrect mixing might be required should the evaluation for adrenal hyperplasia be negative.

406. The answer is d. (*Hay et al, pp 124-125. Kliegman et al, pp 2742-2743. Rudolph et al, p 294.*) Gynecomastia is a common occurrence in adolescent boys, especially during Tanner stage 2 or 3. It can occur unilaterally or bilaterally, and can affect one breast more significantly than the other. It is thought to be caused by a temporary reduction in the testosterone to estradiol ratio. Spontaneous regression usually occurs; it rarely lasts for more than 2 years. In the child, who otherwise has a normal physical examination and no significant past medical history, reassurance of the benign nature of the condition is all that is required for most cases. Rarely, the gynecomastia is significant; antiestrogen agents can be utilized or surgery can be considered. Other, more serious causes for this condition include Klinefelter syndrome, hyperthyroidism, hormone-producing tumors, and drugs (including marijuana and anabolic steroids). A thorough history and physical examination can help eliminate these relatively unusual causes.

407. The answer is a. (*Kliegman et al, p 642. Rudolph et al, pp 564-565.*) The infant described in the question has alkaptonuria (alcaptonuria is an alternate spelling), an autosomal recessive disorder caused by a deficiency of homo-gentisic acid oxidase. The diagnosis is made in infants when their urine turns dark brown or black on exposure to air because of the oxidation of homo-gentisic acid. Affected children are asymptomatic. In adults, ochronosis—the deposition of a bluish pigment in cartilage and fibrous tissue—develops; symptoms of arthritis may appear later. No specific treatment is available for patients who have alkaptonuria, although supplemental ascorbic acid may delay the onset of the disorder and reduce clinical symptoms. The other deficiencies listed in the question are found in PKU, histidinemia, maple syrup urine disease, and isovaleric acidemia, respectively.

408. The answer is e. (*Hay et al, pp 654-656. Kliegman et al, pp 1939-1940. Rudolph et al, pp 1507-1508.*) Wilson disease is an autosomal recessive disorder characterized by liver disease (usually seen in childhood), neuro-logic and behavioral disturbances (seen in adolescence), renal tubular dysfunction (Fanconi syndrome), and eye findings (Kayser-Fleischer rings). Its multisystem manifestations are caused by the deposition of copper in various tissues (resulting in low serum levels), and therapy is aimed at the prevention of accumulation of copper. Defective metabolism of the copper-binding protein ceruloplasmin (usually reduced) has been demonstrated by some.

Indian childhood cirrhosis is a non-treatable, fatal condition found in rural India, affecting children aged 1-3 years with hepatomegaly, fever, anorexia, and jaundice. It rapidly progresses to cirrhosis and liver failure. Serum immunoglobulin levels and hepatic copper concentrations are elevated. α_1-Antitrypsin deficiency, which causes liver disease through accumulation of an abnormal protein, is caused by a single amino acid substitution on chromosome 14. It has a variable presentation, but in infancy the following are common: cholestasis; bleeding into the CNS, GI tract, or at the umbilical stump; and elevation of transaminase concentrations. In childhood, a picture of chronic hepatitis with cirrhosis and portal hypertension is seen, but the neurologic and behavior changes typical of Wilson disease are not seen. Menkes syndrome presents in the first months of life and includes hypothermia, hypotonia, and myoclonic seizures. These children have chubby, rosy cheeks and kinky, colorless, and friable hair. Severe intellectual disability is always seen. Low serum copper and ceruloplasmin levels are found, with a copper absorption/transport problem being the cause. Dubin-Johnson syndrome is inherited as an autosomal recessive condition with patients being unable to excrete conjugated bilirubin. Such patients present during adolescence or early adulthood, sometimes earlier. Morbidity due to condition is unusual.

409. The answer is e. (*Kliegman et al, pp 773-788. Rudolph et al, p 2129.*) Hypoglycemia with hyperinsulinemia but without evidence of C-peptide suggests that the insulin is exogenous; these findings occurring while the patient is in the hospital would suggest that the current caretaker is injecting insulin into the baby causing hypoglycemia. The caretaker (more commonly the mother) may be suffering from Munchausen syndrome by proxy (MSBP, also known as factitious disorder imposed on another, or FDIA), a disorder in which a parent induces illness in the child or reports symptoms repeatedly to represent the child as ill. There is usually no obvious secondary gain for the parent, as there is with the diagnosis of malingering. Protective services should always be notified about suspected MSBP cases, as there are sometimes fatalities.

Nesidioblastosis, Beckwith-Wiedemann, and galactosemia can all cause hypoglycemia, but do not fit the story and the laboratory values. Pancreatitis can cause hyperglycemia.

410. The answer is d. (*Hay et al, p 1041. Kliegman et al, pp 3384-3389. Rudolph et al, pp 722-725.*) The adolescent in the question has clinical features of Marfan syndrome and a cardiac examination consistent with mitral valve prolapse. Of the choices listed, dilation of the aortic root might be expected. Marfan syndrome is a genetic disorder transmitted as an autosomal dominant trait with variable expression. Vascular complications can be serious if not identified early; aortic dissection can lead to sudden death. None of the other cardiac abnormalities are typically found with Marfan syndrome.

411. The answer is d. (*Hay et al, pp 283-284. Kliegman et al, pp 331-341. Rudolph et al, pp 2098-2101.*) The x-ray demonstrates a fracture of the femur, and also a significant decreased bone mineralization. The infant in the question (exclusively breast-fed, no vitamin D supplementation, northern climate with limited sun exposure, African American mother) is at risk for simple (nutritional) rickets. Nutritional rickets is caused by a dietary deficiency of vitamin D and lack of exposure to sunlight.

Intestinal absorption of calcium and phosphorus is diminished in vitamin D deficiency. Transient hypocalcemia stimulates the secretion of parathyroid hormone and the mobilization of calcium and phosphorus from bone; enhanced parathyroid hormone activity leads to phosphaturia and diminished excretion of calcium. In children with nutritional rickets, the concentration of serum calcium usually is normal and the phosphate level is low. Increased serum alkaline phosphatase is a common finding. The excretion of calcium in the urine is increased only after therapy with vitamin D has been instituted.

The American Academy of Pediatrics (AAP) currently recommends all breast-fed infants be given 400 IU/day of supplemental vitamin D starting in the first few days of life and continuing until the child takes in sufficiency other sources of vitamin D (such as fortified foods or cow's milk).

412. The answer is a. (*Hay et al, p 1070. Kliegman et al, pp 2481-2482. Rudolph et al, pp 211-214.*) The clinical findings on the patient suggest a thyroid nodule, and the family history of some type of "throat cancer" suggests a familial condition. While the majority of medullary thyroid carcinoma cases are sporadic, this family history suggests a multiple endocrine neoplasia (MEN) syndrome. Pheochromocytoma (hypertension) is common to both forms of MEN. Part of the diagnostic evaluation is the finding of elevated serum calcitonin and CEA level. Hyperparathyroidism associated with MEN may result in hyperparathyroidism with resultant hypercalcemia, hypophosphatemia, hypocalciuria, and hyperphosphaturia.

413. The answer is b. (*Hay et al, pp 959-963. Kliegman et al, p 892. Rudolph et al, pp 216-217, 2089-2090.*) Hypocalcemia of newborns can be divided into two groups: early (during the first approximately 72 hours of life) and late (after approximately 72 hours). The most common type of early neonatal hypocalcemia is the so-called idiopathic hypocalcemia.

Contributors to the early onset hypocalcemia include maternal illness (diabetes, preeclampsia, and hyperparathyroidism), neonatal distress (perinatal asphyxia) or sepsis, low birth weight because of prematurity, or hypomagnesemia. Transient or permanent hypoparathyroidism and high phosphate intake are the most common factors associated with late hypocalcemia. The bicarbonate and glucose levels in the question are normal, while the elevated magnesium level may cause sedation and apnea but not tetany and seizures. Intracranial hemorrhages are less common in a newborn of this gestational age, and usually do not present with tetany.

414. The answer is a. (*Hay et al, pp 27-28. Kliegman et al, pp 773-788. Rudolph et al, pp 211-214*). Glucose levels in a newly delivered infant are maintained from hepatic glycogen (the source of glucose via glycogenolysis), muscle (a source of amino acids for gluconeogenesis), and lipid stores (a source of fatty acids for lypolysis). Small-for-gestation age infants have low reserves of each of these nutrients. Additionally such infants have a relatively large body surface area that is often exposed to a cool environment increasing the demand for glucose. Low reserves and increased demand put such infants at increased risk for hypoglycemia. The adrenal and pituitary glands are not primary factors in maintaining glucose in the first hours of life. Excess fetal insulin can result in hypoglycemia, most commonly in an infant born to diabetic mothers (IODM). In this situation the high maternal levels of glucose cross the placenta resulting in the infant's pancreas excreting insulin in response; upon cutting the umbilical cord the "excess" insulin may result in a rapid drop in the infant's serum glucose level. Infants do not have glucagon deficiency.

415. The answer is c. (*Hay et al, p 1161. Kliegman et al, pp 600-602. Rudolph et al, pp 683, 2144.*). The findings in the father are suspicious for Huntington disease, a genetic condition caused triplet repeat expansions. Other common conditions caused by triplet repeat expansion include fragile X syndrome and myotonic dystrophy. The classic condition caused by a maternal defect in chromosome 15 is Angelman syndrome (happy puppet syndrome) which includes developmental delay, autism, seizures, tongue thrusting, and paroxysmal laughter. The classic condition caused by a paternal defect in chromosome 15 is Prader-Willi, a disorder consisting of profound hypotonia and poor feeding in the newborn period often requiring a feeding tube and in older children hypogonadism, hyperphagia, intellectual disability, and profound appetite resulting in obesity and sleep apnea. Examples of sex chromosome imbalance include Turner (45, XO) and Klinefelter (47, XXY) syndromes.

416. The answer is b. (*Hay et al, pp 1157-1158. Kliegman et al, pp 3380-3384. Rudolph et al, pp 720-721.*) The child has fractures with minor trauma that heal well, a high-threshold to pain, and azure (blue) sclera on examination.

The question suggests osteogenesis imperfect type IA, a mild-enough condition that may present with repeated fractures with mild trauma and blue sclera. The cause is a mutation in the COL1A1 gene that is responsible for type I collagen. Physical abuse must be considered in any pediatric patient with injury, but his findings of abnormal sclera hint at a different diagnosis. Similarly, normally developing children have fractures, but repeated fractures suggest further investigation is warranted. Isolated dietary deficiency of vitamin D in previous centuries was common; it is currently extraordinarily rare in developed countries outside the newborn period. Impaired renal production of 1, 25-dihydroxycholecalciferol is seen in chronic renal failure; growth in such children is impaired.

417. The answer is b. (*Hay et al, pp 1052, 1147. Kliegman et al, pp 771-772, 2887, 3159-3160. Rudolph et al, p 700.*) The sibling of the 3-month-old has classic features of Bloom syndrome, an autosomal recessive condition common in Ashkenazi Jews. The erythema and telangiectasia develop in early childhood as a butterfly rash on the face which becomes more prominent with sunlight exposure. These children have intrauterine growth retardation, poor feeding, reflux, and distinctive facial features including prominent nose and ears, as well as a small and narrow face.

Systemic lupus erythematosus is a multisystem condition that, in addition to the classically described butterfly rash, can manifest as unexplained fever, fatigue, anemia, arthralgia, oral lesions, kidney disease, and altered mental status. The constellation of immunodeficiency (sinopulmonary infections) and progressive cerebellar ataxia after children begin to walk with associated findings of dilated small vessels on the bulbar conjunctiva, ears, neck, and popliteal and antecubital fossae is the autosomal recessive immunodeficiency ataxia-telangiectasia. Erythropoietic protoporphyria is an autosomal recessive disease that presents as pain, redness, swelling, and itching quickly after exposure to sunlight. Chronic skin changes include lichenification of exposed surfaces. Children with Cockayne syndrome present after about a year of age with a butterfly facial rash after sun exposure, but also thin, atrophic, and hyperpigmented skin on the face. They have intellectual disability, microcephaly and large hands and feet with long limbs. The condition is inherited in an autosomal recessive pattern.

418. The answer is a. (*Hay et al, pp 1111-1112. Kliegman et al, pp 715-727. Rudolph et al, pp 601-602.*) The case is a classic description of a child with the autosomal recessive condition of von Gierke disease (deficiency of glucose-6-phosphatase activity). Hypoglycemia, seizures, and lactic acidosis in the newborn period along with the examination findings as described. The "milky" blood is due to dramatic hyperlipidemia. Infantile Pompe disease, an autosomal recessive condition, classically present in the first weeks of life with hypotonia, weakness, feeding challenges, macroglossia, hepatomegaly, and cardiomyopathy that leads to death in the first year of life. Currently enzyme replacement infusions (alglucosidase alfa [Myozyme or Lumizyme]) reduce risk of death and need for ventilation among patients identified and treated early. McArdle disease present later in childhood or in early adulthood with muscle weakness, exercise intolerance muscle cramps and pain, myoglobinuria, and elevated serum creatine kinase. It is caused by an autosomal recessive deficiency of muscle phosphorylase activity. Hers disease is a liver phosphorylase deficiency that usually has a benign course but may present with hepatomegaly and growth retardation early in childhood. Hypoglycemia and hyperlipidemia can be seen; lactic acid levels typically are normal. It is inherited in an autosomal recessive pattern. Tarui disease is caused by a deficiency of muscle phosphofructokinase, an autosomal recessively inherited condition notable for exercise intolerance with nausea, vomiting, severe muscle pain, and myoglobinuria.

419 to 424. The answers are 419-m, 420-b, 421-n, 422-h, 423-i, 424-d. (*Hay et al, pp 144, 760-761, 1065-1067, 1075, 1091-1093, 1097-1105, 1151, 1161. Kliegman et al, pp 602-603, 610-616, 2521-2528, 2618-2622, 2665-2674, 2693-2694, 2723-2725, 2739-2741. 2793-2786. Rudolph et al, pp 123, 126, 296-299, 692-694, 701, 1722-1725, 2037-2038, 2055-2056, 2076, 2083-2084, 2086-2093, 2119-2125.*) Patients with type 2 diabetes mellitus have insulin resistance in their skeletal muscles, increased hepatic glucose production, and decreased insulin secretion in response to elevated levels of glucose. They also develop hyperlipidemia and many complications of chronic hyperglycemia. Acanthosis nigricans, as described in the question, is a common finding in type 2 diabetes.

The Prader-Willi syndrome is a disorder consisting of profound hypotonia, hypogonadism, hyperphagia after the newborn period, intellectual disability, and obesity. A deletion of a portion of chromosome 15 has been found in approximately 70% of patients. Children affected by this syndrome exhibit little movement *in utero* and are hypotonic during the neonatal period. Clinical features may be subtle but include narrow head, almond-shaped eyes, and downturned mouth. Significant feeding difficulties that may require tube feedings in the newborn period and failure to thrive can be the presenting complaints in the first year; later, obesity becomes the most common presenting complaint. The enormous food intake of affected children is thought to be caused by a defect in the satiety center in the hypothalamus. Stringent caloric restriction is the only known treatment.

Williams syndrome is thought to be caused by a deletion involving the elastin gene on chromosome 7q11.23. Phenotypic features include an elfin-life face (broad forehead, flat nasal bridge, long upper lip, and round cheeks) as well as intellectual disability and an engaging personality. A history of hypercalcemia in infancy is common. Supravalvular aortic stenosis is an associated finding.

Pseudohypoparathyroidism is a collective term for a variety of diseases. Affected patients have biochemical findings (low serum calcium and high serum phosphorus levels) similar to those associated with hypoparathyroidism, but they also have high levels of endogenous parathyroid hormone; in addition, exogenous parathyroid hormone fails to increase their phosphate excretion or raise their serum calcium level. The defects in these patients appear to be at the hormone receptor site or in the adenylate cyclase-cyclic AMP system. The symptoms of pseudohypoparathyroidism are caused by hypocalcemia. Affected children are short, round-faced, and have mild intellectual disability. Metacarpals and metatarsals are shortened, and subcutaneous and basal ganglia calcifications as well as cataracts can be present. The current treatment consists of large doses of vitamin D and reduction of the phosphate load.

Polycystic ovary disease classically presents at or shortly after puberty with obesity, hirsutism, and secondary amenorrhea. Later, these women have anovulatory infertility. The cause of this condition is not entirely clear.

Kallmann syndrome, the most common form of hypogonadotropic hypogonadism, has anosmia or hyposmia as a presenting feature. This syndrome has a variety of inheritance patterns, all resulting in delayed or incomplete puberty. Laurence-Moon-Biedl (Bardet-Biedl) syndrome is transmitted as an autosomal recessive trait. Obesity, intellectual disability, hypogonadism, polydactyly, and retinitis pigmentosa with night blindness are the principal findings in affected children. There is no known effective treatment. Myriad features are found with Down (trisomy 21) syndrome including findings at birth of typical facies (flat face, upwardly slanting palpebral fissures, epicanthal folds, brachycephaly, microcephaly, small ears), protuberant tongue, poor tone, short neck with redundant skin, short fifth digit, single transverse palmar crease, and high risk of heart defect. Feeding challenges are common, but the dysmorphic features of Down syndrome distinguish the condition from Prader-Willi. Leptin is a hormone secreted by adipose tissue that suppresses appetite through its action on the hypothalamus. Congenital leptin deficiency due to a defect in the leptin gene results in hyperphagia and the early-onset obesity. Affected individuals often have hyperinsulinemia and advanced bone age; most have hypogonadotropic hypogonadism. Food intake is decreased when patients are treated with exogenous leptin. Obesity has also been reported with a defect in the leptin receptor. The initial complaint in Cushing syndrome may be obesity. Accumulation of fat in the face, neck, and trunk causes the characteristics "buffalo hump" and "moon" facies. Characteristic features include growth failure, muscle wasting, thinning of the skin, plethora, and hypertension. The bone age of affected patients is retarded, and osteoporosis can be present. The disorder results from an excess of glucocorticoids that may be caused by a primary adrenal abnormality (adenoma or carcinoma) or secondary hypercortisolism, which may be due to to excess adrenocorticotropin. Exogenous glucocorticoids administered in supraphysiologic doses for a prolonged period of time will produce a similar picture in normal subjects.

Cohen syndrome (aka Pepper syndrome) infants are small for gestation age, have poor tone, a weak and high-pitched cry, and may develop feeding and breathing problems in the first few days of life. Later they have developmental delay along with physical features of large ears, prominent nasal root, low hairline, high-arched eyelids, long eyelashes, elevated palate, shortened philtrum, and prominent central incisors. It is less common than Prader-Willi syndrome. Maternal uniparental disomy of chromosome 14 is a rare condition that results in a condition quite similar to Prader-Willi although typical chromosome 15 abnormalities are not found. Infants with congenital hypothyroidism typically appear normal at birth, although they may have an enlarged head and fontanels. Over the next weeks symptoms of prolonged jaundice, hypothermia, feeding challenges, hypersomnolence, enlarged tongue, and weak cry develop. Congenital hypothyroidism is rare in developed areas where newborn screening is practiced. In older children acquired hypothyroidism may present with goiter, weight gain, myxedematous changes in the skin, cold intolerance, lethargy, increased sleep, and constipation. Nephrotic syndrome is caused by increased permeability of the glomerular capillary wall leading to proteinuria and hypoalbuminemia. Affected patients will have generalized edema with weight gain, hyperlipidemia, increased susceptibility to infections and hypercoagulability.

425 to 428. The answers are 425-e, 426-e, 427-d, 428-a. (*Hay et al, pp 692-693, 952-953, 974-980, 997-998. Kliegman et al, pp 492-496, 1883-1884, 1924-1928. Rudolph et al, pp 601-602, 2025-2027, 2048-2056.*)

In the absence of vasopressin (central diabetes insipidus [DI]), renal collecting tubules are impermeable to water, resulting in the excretion of hypotonic urine. Patients with DI present with polyuria and polydipsia. Net loss of water leads to dehydration and hemoconcentration and, therefore, to relatively high serum concentrations of sodium and potassium. The most common causes for central DI include idiopathic DI, tumors, neurosurgery, and head trauma.

Patients with nephrogenic DI have similar laboratory findings. This genetic disorder is unresponsive to antidiuretic hormone (ADH). These patients are unable to concentrate their urine and present in the neonatal period with hypernatremic dehydration.

In hyperaldosteronism, renal tubular sodium-potassium exchange is enhanced. Hypokalemia, hypernatremia, hyperchloremia, and alkalosis are the usual findings. Primary hyperaldosteronism (Conn syndrome) is very rare in children.

Addison disease is associated with a combined deficiency of glucocorticoids and mineralocorticoids. Resorption of sodium and excretion of potassium and hydrogen ions are impaired at the level of the distal renal tubules. Sodium loss results in loss of water and depletion of blood volume. Persons with compensated Addison disease can have relatively normal physical and laboratory findings; Addisonian crisis, however, characteristically produces hyponatremia, hyperkalemia, and shock. The pathophysiology of the serum electrolyte abnormalities in this disorder is the same as in the salt-losing variety of adrenogenital syndrome.

Option B might be seen in patients with a condition such as deficiency of glucose-6-phosphatase (von Gierke disease) who, as a rule, have profound hyperlipidemia. Increased triglyceride concentration in the serum decreases the volume of the aqueous compartment. Because electrolytes are present only in the aqueous compartment of the serum but are expressed in milliequivalents per liter of serum as a whole, the concentrations of sodium and potassium can be factitiously low in these patients. Option F represents normal electrolytes, and for none of the scenarios presented would normal sodium and potassium be expected.

429 to 435. The answers are 429-g, 430-b, 431-i, 432-l, 433-m, 434-d, 435-j. (*Hay et al, pp 114-115, 860, 1097-1105, 1151-1154, 1156-1157,*

1168-1169. Kliegman et al, pp 611-616, 621-623, 811-813, 3179-3184, 3884-3889. Rudolph et al, pp 692-697, 701, 722-726, 732-739, 1568-1569, 1780, 2068-2070.) Ehlers-Danlos syndrome is characterized by thin fragile skin, easy bruising, and joint hypermobility. Mitral valve prolapse has been reported. There are several different variants.

Trisomy 21, also known as Down syndrome, is easily recognized in older children and adults, but may be more difficult to diagnose in infancy. Characteristics include upslanting palpebral fissures with epicanthal folds, hypotonia, small ears, and a single transverse palmar crease. About half of patients with Down syndrome will have some type of cardiac abnormality.

Holt-Oram syndrome is characterized by abnormalities in the upper extremities, hypoplastic radii, thumb abnormalities, and cardiac anomalies. Occasionally the pectoralis major muscle is missing in Holt-Oram, and as such it needs to be considered when discussing Poland syndrome.

Mothers who consume alcohol during pregnancy put their infant at risk of fetal alcohol syndrome. Key features include growth retardation, short palpebral features, short nose, thin upper lip, intellectual disability, heart defects, and behavioral abnormalities.

Turner syndrome is characterized by short stature, low ears, a wide chest with widely spaced nipples, broad-based neck, low hairline, extremity edema, and congenital heart defects (typically coarctation or bicuspid aortic valve). Intelligence is normal.

Trisomy 18 (Edwards syndrome) babies are small with low-set ears, a prominent occiput, a short sternum, a closed hand with overlapping fingers, cardiac defects, rocker-bottom (rounded) feet, cleft lip and/or palate, and renal and genital abnormalities. Mortality is 50% in the first week and 90% in the first year.

Infants born to diabetic mothers are frequently macrosomic and may become hypoglycemic. However, they can have many other problems as well, including cardiac septal hypertrophy, congenital heart disease, caudal regression, vertebral defects, and a single umbilical artery.

Isotretinoin exposure results in severe fetal anomalies including facial and ear abnormalities (anotia, microtia, microphthalmia, cleft lip, and facial dysmorphia) and severe CNS malformations. Fragile X syndrome classically is described as causing intellectual disability, autistic behavior, macroorchidism (esp. after puberty), and facial features of elongated face, large ears, and high-arched palate. Phenytoin exposure in utero classically causes microcephaly as well as nail and digit hypoplasia; gum hyperplasia is described in older children taking this medication. Marfan syndrome classically is described as a tall patient with abnormally long arms, thin digits, aortic root dilation, and dislocation of the lens. Valproic acid exposure in utero is associated with spina bifida, atrial septal defect, cleft palate, polydactyly, intellectual disability, and autism. Exposure to tetracycline in utero can cause skeletal growth retardation as well as pigmentation and loss of enamel of the teeth. Staining of the teeth is well described in children less than about 8 years of age who receive tetracycline. Klinefelter syndrome is the most common cause of hypogonadism and infertility in men. Findings include puberty at a normal age, but small testes, poor development of secondary sex characteristics, gynecomastia, tall stature, and infertility. Learning disability is common. Lithium exposure in utero can cause macrosomia and Ebstein anomaly. ACE-inhibitors may result in fetal growth retardation, oligohydramnios, and a Potter-like syndrome.

The Adolescent

Questions

436. A 15-year-old girl presents to your office for an annual visit. Menarche was at age 14, and for the last year she has had menses every 30 days. She has had no significant medical problems, and denies smoking, drinking alcohol, and taking other drugs. She does well in school and is involved in track and field. In further conversations with her, which of the following adolescent developmental milestones is mostly likely to be noted?

a. Preoccupation with her changing body
b. Conflicts with her family over control and independence
c. Ability to distinguish law from morality
d. Inability to perceive long-term outcomes for current decisions
e. Predominance of same-sex peer affiliations

437. A 12-year-old boy has scant, long, slightly pigmented pubic hairs; slight enlargement of his penis; and a pink, textured, and enlarged scrotum. He is most likely at which sexual maturation rating (SMR, also called Tanner) stage?

a. SMR 1
b. SMR 2
c. SMR 3
d. SMR 4
e. SMR 5

438. A 16-year-old boy is seen for his annual sports physical. He denies recent illnesses or injuries. He is about to enter the 10th grade after completing summer school having been suspended for getting into two fights during the later part of the year; overall he reports his grades to be "average". He denies drinking, smoking, and other drug use. He reports he is not sexually active. He plays football and is the backup quarterback for the local high school team. On physical examination the temperature is 37°C (98.6°F), heart rate is 80 beats per minute, respiratory rate is 16 breaths per minute, and blood pressure is 130/85 mm Hg. He is pleasant and cooperative. Head is without trauma; hair is oily. Neck is supple. The mucous membranes are pink, moist, and without lesions. Dentition is good. Pupils are equally round and reactive; fundoscopic examination is normal. The chest is clear with gynecomastia. Heart has a normal S1 and S2 without murmur and normal splitting. The abdomen is soft and nontender; no hepatosplenomegaly is noted. He is SMR 5; testes size about 10 cm^3. Neurologic examination is nonfocal. Skin is oily with pustules on face and upper back. Which of the following is likely to explain this clinical scenario?

a. Ingestion of creatine
b. Oxandrolone use
c. Chronic marijuana use
d. Inhalation of toluene
e. Ingestion of methylenedioxymethamphetamine

439. A 15-year-old girl is brought to the pediatric emergency room by the lunchroom teacher, who observed her sitting alone and crying. On questioning, the teacher learned that the girl had taken five unidentified tablets after having had an argument with her mother about a boyfriend of whom the mother disapproved. Her physical examination is normal. Her urine pregnancy test is negative, her urine drug screen is negative, and her serum alcohol, aspirin, and acetaminophen levels are nondetectable.

Which of the following is the most appropriate course of action?

a. Hospitalize the teenager in the adolescent ward.
b. Get a psychiatry consultation.
c. Get a social service consultation.
d. Arrange a family conference that includes the boyfriend.
e. Prescribe an antidepressant and arrange for a prompt clinic appointment.

440. A 15-year-old girl is seen in your clinic with a sprained ankle, which occurred the previous day while she was exercising. She denies recent illnesses or injuries. She had menarche at age 12, had regular cycles from age 13, but has had irregular cycles for the last 6 months. She is about to enter the 9th grade and reports excellent school performance. She denies drinking, smoking, and other drug use. She reports she is not sexually active. She participates in the drill team and in gymnastics. On physical examination the temperature is 35.5°C (96°F), heart rate is 60 beats per minute, respiratory rate is 16 breaths per minute, and blood pressure is 100/60 mm Hg. She is pleasant and cooperative. Head is without trauma; hair is somewhat thin. Neck is supple. The mucous membranes are pink, moist, with a swollen, reddened, and irritated-looking uvula. Dentition is poor with decay on the anterior teeth. Pupils are equally round and reactive; fundoscopic examination is normal. The chest is clear. Heart has a normal S1 and S2 without murmur and normal splitting. The abdomen is soft and nontender; no hepatosplenomegaly is noted. She is SMR 5. Neurologic examination is nonfocal. Extremities are thin and hirsute. They are without trauma except for slight swelling on the right ankle. Which of the following is the most appropriate next step in the management of this girl?

a. Human immunodeficiency virus (HIV) testing
b. Radiograph of ankle
c. Thyroid function panel
d. Comparison of current and past weights
e. Pregnancy testing

441. A 17-year-old sexually active girl comes to your office complaining of acne that is unresponsive to the usual treatment regimen. Physical examination reveals severe nodulocystic acne of her face, upper chest, and back. You consider prescribing isotretinoin (Accutane), but you are concerned about side effects. Reviewing the literature, you find which of the following to be true about isotretinoin?

a. Its efficacy can be profound and permanent.
b. It is safe during pregnancy and breast-feeding.
c. Most patients experience excessive tearing and salivation.
d. Severe arthritis necessitating cessation of the drug occurs in about 15% of patients.
e. Significant decrease in serum triglyceride levels are noted in 25% of patients.

442. A 15-year-old patient presents with the complaint of a rash, as pictured. Which of the following statements is correct concerning the management of this common condition?

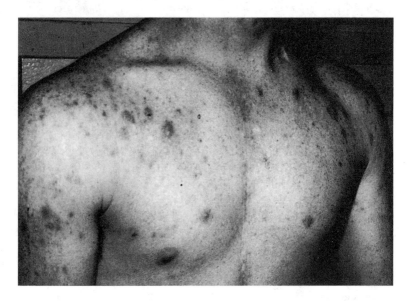

a. Fried foods must be avoided.
b. Frequent scrubbing of the affected areas is key.
c. Topical antibiotics are of no value.
d. Topical benzoyl peroxide is a mainstay of treatment.
e. This rash is solely a disease of the adolescent.

443. A 15-year-old athlete is in your office for his annual physical examination before the start of football season. He has no complaints and has suffered no injuries. On physical examination the temperature is 37°C (98.6°F), heart rate is 100 beats per minute, respiratory rate is 16 breaths per minute, and blood pressure is 110/75 mm Hg. He is in no distress and appears fit. Head is without trauma. Neck is supple. The mucous membranes are pink, moist, and without lesions; dentition is good. Pupils are equally round and reactive; fundoscopic examination is normal. The chest is clear. Heart has a diffuse point of maximal impulse (PMI) with a prominent ventricular lift. He has a normal S1 and S2, with an S4 gallop. No murmur is heard when sitting or squatting, but a late systolic crescendo-decrescendo murmur along the middle left sternal border is heard when he stands. The abdomen is soft and nontender; no hepatosplenomegaly is noted. Genitalia are SMR 4. Neurologic examination is nonfocal. Extremities and joints are normal. For which of the following conditions is this examination most consistent?

a. Wolff-Parkinson-White (WPW) syndrome
b. Valvular aortic stenosis
c. Valvular pulmonic stenosis
d. Myocarditis
e. Hypertrophic cardiomyopathy

Questions 444 and 445 are for the same clinical vignette.

You are the sideline physician for a local high school football team. During a district playoff game, the starting quarterback is sacked for a loss on third down. As the punter heads out onto the field, the quarterback is slow to come to the sidelines. He seems confused and dazed. Aside from his confusion, his examination is normal. After 10 minutes, he is lucid and wants to get back into the game.

444. Based on published guidelines, which of the following is your correct course of action?

a. Allow the player back in the game.
b. Hold the player out for at least 30 minutes.
c. Hold the player out for the rest of the game.
d. Hold the player out for this game and the next game.
e. Send the player to a hospital for evaluation.

445. After the game, the parents ask when he can return to practice. Based on published guidelines, when may this player return to play (RTP)?

a. May return to practice the following day
b. May RTP next week
c. Cannot RTP until next season
d. After being cleared by the trainers using the ImPACT concussion evaluation system
e. After being cleared by a licensed health care provider familiar with concussion

446. A 16-year-old hockey player has sustained a cervical spine injury, has seemingly recovered, and arrives at your office for clearance to RTP. Which of the following is an absolute contraindication to his returning to play?

a. Healed C1 or C2 fracture with normal cervical range of motion
b. Spina bifida occulta
c. C1 + C2 fusion
d. Three or more stingers
e. Single episode of transient quadriparesis

447. An 18-year-old girl is in your office for a 3-day history of a painful rash on her back. She reports she first had the pain in an area under her scapula and did not feel nor see any abnormalities. Over the last day she has noticed a red "rash" in the area. She reports other symptoms including fever, fatigue, and change in appetite. Her past medical history includes successful kidney transplant after renal failure caused by hemolytic uremic syndrome. On physical examination she has a linear patch of redness under the scapula with groups of vesicles on an erythematous base. Which of the following is the most likely mechanism of her condition?

a. Bite of an insect
b. Exposure to a spirochete
c. Contact with a plant irritant
d. Reactivation of a dorsal root ganglia viral infection
e. Infection with a parasite

448. A 15-year-old boy is in the office for a preparticipation sports physical examination before he begins playing with the varsity football team at his school. Although he is a skilled receiver, he will be one of the smallest players on the field and is concerned about the potential for injury. He asks how to bulk up. Appropriate advice to increase muscle mass includes which of the following?

a. Taking extra vitamins
b. Doubling protein intake
c. Using anabolic steroids
d. Increasing muscle work
e. Taking ergogenic medication

449. An 18-year-old college student is seen in the student health clinic for urinary frequency, dysuria, and urethral discharge. Which of the following tests is likely to confirm the etiology of his symptoms?

a. Identification of viral DNA by polymerase chain reaction (PCR)
b. Clean catch urine with more than 10^5 gram-negative, lactose-fermenting rods
c. Positive results on a nucleic acid amplification test (NAAT)
d. Rapid plasma reagin (RPR) test results of 1:4
e. Reactive enzyme immunoassay (EIA) with confirmatory immunoblot or immunofluorescence assay

450. A 19-year-old college student returns from spring break in Fort Lauderdale, Florida, with complaints of acute pain and swelling of the scrotum. Physical examination reveals an exquisitely tender, swollen right testis that is rather difficult to examine. The cremasteric reflex is absent, but there is no swelling in the inguinal area. The rest of his genitourinary examination appears to be normal. A urine dip is negative for red and white blood cells. Which of the following is the appropriate next step in management?

a. Administration of antibiotics after testing for *Chlamydia* and gonorrhea
b. Reassurance and warm compresses
c. Intravenous fluid administration, pain medications, and straining of all voids
d. Ultrasound with blood flow studies of the scrotum
e. Laparoscopic exploration of both inguinal regions

451. A 16-year-old girl presents with lower abdominal pain and fever. On physical examination, a tender adnexal mass is felt. Further questioning in private reveals the following: she has a new sexual partner; her periods are irregular; and she has a vaginal discharge. Which of the following test results is most likely to be seen in this scenario?

a. Appendiceal fecalith on plain radiograph of abdomen
b. Thickened and fluid-filled fallopian tubes with free pelvic fluid on ultrasound
c. 4-cm fluid-filled mass arising from the left ovary
d. Multicystic lesions throughout the right kidney
e. Calcified mass in left ureter with proximal ureter dilatation and mild hydronephrosis

452. A 17-year-old boy is seen for a yearly visit. He has been in good health and reports no serious illness in the previous year other than occasional upper respiratory infections. He denies weight loss, fever, cough, abdominal pain, and changes in stool or urine patterns. He is a senior in high school, makes "average" grades, and participates in basketball and track. He denies smoking cigarettes but admits to marijuana use twice in the previous year and "occasional drinking" of alcohol on weekends. He is sexually active with five total partners, and reports using condoms on most encounters. On physical examination the temperature is 37°C (98.6°F), heart rate is 90 beats per minute, respiratory rate is 16 breaths per minute, and blood pressure is 110/68 mm Hg. He is in no distress and appears fit. Head is without trauma. Neck is supple. The mucous membranes are pink, moist, and without lesions; dentition is good. Pupils are equally round and reactive; fundoscopic examination is normal. The chest is clear. Heart has normal S1 and S2. No murmur is heard. The abdomen is soft and nontender; no hepatosplenomegaly is noted. Genitalia are SMR 5. A 1-cm hard nodule is felt on the posterior aspect of the right testis. Neurologic examination is nonfocal. Extremities and joints are normal. Which of the following is the appropriate next step in his care?

a. Urine NAAT for *Chlamydia* and gonococcus
b. Ultrasound of testes
c. Reassurance and observation
d. Measurement of serum α-fetoprotein
e. Measurement of serum β-human chorionic gonadotropin

Questions 453 to 455

Listed later are various clinical vignettes in which the patient has genital lesions. Match each vignette with the appropriate diagnostic test or therapy. Each lettered option may be used once, more than once, or not at all.

a. Apply clotrimazole to the affected area four times daily until resolution.
b. Confirm findings with the fluorescent treponemal antibody absorption (FTA-ABS) test.
c. Begin a 10 course of oral trimethoprim-sulfamethoxazole.
d. Perform PCR of a lesion specimen.
e. Apply 1% hydrocortisone cream to affected area and avoid latex condoms.
f. Complement fixation of a serum samples demonstrating antibody titers of more than 1:64.
g. Apply mupirocin to the affected area three times daily and wash with antibacterial soap.
h. Perform immunochromatography on a lesion specimen.

453. A 16-year-old girl is seen for a new-onset ulcer on her labia. She has had three sexual partners in the previous 18 months and reports inconsistent use of condoms. On physical examination she has a painless ulcer on her labia. Laboratory data show a positive RPR of 1:64.

454. A 19-year-old woman is seen in the student health center. She has had a new sexual partner for the last 4 weeks and reports "almost always using condoms." She reports that she had a few small, painless lesions on her left labia about 2 weeks prior, but these have resolved. Now she has fever, headache, chills, muscle aches, and swollen left inguinal "glands." On examination she has an enlarged, tender left-sided inguinal node.

455. A 19-year-old man reports to the adolescent clinic with the complaint of recurrent episodes of painful "sores" on the head of his penis for the last 3 years. His sexual debut was at 15 years of age, he has had eight total partners, and he reports inconsistent condom use. On examination he has several small, erythematous vesicles and ulcers on his glans. Regional nodes are slightly enlarged.

The Adolescent

Answers

436. The answer is b. (*Hay et al, pp 127-128. Kliegman et al, p 927. Rudolph et al, pp 271-272.*) The adolescent in the question seems to be developing normally. At her age (14-17 years) and her sexual maturity rating (likely to be 3-5 since she is menstruating regularly), conflict with her family over control and independence is likely to be an ongoing issue; this is a common feature of middle adolescence. Preoccupation with her changing body, predominance of same-sex peer affiliations, and inability to perceive long-term outcomes for current decisions are features of early adolescence (aged about 10-13 years with sexual maturity rating of 1-2). Late adolescence (ages about 18-21 years with sexual maturation scale of 5) includes the ability to distinguish law from morality.

437. The answer is b. (*Hay et al, pp 113-114. Kliegman et al, p 929. Rudolph et al, pp 265-266.*) Normal sexual maturation during puberty follows a consistent pattern. The first sign of puberty in boys is scrotal and testicular growth; penis growth usually occurs about a year after. Pubic hair growth is more variable. In girls, the first sign of puberty is the development of breast buds. The SMRs are not synchronized. In that a girl with SMR 3, pubic hair does not always have SMR 3 breasts.

The description in the question is typical of SMR 2 in boys: sparse, thin, and long pubic hair with slight penile enlargement. In SMR 3, pubic hair becomes darker and begins to curl, and the penis lengthens. In SMR 4, the genitalia is starting to resemble adult pubic hair but without complete coverage, and the penis continues to grow. At SMR 5, pubic hair extends to the inner thigh and is in the typical adult configuration.

Girls have sparse pubic hair to start SMR 2 as well, and progress over time to full pubic coverage with medial thigh extension in SMR 5. Breasts start with buds in SMR 2, and progress to larger breasts and areola without a separate areolar contour in SMR 3. Breasts at SMR 4 will have elevation of the areola, but by SMR 5 the areola is part of the general breast contour.

438. The answer is b. (*Hay et al, pp 145-158. Kliegman et al, pp 947-962, 3356-3357. Rudolph et al, pp 278-282.*) About 6.6% of high school boys report use of performance-enhancing steroids. In addition to the desired increase in muscle mass and strength, untoward effects include infertility, gynecomastia, hypertension, atherosclerosis, aggression, depression, acne, and physeal closure. The goal of creatine use is to gain muscle mass and strength, although in doing so the adolescent is at risk for dehydration, muscle cramps, GI distress, and damaged kidney function. Inhalants of volatile organic compounds, often viewed as "safe" can result in arrhythmia and death, and chronic use can result in brain damage, peripheral neuropathies, and spasticity. Marijuana causes elation and euphoria, short-term memory impairment, distorted time perception, and flashbacks. Methylenedioxymethamphetamine (more commonly known as MDMA, or even more commonly E, X, XTC, or Ecstasy) is a "club drug" for all-night parties, and typically causes euphoria and increased energy.

439. The answer is a. (*Hay et al, pp 188-190. Kliegman et al, pp 159-162. Rudolph et al, pp 356-360.*) The adolescent who has attempted suicide should be hospitalized so that a complete medical, psychological, and social evaluation can be performed and an appropriate treatment plan developed. Hospitalization also emphasizes the seriousness of the adolescent's action to her and her family and the importance of cooperation in carrying out the recommendations for ongoing future therapy. The treatment plan may include inpatient psychiatric hospitalization, continued counseling or supportive therapy with a pediatrician, outpatient psychotherapy with a psychiatrist or other mental health worker, or family therapy.

440. The answer is d. (*Hay et al, pp 159-170. Kliegman et al, pp 90-96. Rudolph et al, pp 288-292.*) The young girl in the question could have any number of problems, and all of the answers could ultimately prove to be helpful. As a first step, however, a close look at her weight in comparison to previous ones is in order; she has some physical examination findings seen with bulimia (dental decay, irritated uvula), and others seen with anorexia nervosa (lanugo, thinning hair, low resting heart rate, hypothermia, secondary amenorrhea). Parents may not appreciate the magnitude of weight loss until it reaches 10% or more of body weight, because girls will not undress in their parents' presence and because the facial contours are the last parts to be affected. Bulimia usually appears in mid adolescence rather than early adolescence and is characterized by sessions of gorging, often in secret and often involving a single favored snack food such as ice cream, cake, or candy, although it may also be manifested as immoderate eating at mealtimes. This gorging is followed by secret bouts of self-induced vomiting. Some bulimics also use laxatives and purgatives. Physical consequences of bulimia include esophageal varices and hemorrhage; dental decay, especially of anterior teeth (because of exposure of enamel to gastric HCl); and a swollen, reddened, irritated uvula (also from chronic HCl exposure). Physical consequences of anorexia include profound weight loss (25%-30% or more of body weight), dehydration, facial and arm hirsutism, loss of hair of the head, bradycardia, cardiac conduction problems, reduced cardiac output, hypothermia, impaired renal function, multiple malnutrition effects (including avitaminoses), a primary or secondary amenorrhea, and osteoporosis. Significant mortality in treatment-resistant cases is seen.

441. The answer is a. (*Hay et al, pp 387-389. Kliegman et al, pp 3235-3238. Rudolph et al, pp 1287-1288.*) Isotretinoin (13-*cis*-retinoic acid; Accutane) has proved to be very effective in the treatment of refractory nodulocystic acne. The effects of treatment appear to be long-lasting. Precautions regarding its use, however, are essential. Because of its teratogenic effects (isotretinoin syndrome), the drug is absolutely contraindicated during pregnancy and within 4-6 weeks of becoming pregnant. Dry skin, eyes, and mucous membranes are the most frequent complications of therapy. Other associated problems include musculoskeletal pain and hyperostosis, inflammatory bowel disease, pseudotumor cerebri, and corneal opacities. Patients on isotretinoin therapy can often develop abnormal liver function tests, elevated triglyceride and cholesterol levels, and lowered levels of high-density lipoproteins. Some have suggested that an increased risk of suicide is related to its use, although this link is less well established.

442. The answer is d. (*Hay et al, pp 387-389. Kliegman et al, pp 3228-3235. Rudolph et al, pp 1287-1288.*) Acne is a skin disorder that affects virtually all adolescents and is seen less commonly in older patients. The goals of therapy are to prevent scarring and disfigurement and to avoid loss of self-esteem. Mainstays of therapy are topical retinoids (exfoliant and comedolytic) in the evening and benzoyl peroxide (antibacterial activity) in the morning. Oral tetracycline and topical antibiotics can be necessary to control the inflammatory component of acne. Studies have failed to demonstrate adverse effects of any particular foods on disease activity. Vigorous facial or body scrubbing can traumatize the skin and aggravate the problem.

443. The answer is e. (*Hay et al, p 578. Kliegman et al, pp 2275-2276. Rudolph et al, pp 1906-1907.*) Hypertrophic cardiomyopathy (also known as idiopathic hypertrophic subaortic stenosis [IHSS], hypertrophic obstructive cardiomyopathy [HOCM], or asymmetrical septal hypertrophy [ASH]) should be a significant concern to anyone caring for young athletes. Although uncommon (one study of asymptomatic young adults found echocardiographic evidence of hypertrophic cardiomyopathy in 2 of 1000 patients), the sudden death of an athlete on the playing field generates significant public awareness of the condition. Unfortunately, youth afflicted with hypertrophic cardiomyopathy are frequently asymptomatic. The first hint of the condition may be when the athlete collapses during a practice or game. Thus, potential warning signs are extremely important and should not be missed. As the condition is passed as a Mendelian dominant trait with variable expression, a family history of sudden cardiac death or early myocardial infraction (MI) should be investigated. Similarly, a past history of syncope during exercise or the physical examination described in the question should prompt further evaluation with an echocardiograph. On examination a harsh, diamond-shaped systolic murmur at the left lower sternal border can be noted at the beginning of systole which then ends before the second heart sound begins. Moving from a squatting to a standing position causes pooling of blood in the legs (similar to Valsalva) resulting in decreased venous return to the heart. This then results in decreased left ventricular filling which results in worsened left ventricular outflow tract obstruction and a more prominent murmur.

Wolff-Parkinson-White (WPW) syndrome is a reentrant tachycardia with abrupt onset and termination. WPW syndrome has been associated with hypertrophic cardiomyopathy, but would not present by itself as the vignette presented earlier. Valvular aortic stenosis presents with a left ventricular thrust, a systolic thrill, a prominent aortic ejection click between S_1 and S_2, and a loud rough systolic ejection murmur is heard in the first and second intercostal spaces. Valvular pulmonic stenosis presents with a right ventricular heave and systolic thrill and a prominent ejection click best heard in the left third intercostal space that is more easily identified during expiration. Myocarditis can be acute or chronic, and should display some elements of heart failure.

444 to 445. The answers are 444-c, 445-e. (*Hay et al, pp 804-805. Kliegman et al, pp 3350-3352. Rudolph et al, pp 2159-2161.*) Concussion, or mild traumatic brain injury (mTBI), is a common sports injury occurring an estimated 1.6-3.8 million times each year. Symptoms of concussion include mental confusion, vomiting, headache, irritability, restlessness, amnesia, dizziness, visual changes, or change in personality. Published guidelines require team personnel to use checklists to objectively assess a player who may have sustained a concussion. If concussion is a possibility, an athlete should immediately be removed from play, and should not return to the game or to subsequent practices until evaluated by a licensed health care provider familiar with the diagnosis and management of concussion.

The guidelines make it clear that the return to play (RTP) should be individualized; a specific amount of time after which it is safe to RTP is not listed. Part of that evaluation may include neurocognitive testing. Immediate Post-Concussion Assessment and Cognitive Testing (ImPACT) is one such test. Comparing a postinjury online testing session to a baseline session that was completed at the start of the season can identify subtle cognitive deficiencies that can help guide RTP decisions. However, neurocognitive testing is not a replacement for medical evaluation and treatment.

446. The answer is c. (*Hay et al, pp 900-904. Kliegman et al, p 3353. Rudolph et al, pp 356-360.*) Absolute contraindications to RTP include surgical procedures such as C1 + C2 fusion; cervical laminectomy; and three-level anterior or posterior cervical fusions. Other absolute contraindications include such conditions as multilevel Klippel-Feil anomaly; ankylosing spondylitis; and Arnold-Chiari syndrome. Examples of conditions that are not contraindications to RTP are spina bifida occulta; Klippel-Feil disease not involving C1; healed C1 or C2 fractures with normal range of motion; fewer than three stingers lasting less than 24 hours and with full range of cervical motion; and single episode of transient quadriparesis with return to normal function and normal MRI. Relative contraindications for RTP include three or more stingers with prolonged recovery; more than one episode of transient quadriparesis or episodes lasting longer than 24 hours; and posterior fusion with or without instrumentation.

447. The answer is d. (*Hay et al, pp 1245-1249. Kliegman et al, pp 1579-1586. Rudolph et al, 1160-1164.*) The adolescent has a case of shingles, a reactivation of a varicella infection lying dormant in the dorsal root ganglia. While more commonly seen in adults, shingles are a pediatric condition among those with immunocompromising conditions such as AIDS, malignancy, and transplant. The classic presentation is as described, including pain over a dermatome (occasionally itching or paresthesia) that then develops erythema and the grouped vesicles on an erythematous base. Insect bites (such as fleas or ants) can result in isolated skin lesions but the prodrome of pain followed by vesicles is not expected. Secondary syphilis can cause widespread skin lesions, but localized lesions to one area of the body would be unusual. Poison ivy or oak can cause a localized rash, but the rash and itching occur simultaneously rather than sequentially. Infection with a parasite such as hookworm (the agent that causes cutaneous larva migrans) can cause an intensely pruritic, localized lesion typically found on the foot.

448. The answer is d. (*Hay et al, pp 884-885.*) Increased muscle work (along with increased calories) is the only appropriate way to increase muscle mass. Measurements of skin-fold thickness, performed serially, are a useful way to detect changes in the amount of body fat, so that obesity can be avoided. Protein loading or using drugs, hormones, and vitamins will not be helpful and may be harmful.

449. The answer is c. (*Hay et al, pp 1265-1266, 1274-1275. Kliegman et al, pp 1494-1495. Rudolph et al, pp 923-933.*) Urethritis in an adolescent boy is almost always a sexually transmitted disease (STD), either gonococcal or nongonococcal urethritis (NGU). *Chlamydia trachomatis* is usually the causative agent in NGU. Less frequently, NGU can be caused by *Ureaplasma urealyticum, Trichomonas vaginalis,* and yeast. Herpes simplex can cause an NGU, but it is considerably less likely than *C trachomatis.* Gonococcal culture and Gram stain are easily available; chlamydial culture may not be. NAATs are a less invasive way of diagnosing STDs. Able to be performed on a urine sample, NAATs can produce a response with as little as one strand of target DNA or RNA. Direct monoclonal antibody tests as well as enzyme immunoassay and molecular probe tests are alternative methods for *Chlamydia* identification, although they are less sensitive and less specific than chlamydial culture. Urine ligase testing for *Chlamydia* and gonococcus is available. Serologic testing for syphilis should always be done in high-risk individuals, but in none of its normal presentations is urethral discharge common. Testing for HIV should be offered and safer sexual practices encouraged; HIV does not cause urethral discharge. Urinary tract infection is not associated with a urethral discharge.

450. The answer is d. (*Hay et al, p 1275. Kliegman et al, pp 2592-2598. Rudolph et al, pp 923-933.*) Epididymitis and torsion are high on the differential on this patient. The lack of white and red blood cells on urinalysis suggests that torsion must be considered, a condition that requires immediate attention. Prehn sign, although not totally reliable, is elicited by gently lifting the scrotum toward the symphysis. Relief of the pain points to epididymitis; its worsening, to torsion. Doppler ultrasound (or surgical consultation) is a logical first step in this man's evaluation, demonstrating absence of flow in torsion and increased flow in epididymitis. Alternatively, a radionuclide scan will show diminished uptake in torsion and increased uptake in epididymitis. Treatment for torsion is surgical exploration and detorsion with scrotal orchiopexy. Causative organisms for epididymitis include *Neisseria gonorrhoeae, C trachomatis,* and other bacteria. Treatment with appropriate antibiotics and rest is indicated for epididymitis. However, treating this patient with antibiotics without first excluding testicular torsion is ill-advised; loss of the testis can be expected after 4-6 hours of absent blood flow if the testis has torsed. Strangulated hernia is associated with abdominal pain, vomiting, and other evidence of intestinal obstruction.

451. The answer is b. (*Hay et al, pp 1273-1274. Kliegman et al, p 988. Rudolph et al, pp 923-933.*) Pelvic inflammatory disease (PID) refers to sexually transmitted infections of the female upper genital tract including tuboovarian abscess, endometritis, salpingitis, and pelvic peritonitis. Sexually active teenagers are at great risk of acquiring PID because of their high-risk behavior, exposure to multiple partners, and failure to use contraceptives. The strong likelihood of PID in the patient presented should not preclude consideration of serious conditions requiring surgical intervention, such as appendiceal abscess, ectopic pregnancy, and ovarian cyst. Renal cyst does not present in the manner described. An episode of PID raises the risk of ectopic pregnancy, and about 20% of women become infertile following one episode of PID. Other sequelae include dyspareunia, pyosalpinx, tuboovarian abscess, and pelvic adhesions. Endometriosis is not related to PID.

452. The answer is b. (*Kliegman et al, pp 2597-2598. Rudolph et al, pp 295-296.*) About 98% of painless solid testicular masses are malignant; the first step in management is to confirm the findings on ultrasound which will then guide further therapy which might include measurement of serum α-fetoprotein and β-human chorionic gonadotropin. Observation would be an appropriate choice if the finding was not hard and rather "like a bag of worms", indicating varicocele. Testing for sexually transmitted infections is appropriate for all at-risk adolescents, even if they are asymptomatic. The highest priority for this patient is determination of malignancy or not.

453 to 455. The answers are **453-b, 454-f, 455-d.** (*Hay et al, pp 1400-1442. Kliegman et al, pp 1375-1376, 1470-1478, 1495-1496, 1572-1575. Rudolph et al, pp 923-933.*) In the first patient, syphilis is likely. A scraping from a genital ulcer could be examined under dark-field microscopy for *Treponema pallidum*, but this test is generally unavailable. Confirmation of a positive RPR (high sensitivity, low specificity) with a high specificity, low sensitivity confirmatory test such as FTP-ABS is appropriate.

Inguinal adenopathy that suppurates and causes chronic draining of sinuses is commonly seen in chancroid and can be confused with lymphogranuloma venereum (LGV). Typically, the inguinal adenopathy of chancroid occurs at the same time as the genital ulcer as is seen in the young woman in the second case, while the adenopathy in LGV occurs after the ulcer has healed. LGV is caused by serotypes L1, L2, and L3 of *C trachomatis*. While culture is definitive for the diagnosis of LGV, it is technically difficult and expensive, and yields are poor. A complement fixation titer of more than 1:64 is considered diagnostic for LGV.

Herpes should be suspected in the third patient with recurrent shallow, painful ulcers of the genitourinary tract. Herpes simplex virus polymerase chain reaction (HSV PCR) assay is the preferred diagnostic test.

Chancroid caused by *Haemophilus ducreyi* is difficult to culture. Special chocolate agar medium is only 65% sensitive. Immunochromatography is often used in areas where chancroid is common (sub-African countries; low incidence in the United States) since it is easy and rapidly performed albeit with low sensitivity. Consideration for this diagnosis in the United States is the correct presentation: painful ulcers, regional lymphadenopathy, no evidence of syphilis, and negative HSV testing.

Clotrimazole is the treatment for tinea cruris. Oral trimethoprim-sulfamethoxazole and/or mupirocin might be considered for folliculitis, such as that caused by shaving.

Rapid Fire Questions

1.1 A formula-fed 2-month-old infant has fever, irritability, hepatomegaly, and jaundice on examination. Urinalysis is positive for reducing substances, total serum bilirubin is 6.5 mg/dL, and a blood culture is growing *Escherichia coli*. In addition to treating the positive blood culture with IV antibiotics, management should include which of the following?

a. Change to exclusive breast milk
b. Phototherapy
c. Change to low protein formula
d. CNS imaging
e. Change to soy formula

Answer: e

1.2 Which of the following maternal infections is a contraindication to breast-feeding a healthy term baby?

a. Cytomegalovirus
b. Hepatitis B
c. Active tuberculosis
d. Hepatitis C
e. Genital herpes

Answer: c

1.3 Which nutrient requires specific supplementation in a vegan diet but not necessarily in a vegetarian diet?

a. Vitamin B_{12}
b. Vitamin C
c. Vitamin E
d. Magnesium
e. Potassium

Answer: a

1.4 The developmentally normal child in your office can walk alone, can eat with a spoon and drink from a cup, says "mama" and "dada" and several other single words, and follows one step commands. What is the most likely age of the child?

a. 12 months
b. 18 months
c. 24 months
d. 36 months
e. 48 months

Answer: b

2.1 A large for gestational age newborn has left-sided parietal scalp swelling that crosses suture lines. The skin in the area feels thick and pits with pressure; there is no fluid wave. This infant has which of the following traumatic injuries?

a. Intraventricular hemorrhage (IVH)
b. Caput succedaneum
c. Subdural hemorrhage
d. Cephalohematoma
e. Subgaleal hemorrhage

Answer: b

2.2 The most likely cause of a greyish mucous vaginal discharge in a 1-day-old girl is which of the following?

a. Maternal hormones
b. Müllerian duct malformation
c. Chlamydia
d. Gonorrhea
e. Recto-vaginal fistula

Answer: a

2.3 Which of the following diagnoses is most likely in a 48-hour-old term infant who has been feeding well but has yet to pass a stool?

a. Imperforate anus
b. Ileal atresia
c. Hirschsprung disease
d. Meconium plug
e. Meconium ileus

Answer: d

2.4 A 1-week-old exclusively breast-fed infant has several hours of bilious emesis and mild abdominal distension on examination. Which of the following should be the next step in evaluation and management?

a. Emergent contrast enema
b. Emergent upper gastrointestinal series
c. Initiate acid blockade with ranitidine
d. Change to "sensitive" formula and reassure the parents
e. Outpatient abdominal ultrasound in the morning

Answer: b

3.1 The baseline incidence of congenital heart disease is about 1%. For a family with a child with isolated congenital heart disease, the incidence of heart disease in future children is which of the following?

a. 1%
b. 2%-6%
c. 8%-10%
d. 15%-20%
e. 25%-30%

Answer: b

3.2 Syncope while exercising is sometimes the only clinical clue to which of the following disorders?

a. Congenital heart block
b. Hypertrophic cardiomyopathy
c. Tetralogy of Fallot
d. Still's murmur
e. Patent ductus arteriosus

Answer: b

3.3 A history of congenital hearing loss and syncopal episodes suggests which of the following arrhythmias?

a. Prolonged QT syndrome
b. Supraventricular tachycardia
c. Atrial flutter
d. Ventricular tachycardia
e. Wolff-Parkinson-White (WPW) syndrome

Answer: a

3.4 Which of the following heart conditions is most likely to be associated with an infant who has congenital rubella syndrome?

a. Aortic stenosis
b. Hypoplastic left heart
c. Tricuspid regurgitation
d. Coarctation of the aorta
e. Pulmonary artery stenosis

Answer: e

4.1 Which of the following arterial blood gas results is most consistent with a 12-year-old obese boy who, while sleeping, has loud snoring and a drop in his pulse oximetry readings?

pH	PCO$_2$ (mm Hg)	PO$_2$ (mm Hg)	Base Excess (mEq/L)
a. 6.92	101	19	−15
b. 7.36	60	50	7
c. 7.50	46	76	11
d. 7.41	60	90	10
e. 7.34	58	89	−5

Answer: b

4.2 A term newborn born via scheduled cesarean section after a benign pregnancy develops grunting, flaring, retracting, and hypoxia shortly after birth. What is the most likely cause of the infant's respiratory distress?

a. Primary surfactant deficiency
b. Pneumothorax
c. Group B streptococcal pneumonia
d. Congenital diaphragmatic hernia
e. Transient tachypnea of the newborn

Answer: e

4.3 Which of the following is the likely diagnosis in a patient with acute onset of chest pain, subcutaneous crepitus palpable around the upper chest and neck, and precordial systolic crepitus on auscultation?

a. Pneumothorax
b. Pneumomediastinum
c. Pneumoperitoneum
d. Pneumocephalus
e. Infection with clostridium perfringens

Answer: b

4.4 According to the Infectious Disease Society of America 2011 guideline for community-acquired pneumonia (CAP) in children, which antibiotic should be first-line therapy for previously healthy preschool children with mild to moderate CAP presumed to be bacterial in origin?

a. Amoxicillin
b. Amoxicillin/clavulanic acid
c. Trimethoprim/sulfamethoxazole
d. Cefotaxime
e. Ceftriaxone

Answer: a

5.1 A term newborn takes a bottle slowly and chokes and gags with feeds. Which study should be performed next?

a. Esophageal manometry
b. 24-hour pH probe
c. Upper GI endoscopy
d. Upper GI fluoroscopy (upper GI series)
e. Modified barium swallow

Answer: e

5.2 The congenital gastrointestinal malformation most commonly associated with trisomy 21 is which of the following?

a. Pyloric stenosis
b. Hirschsprung disease
c. Esophageal atresia
d. Duodenal atresia
e. Anal atresia

Answer: d

5.3 A toxic-appearing 14-year-old boy with a recent diagnosis of nephrotic syndrome presents with diffuse abdominal pain, vomiting, fever, tachycardia, and hypotension. His abdomen is rigid and demonstrates rebound tenderness. The next step in the management of this boy is which of the following?

a. Stool culture
b. Urinalysis and culture
c. Diagnostic paracentesis
d. Abdominal ultrasound
e. Prescribe 2 weeks of amoxicillin and bismuth subsalicylate

Answer: c

5.4 A 2-week old is spitting up formula after every four ounce bottle. The infant is now above birthweight. The most likely cause is which of the following?

a. Overfeeding
b. Gastroesophageal reflux disease
c. Pyloric stenosis
d. Duodenal web
e. Esophageal atresia

Answer: a

6.1 Which of the following is most likely to be seen in a child with severe hypertension?

a. Multiple cranial nerve palsy
b. Headache
c. Hyporeflexia
d. Increased urine output
e. Right ventricular hypertrophy

Answer: b

6.2 A child with an *E coli* UTI, fever despite antibiotics, and lobar nephronia diagnosed by CT scan requires which of the following?

a. Prolonged antibiotic therapy
b. Routine treatment with 10-14 days of antibiotics for pyelonephritis
c. Surgical consultation
d. Dimercaptosuccinic acid (DMSA) scan
e. Renal biopsy

Answer: a

7.1 Which of the following conditions is classically described as a normal infant who, in the first month of life, develops a cherry-red lesion on the macula and extreme sensitivity to noise?

a. Niemann-Pick disease, type A
b. Infantile Gaucher disease
c. Tay-Sachs disease
d. Krabbe disease
e. Fabry disease

Answer: c

7.2 Which of the following is the most common site of brain tumor development in a child less than about a year of age?

a. Subtentorial
b. Supratentorial
c. Intraventricular
d. Spinal canal
e. Peripheral nervous system

Answer: b

7.3 Which of the following is the most common site of brain tumor development in a child from about 1 year of age through about 10 years of age?

a. Subtentorial
b. Supratentorial
c. Intraventricular
d. Spinal canal
e. Peripheral nervous system

Answer: a

7.4 Which of the following is the most common site of brain tumor development in a child older than about 10 years of age?

a. Subtentorial
b. Supratentorial
c. Intraventricular
d. Spinal canal
e. Peripheral nervous system

Answer: b

7.5 Which of the following is the most appropriate screening test for a child suspected of having muscular dystrophy?

a. Ultrasound of the lower spine
b. Serum creatinine phosphokinase (CPK) levels
c. MRI of the brain
d. Lumbar puncture
e. Nerve conduction studies

Answer: b

8.1 Which of the following is the most appropriate approach to a patient who may have a rabies exposure (such as a bat found in the child's room)?

a. Treatment of the child is indicated only if symptoms develop.
b. Observation; bats are not a natural reservoir.
c. Begin rabies vaccine series.
d. Begin treatment with acyclovir.
e. Initiate course of ribavirin.

Answer: c

9.1 Which of the following is the most likely answer for anemia in a chubby 1-year old?

a. Excessive cow's milk intake
b. Excessive infant formula intake
c. Sickle cell disease
d. Acute lymphoblastic leukemia
e. Congenital spherocytosis

Answer: a

10.1 Which of the following is the most common reason that a small for gestational age (SGA) newborn would have hypoglycemia at 1 hour of age?

a. Inadequate stores of glycogen and fats
b. Adrenal immaturity
c. Pituitary immaturity
d. Insulin excess
e. Surfactant deficiency

Answer: a

11.1 Teenage pregnancy is associated with which of the following?

a. Twin gestation
b. Low-birth-weight infants
c. Hypotension
d. Excessive maternal weight gain
e. Infants with genetic defects

Answer: b

Bonus Quick Fires

B.1 Of the choices listed, which is the most appropriate for a severe toxicodendron dermatitis (poison ivy or poison oak exposure)?

a. 1% topical steroids
b. Topical calamine lotion
c. 14 days of oral methylprednisolone
d. A "steroid dose pack"
e. Oral diphenhydramine q 6 hours

Answer: c

B.2 Which of the following therapies is recommended for mild stuttering in an otherwise healthy 2-year-old child?

a. Observation
b. Trial of risperidone
c. Trial of olanzapine (Zyprexa)
d. 2 minutes of time-out
e. Referral to speech pathologist

Answer: a

B.3 An underweight 18-month-old child with nasal polyps should be evaluated for which of the following?

a. Adrenal insufficiency
b. Allergies
c. Cystic fibrosis
d. Nasal foreign body
e. Sinusitis

Answer: c

B.4 Which of the following therapies is most appropriate for a 5-year-old child with a 3-day history of a hordeolum (stye) of the left eye?

a. Topical azithromycin
b. Incision and drainage
c. Examination of eye under anesthesia
d. Systemic antibiotics
e. Warm compresses and eye hygiene

Answer: e

Index

Note: Page numbers followed by *f* indicate figures

Trisomy 13, 40, 83, 432, 434, 436, 456, 459
Trisomy 18, 77, 121, 434, 456, 459, 463, 477
Trisomy 21, 77, 127, 162, 432, 459, 474–475, 477, 501. *See also* Down syndrome
Truncal ataxia, 338
Truncus arteriosus, 173
TTFS. *See* Twin-to-twin transfusion syndrome
TTN. *See* Transient tachypnea of the newborn
Tuberculin skin test, 200, 215
Tuberculomas, calcified, 340–341
Tuberculosis, 214–215, 381, 397
Tuberculosis skin test, 192, 202, 423
Tuberculous meningitis, 28, 70, 322, 335, 344
Tuberous sclerosis, 155, 335, 341
Tuberous sclerosis complex, 462
Tularemia, 395
Turner syndrome, 140–141, 181, 289, 457, 477
Twins, 121
Twin-to-twin transfusion syndrome, 150–151
Tympanic membrane, 28
Tympanosclerosis, 71
Typhoid fever, 360
Tyrosinemia, 428
Tyrosinosis, 453

U
Ulcerative colitis, 256, 265
Umbilical granulomas, 72
Umbilical hernia, 262
Undescended testis, 119, 294

Upper brachial plexus injury, 153
Upper respiratory tract infections, 205, 368, 387
Ureteropelvic junction obstruction, 275, 292
Urethritis, 493
Urinary tract infection, 277, 292, 302, 502
Urolithiasis, 291, 302

V
Vaccinations, 106
VACTERL, 143
Vaginal discharge, 271, 281, 486, 498
Vaginal foreign bodies, 73, 288
Valproic acid, 312, 478
Valvular aortic stenosis, 483, 491
Valvular pulmonic stenosis, 483, 491
Vancomycin, 192, 203, 214, 221, 315, 366, 412
Vanillylmandelic acid, 412, 424
Varicella
  description of, 92, 388
  immunization for, 38, 347
  rash associated with, 376
  signs and symptoms of, 376
Varicella-zoster immunoglobulin, 129
Varicella-zoster virus
  description of, 53
  immunization for, 129
Varicocele, 298–299
Vasopressin, 289, 476
Vasovagal syncope, 343
VATER, 40, 83
VCUG. *See* Voiding cystourethrogram
Vegan diet, 497